a LANGE medical book

CURRENT
Practice Guidelines
In Primary Care
2016

Joseph S. Esherick, MD, FAAFP
Director of Medicine
Ventura County Medical Center
Associate Clinical Professor of Family Medicine
David Geffen School of Medicine
Los Angeles, California

Daniel S. Clark, MD, FACC, FAHA
Department of Cardiology
Ventura County Medical Center
Assistant Clinical Professor of Family Medicine
David Geffen School of Medicine
Los Angeles, California

Evan D. Slater, MD
Director, Hematology and Medical Oncology
Ventura County Medical Center
Assistant Clinical Professor of Medicine
David Geffen School of Medicine
Los Angeles, California

Mc
Graw
Hill
Education

New York   Chicago   San Francisco   Athens   London   Madrid
Mexico City   Milan   New Delhi   Singapore   Sydney   Toronto

CURRENT Practice Guidelines in Primary Care, 2016

1 2 3 4 5 6 7 8 9 0   DOC/DOC   19 18 17 16 15

ISBN 978-1-259-58546-3
MHID 1-259-58546-8
ISSN 1528-1612

Notice

Medicine is an ever-changing science. As new research and clinical experience broaden our knowledge, changes in treatment and drug therapy are required. The authors and the publisher of this work have checked with sources believed to be reliable in their efforts to provide information that is complete and generally in accord with the standards accepted at the time of publication. However, in view of the possibility of human error or changes in medical sciences, neither the authors nor the publisher nor any other party who has been involved in the preparation or publication of this work warrants that the information contained herein is in every respect accurate or complete, and they disclaim all responsibility for any errors or omissions or for the results obtained from use of the information contained in this work. Readers are encouraged to confirm the information contained herein with other sources. For example and in particular, readers are advised to check the product information sheet included in the package of each drug they plan to administer to be certain that the information contained in this work is accurate and that changes have not been made in the recommended dose or in the contraindications for administration. This recommendation is of particular importance in connection with new or infrequently used drugs.

This book was set in Times LT Std by Thomson Digital.
The editors were Amanda Fielding and Peter J. Boyle.
The production supervisor was Richard Ruzycka.
Project management was provided by Nikhil, Thomson Digital.
RR Donnelley was printer and binder.

This book is printed on acid-free paper.

McGraw-Hill Education books are available at special quantity discounts to use as premiums and sales promotions, or for use in corporate training programs. To contact a representative please visit the Contact Us pages at www.mhprofessional.com.

This book is dedicated to all of our current and former residents at the Ventura County Medical Center.

Contents

√ denotes major 2016 updates.
+ denotes new topic for 2016.

2. DISEASE PREVENTION

√ denotes major 2016 updates.
+ denotes new topic for 2016.

3. DISEASE MANAGEMENT

√ denotes major 2016 updates.
+ denotes new topic for 2016.

√ denotes major 2016 updates.
+ denotes new topic for 2016.

√ denotes major 2016 updates.
+ denotes new topic for 2016.

√ denotes major 2016 updates.
+ denotes new topic for 2016.

4. APPENDICES

√ denotes major 2016 updates.
+ denotes new topic for 2016.

Preface

Current Practice Guidelines in Primary Care, 2016 is intended for all clinicians interested in updated, evidence-based guidelines for primary care topics in both the ambulatory and hospital settings. This pocket-sized reference consolidates information from nationally recognized medical associations and government agencies into concise recommendations and guidelines of virtually all ambulatory care topics. This book is organized into topics related to disease screening, disease prevention, and disease management for quick reference to the evaluation and treatment of the most common primary care disorders.

The 2016 edition of *Current Practice Guidelines in Primary Care* contains updates or new chapters in over 80 primary care topics. It is a great resource for residents, medical students, midlevel providers, and practicing physicians in family medicine, internal medicine, pediatrics, and obstetrics and gynecology.

Although painstaking efforts have been made to find all errors and omissions, some errors may remain. If you find an error or wish to make a suggestion, please e-mail us at EditorialServices@mheducation.com.

Evan D. Slater, MD
Joseph S. Esherick, MD, FAAFP
Daniel S. Clark, MD, FACC, FAHA

ABDOMINAL AORTIC ANEURYSM

Disease Screening	Organization	Date	Population	Recommendations	Comments	Source
Abdominal Aortic Aneurysm (AAA)	USPSTF ACC/AHA Canadian Society for Vascular Surgery	2014 2006	Men age 65–75 y who have ever smoked	One-time screening for AAA by ultrasonography. No recommendation for or against screening for AAA in men age 65–75 y who have never smoked.	1. Cochrane review (2007): Significant decrease in AAA-specific mortality in men (OR, 0.60, 95% CI 0.47–0.99) but not for women. (*Cochrane Database Syst Rev.* 2007;2:CD002945; http://www.thecochranelibrary.com) 2. Early mortality benefit of screening (men age 65–74 y) maintained at 7-y follow-up. Cost-effectiveness of screening improves over time. (*Ann Intern Med.* 2007;146:699) 3. Surgical repair of AAA should be considered if diameter ≥5.5 cm or if AAA expands ≥0.5 cm over 6 mo to reduce higher risk of rupture. Meta-analysis: endovascular repair associated with fewer postoperative adverse events and lower 30-d and aneurysm-related mortality but not all-cause mortality compared with open repair. (*Br J Surg.* 2008;95(6):677) 4. Asymptomatic AAA between 4.4 and 5.5 cm should have regular ultrasound surveillance with surgical intervention when AAA expands >1 cm y or diameter reaches 5.5 cm. (*Cochrane Database Syst Rev.* 2008. CD001835; http://www.thecochranelibrary.com) 5. Medicare covers one-time limited screening.	http://www.uspreventive servicestaskforce.org/ Page/Topic/recommendation-summary/abdominal-aortic-aneurysm-screening *J Vasc Surg.* 2007;45:1268-1276
	Canadian Society for Vascular Surgery	2008	Men/women at high risk	All men age 65–75 be screened for AAA. Individual selective screening for those at high risk for AAA: a. Women older than age 65 at high risk secondary to smoking, cerebrovascular disease, and family history b. Men younger than 65 with positive family history		*Circulation.* 2006;113(11): e463-e654 *J Vasc Surg.* 2007;45:1268-1276 *Can J Surg.* 2008;51(1):23-34
	USPSTF	2014	Women who have never smoked	Routine screening is not recommended.		
	UPSTF		Women ages 65–75 y who have ever smoked	The USPSTF concludes that the current evidence is insufficient to assess the balance of benefits and harms of screening for AAA in women ages 65 to 75 y who have ever smoked.		http://www.medicare.gov/ coverage/ab-aortic-aneurysm-screening.html
	CMS	2015	Men age 65–75 y who have smoked at least 100	Recommend one-time ultrasound screening for AAA.		
	ESVS	2011	cigarettes in their lifetime or people at risk who have a family history of AAA	Men should be screened with a single scan at age 65 y. Screening should be considered at an earlier age in those at higher risk for AAA.		Moll FL, Powell JT, Fraedrich G, et al. Management of abdominal aortic aneurysms clinical practice guidelines of the European Society for Vascular Surgery. *Eur J Vasc Endovasc Surg.* 2011;(41):S1-S58

ABDOMINAL AORTIC ANEURYSM

Disease Screening	Organization	Date	Population	Recommendations	Comments	Source
Abdominal Aortic Aneurysm (AAA) (continued)	ESC	2014	Male> 65 y Female > 65 y	Ultrasound screening is recommended in all men > 65 y of age. Ultrasound screening may be considered if history of current/past smoking is present. It is not recommended in female non-smokers without family history of AAA. Targeted screening for AAA with ultrasound should be considered in first-degree siblings of a patient with AAA.	Abdominal echocardiography used for mass screening in subgroups at risk was associated with a significant 45% decreased risk of AAA-related mortality at 10 y.	Erbel R, Aboyans V, Boileau C, et al. 2014 ESC guidelines on the diagnosis and treatment of aortic diseases. *Eur Heart J*. doi:10.1093/eurheartj/ehu281 www.escardio.org/guidelines
	ACR–AIUM–SRU	2014	Male ≥ 65 y Female ≥ 65 y with cardiovascular risk factors.	Ultrasound screening is recommended in all men ≥ 65 y and women ≥ 65 y with cardiovascular risk factors. Patients ≥ 50 y with a family history of aortic and/or peripheral vascular aneurysmal disease. Patients with a personal history of peripheral vascular aneurysmal disease. Groups with additional risk include patients with a history of smoking, hypertension, or certain connective tissue diseases (eg, Marfan syndrome).		http://www.acr.org/~/media/ACR/Documents/PGTS/guidelines/US_Abdominal_Aorta.pdf

ACR = American College of Radiology

ALCOHOL ABUSE AND DEPENDENCE

Disease Screening	Organization	Date	Population	Recommendations	Comments	Source
Alcohol Abuse and Dependence	AAFP USPSTF VA/DOD ICSI	2010 2013 2009 2010	Adults older than 18 y of age	Screen all adults in primary care settings, including pregnant women, for alcohol misuse and provide persons engaged in risky or hazardous drinking with brief behavioral counseling interventions to reduce alcohol misuse.	1. Screen annually using validated tool. 2. AUDIT score ≥4 for men and ≥3 for women and SASQ reporting of ≥5 drinks in a day (men) or ≥4 drinks in a day (women) in the past year are valid and reliable screening instruments for identifying unhealthy alcohol use. 3. The TWEAK and the T-ACE are designed to screen pregnant women for alcohol misuse.	http://www.ahrq.gov/clinic/pocketgd1011/pocketgd1011.pdf http://www.icsi.org/preventive_services_for_adults/preventive_services_for_adults_4.html http://www.uspreventive servicestaskforce.org/uspstf/uspsdrin.htm
	VA/DOD	2009	Adults	Provide brief intervention to those who have a positive alcohol misuse screen. Brief interventions during future visits.		http://www.guidelines.gov/content.aspx?id=15676
	AAFP USPSTF ICSI	2010 2013 2010	Adolescents Children and adolescents	Insufficient evidence to recommend for or against screening or counseling interventions to prevent or reduce alcohol misuse by adolescents.	1. AUDIT and CAGE questionnaires have not been validated in children or adolescents. 2. Reinforce not drinking and driving or riding with any driver under the influence. 3. Reinforce to women the harmful effects of alcohol on fetuses.	http://www.uspreventive servicestaskforce.org/uspstf/uspsdrin.htm http://www.icsi.org/preventive_services_for_children_guideline_/preventive_services_for_children_and_adolescents_2531.html

AUDIT, alcohol use disorders identification test; SASQ, single alcohol screening question.

ANEMIA

Disease Screening	Organization	Date	Population	Recommendations	Comments	Source
Anemia	AAFP	2006	Infants age 6–12 mo	Perform selective, single hemoglobin or hematocrit screening for high-risk infants.[a]	Reticulocyte hemoglobin content is a more sensitive and specific marker than is serum hemoglobin level for iron deficiency. One-third of patients with iron deficiency will have a hemoglobin level >11 g/dL.	http://www.aafp.org/online/en/home/clinical/exam.html *Am Fam Physician.* 2013;87:98
	USPSTF	2010	Infants age 6–12 mo	Evidence is insufficient to recommend for or against routine screening, but risk assessment based on diet, socioeconomic status, prematurity, and low birth weight should be done.	Recommend routine iron supplementation in asymptomatic high-risk children age 6–12 mo but not in those who are of average risk for iron-deficiency anemia.	
	USPSTF	2015	Pregnant women	Screen all women with hemoglobin or hematocrit at first pre-natal visit.	1. Insufficient evidence to recommend for or against routine use of iron supplements for nonanemic pregnant women (USPSTF). 2. When acute stress or inflammatory disorders are not present, a serum ferritin level is the most accurate test for evaluating iron deficiency anemia. Among women of childbearing age, a cutoff of 30 ng/mL has sensitivity of 92%, specificity of 98%. (*Blood.* 1997;89:1052-1057). 3. Severe anemia (hemoglobin <6) associated with abnormal fetal oxygenation and transfusion should be considered. In iron-deficient women intolerant of oral iron, intravenous iron sucrose or iron dextran should be given.	http://www.ahrq.gov/clinic/cpgsix.htm *Ann Intern Med.* 2015;162:566
	AAP	2010	Infants and young children 0–3 y	Universal screening of Hgb at 12 mo. If anemic, measure ferritin, C-reactive protein, and reticulocyte hemoglobin content.	Use of transferring receptor 1 (TfR₁) assay as screening for iron deficiency is under investigation. (*Pediatrics.* 2010;126:1040).	http://pediatrics.aappublications.org.libproxy.usc.edu/content/126/5/1040.full

[a]Includes infants living in poverty, Blacks, Native Americans, Alaska natives, immigrants from developing countries, preterm and low-birth-weight infants, and infants whose principal dietary intake is unfortified cow's milk or soy milk. Less than two servings per day of iron-rich foods (iron-fortified breakfast cereals or meats).

ATTENTION-DEFICIT/HYPERACTIVITY DISORDER

Disease Screening	Organization	Date	Population	Recommendations	Comments	Source
Attention Deficit/ Hyperactivity Disorder (ADHD)	AAFP AAP	2000	Children age 6–12 y with inattention, hyperactivity, impulsivity, academic underachievement, or behavioral problems	Initiate an evaluation for ADHD. Diagnosis requires the child meet DSM-IV criteria[a] and direct supporting evidence from parents or caregivers and classroom teacher. Evaluation of a child with ADHD should include assessment for coexisting disorders.	1. The rise in stimulant prescriptions since 1990 plateaued in 2002. (*Am J Psychiatry.* 2006;163:579) 2. Current estimates are that 8.7% of U.S. children/adolescents and 5% of adults meet criteria for ADHD. (*Arch Pediatr Adolesc Med.* 2007;161:857. *Am J Psychiatry.* 2006;163:716) Worldwide prevalence is estimated at 5.3%. (*Am J Psychiatry.* 2007;164:942) 3. The U.S. Food and Drug Administration (FDA) approved a "black box" warning regarding the potential for cardiovascular side effects of ADHD stimulant drugs. (*N Engl J Med.* 2006;354:1445)	*Pediatrics.* 2000;105:1158

[a]DSM-IV Criteria for ADHD:

I: Either A or B.

A: Six or more of the following symptoms of inattention have been present for at least 6 mo to a point that is disruptive and inappropriate for developmental level. *Inattention:* (1) Often does not give close attention to details or makes careless mistakes in schoolwork, work, or other activities. (2) Often has trouble keeping attention on tasks or play activities. (3) Often does not seem to listen when spoken to directly. (4) Often does not follow instructions and fails to finish schoolwork, chores, or duties in the workplace (not due to oppositional behavior or failure to understand instructions). (5) Often has trouble organizing activities. (6) Often avoids, dislikes, or does not want to do things that take a lot of mental effort for a long period of time (such as schoolwork or homework). (7) Often loses things needed for tasks and activities (eg, toys, school assignments, pencils, books, or tools). (8) Is often easily distracted. (9) Is often forgetful in daily activities.

B: Six or more of the following symptoms of hyperactivity-impulsivity have been present for at least 6 mo to an extent that is disruptive and inappropriate for developmental level. *Hyperactivity:* (1) Often fidgets with hands or feet or squirms in seat. (2) Often gets up from seat when remaining in seat is expected. (3) Often runs about or climbs when and where it is not appropriate (adolescents or adults may feel very restless). (4) Often has trouble playing or enjoying leisure activities quietly. (5) Is often "on the go" or often acts as if "driven by a motor." (6) Often talks excessively. *Impulsivity:* (1) Often blurts out answers before questions have been finished. (2) Often has trouble waiting one's turn. (3) Often interrupts or intrudes on others (eg, butts into conversations or games).

II: Some symptoms that cause impairment were present before age 7 y.

III: Some impairment from the symptoms is present in two or more settings (eg, at school/work and at home).

IV: There must be clear evidence of significant impairment in social, school, or work functioning.

V: The symptoms do not happen only during the course of a pervasive developmental disorder, schizophrenia, or other psychotic disorder. The symptoms are not better accounted for by another mental disorder (eg, mood disorder, anxiety disorder, dissociative disorder, or a personality disorder).

BACTERIURIA, ASYMPTOMATIC

Disease Screening	Organization	Date	Population	Recommendations	Comments	Source
Bacteriuria, Asymptomatic	AAFP USPSTF	2010 2008	Pregnant women	Recommend screening for bacteriuria at first prenatal visit or at 12–16 wk' gestation.		http://www.guideline.gov/content.aspx?id=38619
	AAFP USPSTF	2010 2008	Men and nonpregnant women	Recommend against routine screening for bacteriuria.		http://www.uspreventiveservicestaskforce.org/uspstf08/asymptbact/asbactrs.htm

BACTERIAL VAGINOSIS

Disease Screening	Organization	Date	Population	Recommendations	Comments	Source
Bacterial Vaginosis	AAFP USPSTF	2010 2008	Pregnant women at high risk for preterm delivery	Insufficient evidence to recommend for or against routine screening.		http://www.guideline.gov/content.aspx?id=38619 http://www.uspreventiveservicestaskforce.org/uspstf08/bv/bvrs.htm
	AAFP USPSTF	2010 2008	Low-risk pregnant women	Recommend against routine screening.		

BARRETT ESOPHAGUS

Disease screening	Organization	Date	Population	Recommendations	Comments	Source
Barrett Esophagus (BE)	AGA	2011	General population with GERD	Against screening general population with GERD for BE (strong recommendation).	—Despite lack of evidence of benefit of screening general population with GERD for BE, endoscopic screening is common and widespread.	
			High-risk population with GERD (multiple risk factors including age >50, male gender, white, chronic GERD, hiatal hernia, BMI >30, intra-abdominal body fat distribution or tobacco use.)	Screening should be strongly considered in this population, especially patients with multiple risk factors (weak recommendation). If Barrett's found without dysplasia follow-up endoscopy in 1 y then every 3–5 y. (*JAMA.* 2013;310:627)	—40% of patients with BE and esophageal cancer have not had chronic GERD symptoms. —The diagnosis of dysplasia in BE should be confirmed by at least one additional pathologist, preferably one who is an expert in esophageal pathology. (*Gastroenterology.* 2011;140:1084) (*N Engl J Med.* 2014;371:836)	

CANCER, BLADDER

Disease Screening	Organization	Date	Population	Recommendations	Comments	Source
Cancer, Bladder	AAFP	2011	Asymptomatic persons	Recommends against routine screening for bladder cancer (CA) in adults. Evidence is insufficient to assess balance of benefits and harms of screening for bladder CA in asymptomatic adults. (No major organization recommends screening for bladder cancer in asymptomatic adults.)	1. *Benefits:* There is inadequate evidence to determine whether screening for bladder CA would have any impact on mortality. *Harms:* Based on fair evidence, screening for bladder CA would result in unnecessary diagnostic procedures and overdiagnosis (70% of bladder CA is in situ) with attendant morbidity. (NCI, 2008) 2. A high index of suspicion should be maintained in anyone with a history of smoking (4- to 7-fold increased risk[a]), an exposure to industrial toxins (aromatic amines, benzene) or therapeutic pelvic radiation, cyclophosphamide chemotherapy, history of *Schistosoma haematobium* cystitis, hereditary nonpolyposis colon CA (Lynch syndrome), and history of transitional cell carcinoma of ureter (50% risk of subsequent bladder CA). Large screening studies in these high-risk populations have not been performed. 3. Voided urine cytology with sensitivity of 40% but only 10% positive predictive value, urinary biomarkers (nuclear matrix protein 22, telomerase) with suboptimal sensitivity and specificity. Screening by microscopic hematuria has <10% positive predictive value.	http://www.aafp.org/online/en/home/clinical/exam.html
	USPSTF	2011				http://www.ahrq.gov/clinic/uspstf/uspsblad.htm http://www.cancer.gov

[a]Individuals who smoke are 4–7 times more likely to develop bladder CA than are individuals who have never smoked. Additional environmental risk factors: exposure to aminobiphenyls; aromatic amines; azo dyes; combustion gases and soot from coal; chlorination by-products in heated water; aldehydes used in chemical dyes and in the rubber and textile industries; organic chemicals used in dry cleaning, paper manufacturing, rope and twine making, and apparel manufacturing; contaminated Chinese herbs; arsenic in well water. Additional risk factors: prolonged exposure to urinary *S. haematobium* bladder infections, cyclophosphamide, or pelvic radiation therapy for other malignancies.

				CANCER, BREAST		

Disease Screening	Organization	Date	Population	Recommendations[a,b]	Comments	Source
Cancer, Breast	ACS	2015	Women age 20–39 y	Inform women of benefits and limitations of breast self-examination (BSE). Educate concerning reporting a lump or breast symptoms. Clinical breast exam (CBE) every 2–3 y. Breast imaging not indicated for average-risk women.	1. *Benefits of mammography screening:* Based on fair evidence, screening mammography in women age 40–70 y decreases breast CA mortality. The benefit is higher in older women (reduction in risk of death in women age 40–49 y = 15%–20%, 25%–30% in women age ≥50 y). *Harms:* Based on solid evidence, screening mammography may lead to potential harm by overdiagnosis (indolent tumors that are not life-threatening) and unnecessary biopsies for benign disease. It is estimated that 20%–25% of diagnosed breast cancers are indolent and unlikely to be clinically significant. (*CA Cancer J Clin.* 2012;62:5. *Ann Intern Med.* 2012;156:491)	http://www.cancer.org
	ACP	2012	Women age 40–49 y	Perform individualized assessment of breast CA risk; base screening decision on benefits and harms of screening (see Comment 1), as well as on a woman's preferences and CA risk profile. (*Ann Intern Med.* 2012;156:635. *Ann Intern Med.* 2012;156:662)	2. BSE does not improve breast CA mortality (*Br J Cancer.* 2003;88:1047) and increases the rate of false-positive biopsies. (*J Natl Cancer Inst* 2002;94:1445) 3. Twenty-five percent of breast CAs diagnosed before age 40 y are attributable to *BRCA1* or 2 mutations.	*Ann Intern Med.* 2012;156:609. *Ann Intern Med.* 2014;160:864.
	UK-NHS	2012	Women age 40–49 y	Based on current evidence, routine screening is not recommended.	4. The sensitivity of annual screening of young (age 30–49 y) high-risk women with magnetic resonance imaging (MRI) and mammography is superior to either alone, but MRI is associated with a significant increase in false positives. (*Lancet.* 2005;365:1769. *Lancet Oncol.* 2011;378:1804) 5. Computer-aided detection in screening mammography appears to reduce overall accuracy (by increasing false-positive rate), although it is more sensitive in women age <50 y with dense breasts. (*N Engl J Med.* 2007;356:1399) 6. Digital mammography vs. film screen mammography equal in women 50–79 y old but digital more accurate in women 40–49 y old. (*Ann Intern Med.* 2011;155:493). 7. Future cancer screening—circulating tumor DNA (ctDNA)—mutations identified consistent with specific underlying malignancy. Promising preliminary data. (*Nat Med.* 2014;20:548. *J Clin Onc.* 2014;82:5)	http://www.cancerscreening.nhs.uk
	AAFP	2013	Women age ≥40 y	Mammography, with or without CBE, every 1–2 y after counseling about potential risks and benefits.	Evidence is insufficient to recommend for or against routine CBE alone, or teaching or performing a routine BSE; recommend against screening women >75 y old. Breast MRI annually for BRCA 1 and 2 mutation carriers. Consider in women with >20% lifetime risk of breast cancer.	http://www.aafp.org/online/en/home/clinical/exam.html

Disease Screening	Organization	Date	Population	Recommendations[a,b]	Comments	Source
Cancer, Breast (continued)	ACS	2015	Women age ≥40 y	Mammography and CBE yearly; if >20% lifetime risk of breast CA, annual mammogram + MRI. *BRCA1* and *2* mutation-positive women should begin MRI and mammogram screening at age 30 y or younger, depending on family history. Lymphoma survivors with a history of mediastinal radiation should begin mammography and MRI yearly 10 y after radiation. Dense breasts (>50%) by itself is not an indication for MRI screening. New ACS guidelines—mammo once yearly 45–55 y/o; every 2 yrs. >55y/o; clinical breast exam not recommended	1. In high-risk women, probability of breast CA when mammogram is negative = 1.4% (1.2%–1.6%) vs. when mammogram plus MRI are negative = 0.3% (0.1%–0.8%). (*Ann Intern Med.* 2008;148:671) MRI 2–3 times as sensitive as mammogram, but 2-fold increase in false positives—use in selected high-risk population only. (*J Clin Oncol.* 2005;23:8469. *J Clin Oncol.* 2009;27:6124) Tomosynthesis (3-dimensional mammography) under study with increase in sensitivity and specificity and reduction in false positives vs film or digital mammography. There is double the dose of radiation compared to mammogram which may limit its use. (*JAMA.* 2014;311:2499) (*JAMA.* 2014;311:2488) 2. If lifetime risk of breast CA is between 15% and 20%, women should discuss risks/benefits of adding annual MRI to mammography screening. Sensitivity of MRI superior to mammography, especially in higher-risk women age <50 y with dense breasts (increasing breast density increases risk of breast CA and lowers sensitivity of mammogram). A >75% breast density increases risk of breast CA 5-fold. (*J Clin Oncol.* 2010;28:3830. *N Engl J Med.* 2015;372:2243. *Ann Inter Med.* 2015;162:157). 3. Genetic evaluation increasing with more women tested for BRCA 1 and 2 mutations as well as mutations in PALB2, CHEK 2, TP53, PTEN, DNA mismatch repair and others through use of next generation gene sequencing panels. (*Curr Opin Genet Dev.* 2010;20:268. *Genet Med.* 2013;15:733. *N Engl J Med.* 2015;372:2243)	http://www.cancer.org *CA Cancer J Clin.* 2015;65:30 *N Engl J Med.* 2015;372:2353.
	UK-NHS	2012	Women age 50–70 y Women age >70 y	Program-initiated mammography screening of all women every 3 y. Patient-initiated screening covered by National Health Service (NHS).	Annual vs 3-y screening interval showed no significant difference in predicted breast CA mortality, although relative risk reduction among annually screened women had nonsignificant reduction of 5%–11%. (*Eur J Cancer.* 2002;38:1458)	http://www.cancerscreening.nhs.uk
	AAFP	2013	Women with family history associated with increased risk (breast CA age <50 y or ovarian CA at any age) for deleterious mutations in *BRCA1* or *BRCA2* genes[c] (Gail model: *J Natl Cancer Inst.* 1999;91:1541. BRAC PRO model: *Am J Hum Genet.* 1998;62:145)	Refer for genetic counseling and evaluation for *BRCA* testing.	1. In one study, nearly half of *BRCA*-positive women with newly diagnosed breast CA developed malignant disease detected by mammography <1 y after a normal screening mammogram. (*Cancer.* 2004;100:2079) 2. Consider mammography plus MRI screening in high-risk women. (*CA Cancer J Clin.* 2011;61:8-30) 3. Management of an inherited predisposition to breast CA is controversial. (*N Engl J Med.* 2007;357:154). Risk-reducing surgery vs. enhanced surveillance with yearly magnetic resonance imaging (MRI) and mammography.	http://www.aafp.org/online/en/home/clinical/exam.html

CANCER, BREAST						

Disease Screening	Organization	Date	Population	Recommendations[a,b]	Comments	Source
Cancer, Breast (continued)	USPSTF	2015	Women age 50–74 y	—Biennial screening mammography. —BSE teaching not recommended. —Inconclusive data for screening women age >75 y.	These recommendations for women age 40–50 y have been widely criticized and largely ignored by other advisory organizations as inconsistent with available data. Subsequent trial from Norway showed significant benefit in mortality reduction (28%) in the age 40–49 y subset. Analysis of data sets continues, but there has been no major change in practice patterns. (*AJR Am J Roentgenol.* 2011;196:112. *J Am Coll Radiol.* 2010;7:18. *Cancer.* 2011;117:7. *Eur J Cancer.* 2010;46:3137. *CA Cancer J Clin.* 2012;62:129)	http://www.ahrq. gov/clinic/ uspstfix.htm
			Women age 40–50 y	—Decision to begin screening mammography before age 50 y should be individualized according to benefit vs. harm for each unique patient. (*Ann Intern Med.* 2012 156:609. *Ann Intern Med.* 2009;151:727)		
	NCCN	2015	Age 25–40 y (average risk) Age >40 y (average risk) Acquired increased risk—prior thoracic radiation therapy	CBE every 1–3 y—breast awareness education. Annual CBE, annual mammogram. MRI not recommended in average-risk patients. CBE q6–12 mo, annual mammogram and annual MRI beginning 8–10 y after radiation therapy or age 40 y, whichever comes first. Breast MRI should be performed days 7–15 of menstrual cycle to maximize accuracy.	The Canadian National Breast Screening study began in 1980 found no survival benefit for mammography in 40–59 y old women but the study is thought to be flawed by most experts in the United States because of study design. (*BMJ.* 2014;348:g366. *N Engl J Med.* 2014;370:1965). A recent meta-analysis (*JAMA.* 2014;311:1327) from Harvard found an overall reduction of breast cancer mortality of 19% (15% for women in their 40s and 32% for women in their 60s). They were concerned about over diagnosis and other potential harms of screening including false positive findings and unnecessary biopsies. These recent studies have led to an increased in further screening studies based on the predicted individual risk of breast cancer occurrence (*Ann Int Med,* published online 8 Apri., 2014). A woman with mediastinal radiation at age 10–30 y will have a 75-fold increased risk of breast CA at age 35 y vs age-matched controls. Salpingo-oophorectomy will decrease risk of breast CA in *BRCA*₁ and 2 carriers by 50% and decrease risk of ovarian CA by 90%–95%.	www.nccn.org

CANCER, BREAST

Disease Screening	Organization	Date	Population	Recommendations[a,b]	Comments	Source
Cancer, Breast (continued)	NCCN	2015	High risk-lifetime risk of breast CA >20% based on personal and family history (utilize Gail model, BRCAPRO model, or Tyrer-Cuzick model) genetic predisposition (BRCA 1 or 2). (http://www.cancer.gov/bcrisktool/) Also, a history of lobular carcinoma in situ, atypical hyperplasia or history of breast CA. (invasive and DCIS).	Aged <25 y annual CBE, breast awareness education, and referral to genetic counselor. Aged >25 y, annual mammogram and MRI, CBE q6–12 mo, consider risk-reducing strategies (surgery, chemoprevention).	Tamoxifen or raloxifene not studied as de novo chemo prevention in BRCA1 or 2 patients, but tamoxifen will decrease risk of contralateral breast CA by 50% in BRCA-mutated breast CA patients. (*Int J Cancer.* 2006;118:2281) Risk-reducing bilateral mastectomy in BRCA1 and 2 mutation carriers results in a 90% risk reduction in incidence of breast CA and a 90% rate of satisfaction with risk-reducing surgery. (*N Engl J Med.* 2001;345:159. *JAMA.* 2010;304:967)	http://www.ahrq.gov/clinic/uspstf www.nccn.org

[a]Debate about the value of screening mammograms was triggered by a Cochrane review published on October 20, 2001 (*Lancet.* 2001;358:1340-1342). This review cited a number of methodologic and analytic flaws in the large long-term mammography trials. The USPSTF and NCI concluded that the flaws were problematic but unlikely to negate the consistent and significant mortality reductions observed in the trials.

[b]Summary of current evidence: *CA Cancer J Clin.* 2011;61:8-30.

[c]1. Women not of Ashkenazi Jewish heritage:

Two first-degree relatives with breast CA, one of whom received the diagnosis at age ≤50 y.

A combination of ≥3 first- or second-degree relatives with breast CA.

A combination of both breast and ovarian CA among first- and second-degree relatives.

A first-degree relative with bilateral breast CA.

A combination of ≥2 first- or second-degree relatives with ovarian CA.

A first- or second-degree relative with both breast and ovarian CA.

A history of breast CA in a male relative.

2. Women of Ashkenazi Jewish heritage: Any first-degree relative (or second-degree relatives on the same side of the family) with breast or ovarian CA.

CANCER, BREAST				
TABLE A: HARMS OF SCREENING MAMMOGRAPHY				
Harm	**Internal Validity**	**Consistency**	**Magnitude of Effects**	**External Validity**
Treatment of insignificant CAs (overdiagnosis of indolent cancer) can result in breast deformity, lymphedema, thromboembolic events, and chemotherapy-induced toxicities.	Good	Good	Approximately 20%–30% of breast CAs detected by screening mammograms represent overdiagnosis. (*BMJ.* 2009;339:2587) Oncotype DX (a predictive panel of 15 breast CA genes) can reduce the use of chemotherapy by 50% in node-negative hormone receptor-positive patients.	Good
Additional testing (false positives)	Good	Good	Estimated to occur in 30% of women screened annually for 10 y, 7%–10% of whom will have biopsies. This creates anxiety and negative quality of life impact. (*Ann Intern Med.* 2009;151:738. *Ann Intern Med.* 2011;155:481)	Good
False sense of security, delay in CA diagnosis (false negatives)	Good	Good	Approximately 10%–30% of women with invasive CA will have negative mammogram results, especially if young with dense breasts or with lobular or high-grade CAs. (*Radiology.* 2005;235:775) All suspicious lumps should be biopsied even with negative mammogram.	Good
Radiation-induced mutation can cause breast CA, especially if exposed before age 30 y. Latency is more than 10 y, and the increased risk persists lifelong.	Good	Good	In women beginning screening at age 40 y, benefits far outweigh risks of radiation inducing breast CA. Women should avoid unnecessary CT scanning. (*Br J Cancer.* 2005;93:590. *Ann Intern Med.* 2012;156:662)	Good
Source: NCI. 2010—http://www.cancer.gov				

CANCER, CERVICAL

Disease Screening	Organization	Date	Population	Recommendations	Comments	Source
Cancer, Cervical	ACS	2015	Women age <21 y old: no screening[a] Women between age 21 and 29 y old Average risk women 30–65 y old	Cytology alone (PAP smear) every 3 y until age 30 y. Human papillomavirus (HPV) DNA testing not recommended if age <30 y (majority of young patients will clear the infection). HPV and cytology "cotesting" every 5 y (preferred) or cytology alone every 3 y (acceptable). If HPV positive/cytology negative—either 12-mo follow-up with cotesting or test for HPV 16 or 18 genotypes with referral to colposcopy if positive. Continue to screen more frequently if high-risk factors present.[b-d] 10% of women aged 30–34 will have normal cytology but a positive HPV test and will need more frequent testing. In women 60–65 years old only 2.5% will have negative cytology but positive HPV testing.	1. Cervical CA is causally related to infection with HPV (>70% associated with either HPV-18 or HPV-16 genotype) (see new ACIP HPV Recommendations, Appendix VIII). 2. Immunocompromised women (organ transplantation, chemotherapy, chronic steroid therapy, or human immunodeficiency virus [HIV]) should be tested twice during the first year after initiating screening and annually thereafter. (*CA Cancer J Clin.* 2011:61:8. *Ann Intern Med.* 2011:155:698) 3. Women with a history of cervical CA or in utero exposure to diethylstilbestrol (DES) should continue average-risk protocol for women age <30 y indefinitely. 4. HPV vaccination of young women is now recommended by ACIP, UK-NHS, and others. Cervical CA screening recommendations have not changed for women receiving the vaccine because the vaccine covers only 70% of HPV serotypes that cause cervical CA. (*MMWR.* 2007:56(RR-2):1–24. *CA cancer J Clin.* 2014:64:30. *N Engl J Med.* 2015:372:711) 5. Long-term use of oral contraceptives may increase risk of cervical CA in women who test positive for cervical HPV DNA (*Lancet.* 2002:359:1085). Smoking increases risk of cervical CA 4-fold. (*Am J Epidemiol.* 1990:131:945) 6. A vaccine against HPV-16 and -18 significantly reduces the risk of acquiring transient and persistent infection. (*N Engl J Med.* 2002:347:1645. *Obstet Gynecol.* 2006:107(1):4) 7. *Benefits:* Based on solid evidence, regular screening of appropriate women with the Pap test reduces mortality from cervical CA. Screening is effective when starting at age 21 y. *Harms:* Based on solid evidence, regular screening with the Pap test leads to additional diagnostic procedures and treatment for low-grade squamous intraepithelial lesions (LSILs), with uncertain long-term consequences on fertility and pregnancy. Harms are greatest for younger women, who have a higher prevalence of LSILs. LSILs often regress without treatment. False positives in postmenopausal women are a result of mucosal atrophy. (NCI, 2008) 8. There is basically now no significant differences in guidelines for screening for cervical cancer in average risk women among ACOG, ACS, USPSTF.	http://www.cancer.org http://www.survivorship guidelines.org *CA Cancer J Clin.* 2012; 62:147–172 *N Engl J Med.* 2013:369: 2324.
	ACS	2015	Age >65 y after hysterectomy	No screening following adequate prior screening. No screening in women without a cervix and no history of CIN2 or worse in last 20 y or cervical CA ever.		
	USPSTF	2015	Women aged 21–29 y Women aged 30–65 y Women younger than 21 y Women younger than age 30 y	Screen with cytology (PAP smear) every 3 y. Screen with cytology every 3 y or cotesting (cytology/HPV testing) every 5 y. Do not screen. Do not screen with HPV testing (alone or with cytology).		http://www .uspreventive servicestaskforce.org/ *Ann Intern Med.* 2012:156:880

Disease Screening	**Organization**	**Date**	**Population**	**Recommendations**	**Comments**	**Source**

CANCER, CERVICAL

Disease Screening	Organization	Date	Population	Recommendations	Comments	Source
Cancer, Cervical (continued)	UK-NHS UK-NHS	2011 2011	Women age <25 y Women age 25–49 y Women age 50–64 y	Routine screening is not recommended. Routine screen every 3 y—triage to HPV testing if borderline changes or mild dyskaryosis; if HPV positive refer for colposcopy. Routinely screen every 5 y with conventional cytology—HPV triage if borderline abnormal findings.	UK-NHS initiated an HPV immunization program for girls age 12–13 y in September 2008. UK-NHS contacts all eligible women who are registered with a primary care doctor.	http://www.cancerscreening.nhs.uk http://www.cancerscreening.nhs.uk
	UK-NHS	2011	Women age ≥65 years	Screen women who have not been screened since age 50 y or who have had recent abnormal test results—if all previous cervical cancer screening has been negative, cease screening	Stop screening after age 65 y if there are three consecutive normal test results.	http://www.cancerscreening.nhs.uk
	ACOG	2009	Begin at age 21 y independent of sexual history	Every 2 y from ages 21 to 29.	Women age ≥30 y can extend interval to every 2–3 y if three consecutive negative screens, no history of cervical intraepithelial neoplasia 2 or 3, not immunocompromised, no HIV, and not exposed to DES. No more often than 3 y if cervical cytology and HPV testing combined.	ACOG Practice bulletin: *Obstet Gynecol.* 2009;114:1409
	USPSTF	2015	Women age >65 y	Recommends against routine screening if woman has had adequate recent screening and normal Pap smear results and is not otherwise at high risk for cervical CA.[c]	Beyond age 70 y, there is little evidence for or against screening women who have been regularly screened in previous years. Individual circumstances, such as the patient's life expectancy, ability to undergo treatment if CA is detected, and ability to cooperate with and tolerate the Pap smear procedure, may obviate the need for cervical CA screening.	http://www.ahrq.gov/clinic/uspstf/uspscerv.htm
	ACS	2015	Women age ≥70 y	Discontinue screening if ≥3 normal Pap smear results in a row and no abnormal Pap smear results in the last 10 y.[d]		http://www.cancer.org
	ACS ACOG USPSTF	2008 2009 2012	Women without a cervix and no history of high-grade precancer or cervical cancer	Recommends against routine Pap smear screening in women who have had a total hysterectomy or removal of the cervix for benign disease and no history of abnormal cell growth.		http://www.cancer.org http://www.ahrq.gov/clinic/uspstf/uspscerv.htm ACOG practice bulletin-109 12/09

[a]Sexual history in patients <21 y old not considered in beginning cytologic screening, which should start at age 21.

[b]New tests to improve CA detection include liquid-based/thin-layer preparations, computer-assisted screening methods, and HPV testing (*Am Fam Physician.* 2001;64:729. *N Engl J Med.* 2007;357:1579. *JAMA.* 2009;302:1757).

[c]High-risk factors include DES exposure before birth, HIV infection, or other forms of immunosuppression, including chronic steroid use.

[d]Women with a history of cervical CA, DES exposure, HIV infection, or a weakened immune system should continue to have screenings as long as they are in >5-y life expectancy.

CANCER, COLORECTAL

Disease Screening	Organization	Date	Population	Recommendations	Comments	Source
Cancer, Colorectal	ACS USMTFCC[a] ACR	2013 2012		See Table on page 20. Tests that find polyps and CA are preferred.	Although colonoscopy is the de facto gold standard for colon CA screening, choice of screening technique depends on risk, comorbidities, insurance coverage, patient preference, and availability. Above all, do something to screen for colon CA.	CA Cancer J Clin. 2013;63:87-105 CA Cancer J Clin. 2012;62:124-142
	AAFP USPSTF	2015 2008	Age ≥50 y at average risk[b]	Screen with one of the following strategies[c,e]: 1. Fecal occult blood test (gFOBT-guaiac based or iFOBT-immunochemical based—iFOBT is preferred) annually[f] 2. Flexible sigmoidoscopy every 5 y 3. FOBT annually plus flexible sigmoidoscopy every 5 y 4. Colonoscopy every 10 y[g] 5. CT colonoscopy 6. Multitargeted stool DNA testing (cologuard)—now approved—92% colon cancers detected in asymptomatic average risk persons but < 50% of polyps detected, 10% false positives and cost $600/test. (JAMA. 2014;312:2566) 7. Follow-up colonoscopy – normal or small hyperplastic polyps—10 y – 1 or 2 < 10 mm tubular adenomas—5–10 y – small serrated polyps without dysplasia—5 y – 3–10 tubular adenomas, a tubular adenoma, or serrated polyp > 10 mm, adenoma with high-grade dysplasia—3 y	1. The USPSTF "strongly recommends" colorectal cancer (CRC) screening in this group up to age 75 y; screening patients >75 y old is not recommended. 2. Flexible sigmoidoscopy and one-time FOBT mandating a colonoscopy if either yields positive results will miss 25% of significant proximal neoplasia. This strategy should include yearly FOBT. (N Engl J Med. 2001;345:555. N Engl J Med. 2012;366:2345) 3. FOBT alone decreased CRC mortality by 33% compared with those who were not screened. (Gastroenterology. 2004;126:1674) 4. Accuracy of colonoscopy is operator dependent—rapid withdrawal time, poor prep, and lack of experience will increase false negatives. (N Engl J Med. 2006;355:2533. Ann Intern Med. 2012;156:692) 5. Multi-targeted DNA stool testing vs. iFOBT with more cancers detected (92.3% vs 73.8%) but more false positives with DNA test. (N Engl J Med. 2014;370:187-1297. N Engl J Med. 2014;370:1298-1306) 6. Percentage of U.S. adults receiving some form of CRC screening increased from 44% in 1999 to 63% in 2008. The goal is 80% by 2018. (CA Cancer J Clin. 2015;65:30. Arch Intern Med. 2011;171:647. Arch Intern Med. 2012;172:575) 7. Colonoscopy vs. iFOBT testing in CRC with similar detection of cancer but more adenomas identified in colonoscopy group. (N Engl J Med. 2012;366:697. N Engl J Med. 2012;366:687)	http://www.aafp.org/online/en/home/clinical/exam.html http://www.cancer.org Gastrointest Endosc. 2006;63:546
	ACOG	2007	Women at average risk age ≥50 y	Preferred method: • Colonoscopy every 10 y Other appropriate methods: • FOBT annually • Flexible sigmoidoscopy every 5 y • FOBT annually plus flexible sigmoidoscopy every 5 y • Double-contrast barium enema every 5 y		Ann Intern Med. 2012;156:378 Gastroenterology. 2003;124:544 http://www.ahrq.gov/clinic/uspstf/uspscolo.htm ACOG Committee Opinion. No. 357. Nov 2007 N Engl J Med. 2013;369:1095
	UK-NHS	2007	Adults age 60–69 y Adults age ≥70 y	Program screened every 2 years with FOBTc Patient-initiated screening covered by NHS		http://www.cancerscreening.nhs.uk/bowel/index.html
	ACS USMTFCC[a]	2008	Persons at increased risk based on family history but without a definable genetic syndrome	Group I: Screening colonoscopy at age 40 y, or 10 y younger than the earliest diagnosis in the immediate family, and repeated every 5 y.[h] Group II: Follow average-risk recommendations, but begin at age 40 y.		CA Cancer J Clin. 2008;58:130

CANCER, COLORECTAL

Disease Screening	Organization	Date	Population	Recommendations	Comments	Source
Cancer, Colorectal (continued)			Very-high-risk hereditary nonpolyposis colorectal cancer (HNPCC or Lynch syndrome); 5% of patients with CRC will have HNPCC. Evaluate if Bethesda or Amsterdam criteria met[b]. Evaluate if the patient <50 y old or Bethesda or Amsterdam criteria met[b]	Colonoscopy every 2 y beginning at age 20–25 y then yearly at age 40 y.[b]	8. In follow-up with curable CRC, CEA every 3 mo for 2 y followed by every 6 mo for 3 y was equivalent to CT scans every 6 mo for 2 y and then every 12 mo for 3 y in discovering recurrence of CRC and length of overall survival. (*JAMA.* 2014;311:263) Increased risk of non-CRC (endometrial, ovary, upper gastrointestinal, pancreas, renal pelvis, ureter, breast) requires systematic screening. (*J Clin Oncol.* 2000;18:11. *J Clin Oncol.* 2012;30:1058) 9. NCCN recommends screening for Lynch syndrome in all patients with CRC <70 y/o. Do DNA mismatch repair analysis or immunohistochemistry followed by PCR study to confirm.	*Am J Gastroenterol.* 2009;104:739 *J Clin Oncol.* 2003;21:2397 *Gut.* 2003;57:704 *JAMA.* 2006;296:1507
			Classic familial adenomatous polyposis (FAP)	At-risk children should be offered genetic testing at age 10–12 y. Flexible sigmoidoscopy or colonoscopy every 12 mo starting at age 10–12 y. Elective colectomy based on number and histology of polyps—usually done by early 20s; upper endoscopy every 5 y if no gastric or duodenal polyps starting in early 20s.	Extraintestinal tumors in FAP include hepatoblastoma (AFP screening recommended in families with this tumor), adrenal tumors, osteomas, brain tumors, skin CA, and thyroid CA.	

[a] U.S. Multisociety Task Force on Colorectal Cancer (ACG, ACP, AGA, ASGE).

[b] Risk factors indicating need for earlier/more frequent screening: personal history of CRC or adenomatous polyps or hepatoblastoma, CRC or polyps in a first-degree relative age <60 y or in 2 first-degree relatives of any age, personal history of chronic inflammatory bowel disease, and family with hereditary CRC syndromes (*Ann Intern Med.* 1998;128(1):900. *Am J Gastroenterol.* 2009;104:739. *N Engl J Med.* 1994;331(25):1669. *N Engl J Med.* 1995;332(13):861). Additional high-risk group: history of ≥30 Gy radiation to whole abdomen; all upper abdominal fields; pelvic, thoracic, lumbar, or sacral spine. Begin monitoring 10 years after radiation or at age 35 y, whichever occurs last (http://www. survivorshipguidelines.org). Screening colonoscopy in those age ≥80 y results in only 15% of the expected gain in life expectancy seen in younger patients (*JAMA.* 2006;295:2357). ACG treats African Americans as high-risk group. See separate recommendation above.

[c] A positive result on an FOBT should be followed by colonoscopy. An alternative is flexible sigmoidoscopy and air-contrast barium enema.

[d] FOBT should be performed on 2 samples from 3 consecutive specimens obtained at home. A single stool guaiac during annual physical examination is not adequate.

[e] USPSTF did not find direct evidence that a screening colonoscopy is effective in reducing CRC mortality rates.

[f] Use the guaiac-based test with dietary restriction, or an immunochemical test without dietary restriction. Two samples from each of three consecutive stools should be examined without rehydration. Rehydration increases the false-positive rate.

[g] Population-based retrospective analysis: risk of developing CRC remains decreased for >10 y following negative colonoscopy findings (*JAMA.* 2006;295:2366). *Group I:* First-degree relative with colon CA or adenomatous polyps at age <60 y or 2 first-degree relatives with CRC or adenomatous polyps at any time. *Group II:* First-degree relative with CRC or adenomatous polyps at age ≥60 y or 2 second-degree relatives with CRC. Revised Bethesda criteria for testing for HNPCC (Lynch syndrome)—screen for tumor microsatellite instability if CRC diagnosed in a patient age <50 y, presence of synchronous, metachronous CRC or other HNPCC defining tumor at any age. CRC with microsatellite unstable-type histology (mucinous, signet ring, infiltrating lymphocytes) in patients age <60 y. CRC diagnosed in 1 or more first-degree relatives with HNPCC-related tumor with one of the cancers diagnosed at age <50 y. CRC diagnosed younger than age 50 y. CRC diagnosed in 2 or more first-degree or second-degree relatives with HNPCC-related tumors regardless of age. Confirmation of HNPCC is made by genetic evaluation of the involved genes (*J Natl Cancer Inst.* 2004;96:261).

CANCER, COLORECTAL

The following options are acceptable choices for CRC screening in average-risk adults beginning at age 50 y. As each of the following tests has inherent characteristics related to prevention potential, accuracy, costs, and potential harms, individuals should have an opportunity to make an informed decision when choosing one of the following options.

In the opinion of the guidelines development committee, *colon CA prevention* should be the primary goal of CRC screening. Tests that are designed to detect both early CA and adenomatous polyps should be encouraged if resources are available and patients are willing to undergo an invasive test.

Tests That Detect Adenomatous Polyps and Cancer

Test	Interval	Key Issues for Informed Decisions
FSIG with insertion to 40 cm or to the splenic flexure	Every 5 y	Complete or partial bowel prep is required.
		Because sedation usually is not used, there may be some discomfort during the procedure.
		The protective effect of sigmoidoscopy is primarily limited to the portion of the colon examined. NCI study of 77,000 patients showed a significant decrease in CRC incidence (both distal and proximal) and a 50% reduction in mortality (distal only). (*J Natl Cancer Inst.* 2012;104:1).
		Patients should understand that positive findings on sigmoidoscopy usually result in a referral for colonoscopy.
Colonoscopy	Every 10 y	Complete bowel prep is required.
		Procedural sedation is used in most centers; patients will miss a day of work and will need a chaperone for transportation from the facility.
		Risks include perforation and bleeding, which are rare but potentially serious; most of the risk is associated with polypectomy (*Ann Intern Med.* 2009;150;1).
DCBE	Every 5 y	Complete bowel prep is required.
		If patients have one or more polyps ≥6 mm, colonoscopy will still be needed for biopsy or polyp removal; follow-up colonoscopy will require complete bowel prep.
		Risks of DCBE are low; rare cases of perforation have been reported—radiation exposure is a concern. USPSTF does not recommend DCBE because of lower sensitivity than other methods (*N Engl J Med.* 2007;357:1403).
CT Colonoscopy (CTC)	Every 5 y	Complete bowel prep usually required. (*Ann Intern Med.* 2012;156:692)
		If patients have one or more polyps ≥6 mm, colonoscopy will be recommended; if same-day colonoscopy is not available, a second complete bowel prep will be required before colonoscopy.
		Risks of CTC are low; rare cases of perforation have been reported.
		Extracolonic abnormalities may be identified on CTC that could require further evaluation (7%–15% of CT examinations). Not as sensitive as colonoscopy for polyps <1 cm, especially for polyps ≤6 mm flat and serrated polyps.

TESTS THAT PRIMARILY DETECT CANCER

Test	Interval	Key Issues for Informed Decisions
gFOBT with high sensitivity for CA	Annual	Depending on manufacturer's recommendations, 2–3 stool samples collected at home are needed to complete testing; a single stool gathered during a digital examination in the clinical setting is not an acceptable stool test and should not be done.
FIT (iFOBT) with high sensitivity for CA	Annual	
		Specificity of iFOBT superior to gFOBT but more expensive. Positive test results are associated with an increased risk of colon CA and advanced neoplasia; colonoscopy should be recommended if the test results are positive.
		If the test result is negative, it should be repeated annually.
		Patients should understand that one-time testing is likely to be ineffective.
sDNA with high sensitivity for CA	Interval uncertain	An adequate stool sample must be obtained and packaged with appropriate preservative agents for shipping to the laboratory.
		New data (*N Engl J Med.* 2014;370:1287) impressive and is being more widely used. The unit cost of the currently available test is significantly higher than that of other forms of stool testing ($600 vs $23).
		If the test result is positive, colonoscopy will be recommended.
		If the test result is negative, the appropriate interval for a repeat test is uncertain. sDNA testing is becoming more widely used at this time. (*Ann Intern Med.* 2008;149:441) (*N Engl J Med.* 2014;370:1350).

CA, cancer; CRC, colorectal cancer; CT, computed tomography; CTC, computed tomography colonography; DCBE, double-contrast barium enema; FIT, fecal immunochemical test; FSIG, flexible sigmoidoscopy; gFOBT, guaiac-based fecal occult blood test; sDNA, stool DNA.

Disease Screening	Organization	Date	Population	Recommendations	Comments	Source
CANCER, ENDOMETRIAL						
Cancer, Endometrial	ACS	2008	All postmenopausal women	Inform women about risks and symptoms of endometrial CA and strongly encourage them to report any unexpected bleeding or spotting. This is especially important for women with an increased risk of endometrial CA (history of unopposed estrogen therapy, tamoxifen therapy, late menopause, nulliparity, infertility or failure to ovulate, obesity, diabetes, or hypertension).	1. *Benefits:* There is inadequate evidence that screening with endometrial sampling or transvaginal ultrasound (TVU) decreases mortality. *Harms:* Based on solid evidence, screening with TVU will result in unnecessary additional exams because of low specificity. Based on solid evidence, endometrial biopsy may result in discomfort, bleeding, infection, and, rarely, uterine perforation. (NCI, 2008) 2. Presence of atypical glandular cells on Pap test from postmenopausal (age >40 y) women not taking exogenous hormones is abnormal and requires further evaluation (TVU and endometrial biopsy). Pap test is insensitive for endometrial screening. 3. Endometrial thickness of <4 mm on TVU is associated with low risk of endometrial CA. (*Am J Obstet Gynecol.* 2001;184:70) 4. Most cases of endometrial CA are diagnosed as a result of symptoms reported by patients (uterine bleeding), and a high proportion of these cases are diagnosed at an early stage and have high rates of cure. (NCI, 2008) 5. Tamoxifen use for 5 y raises the risk of endometrial CA 2- to 3-fold, but CAs are low stage, low grade, with high cure rates. (*J Natl Cancer Inst.* 1998;90:1371)	http://www.cancer.org
	ACS	2008	All women at high risk for endometrial CA[a] (patients with known or high suspicion for HNPCC mutation carrier)	Annual screening beginning at age 35 y with endometrial biopsy. In 2015 54,800 women will be diagnosed with endometrial cancer with 10,100 deaths.	1. Variable screening with ultrasound among women (age 25–65 y; *n* = 292) at high risk for HNPCC mutation detected no CAs from ultrasound. Two endometrial cancers occurred in the cohort that presented with symptoms. (*Cancer.* 2002;94:1708) 2. The Women's Health Initiative (WHI) demonstrated that combined estrogen and progestin did not increase the risk of endometrial CA but did increase the rate of endometrial biopsies and ultrasound exams prompted by abnormal uterine bleeding. (*JAMA.* 2003:290)	http://www.cancer.org

[a]High-risk women are those known to carry HNPCC-associated genetic mutations, or at high risk to carry a mutation, or who are from families with a suspected autosomal dominant predisposition to colon CA (45%–50% lifetime risk of endometrial CA).

				CANCER, GASTRIC	
Disease Screening	**Organization**	**Date**	**Population**	**Recommendations**	**Comments**	**Source**
Cancer, Gastric	NCI	2015	Average-risk population	There are currently no recommendations regarding screening for gastric CA.	1. Endoscopic screening for gastric CA in moderate- to high-risk population subgroups is cost-effective (Japan, South America). (*Clin Gastroenterol Hepatol.* 2006;4:709)	
Adenocarcinoma of gastroesophageal junction	ASGE	2011	Diagnosis— Barrett esophagus with or without gastroesophageal reflux disease (*N Engl J Med.* 2014;371:836)	—No dysplasia—scope every 3 y —Mild dysplasia—scope in 6 mo, then yearly High-grade dysplasia—surgery or endoscopic therapy (*Gastrointest Cancer Res.* 2012;5:49).	2. Patients at increased risk for gastric CA should be educated about risk and symptoms (*Helicobacter pylori*, pernicious anemia, HNPCC, postpartial gastrectomy). 3. *Benefits:* There is fair evidence that screening would result in no decrease in gastric CA mortality in the United States. *Harms:* There is good evidence that esophagogastroduodenoscopy screening would result in rare but serious side effects, such as perforation, cardiopulmonary events, aspiration pneumonia, and bleeding. (NCI, 2008)	*Gastrointest Endosc.* 2006;63:570

CANCER, LIVER

Disease Screening	Organization	Date	Population	Recommendations	Comments	Source
Cancer, Liver (Hepatocellular Carcinoma [HCC])	AASLD[b]	2010 update	Adults at high risk for HCC,[a] especially those awaiting liver transplantation, should be entered into surveillance programs	Surveillance with ultrasound at 6-mo intervals.	1. Alfa-fetoprotein (AFP) alone should not be used for screening unless ultrasound is not available (low sensitivity —60% positive). 2. *Benefits:* Based on fair evidence, screening would result in a decrease in HCC-related mortality. *Harms:* Based on fair evidence, screening would result in rare, but serious, side effects associated with needle biopsy, such as needle-track seeding, hemorrhage, bile peritonitis, and pneumothorax. (NCI, 2008. *Ann Intern Med.* 2012;156:387)	*Hematology.* 2005;42:1208
	British Society of Gastroenterology[b]	2003	Adults	Surveillance with abdominal ultrasound and AFP every 6 mo should be considered for high-risk groups.[a] This is low strength recommendation for screening. It identifies early stage HCC but whether overall survival is improved is not known. (*Ann Intern Med.* 2014;161:261)		*Gut.* 2003;52 (suppl III):iii http://www.bsg.org.uk/

[a]*HBsAg⁺ persons (carriers):* Asian males age ≥40 y; Asian females age ≥40 y; all cirrhotics; family history of HCC; Africans age >20 y. *Non-hepatitis B carriers:* hepatitis C; alcoholic cirrhosis; genetic hemochromatosis; primary biliary cirrhosis, alfa-1-antitrypsin deficiency with cirrhosis, hepatitis C with cirrhosis; hemochromatosis with cirrhosis.
[b]Only two organizations recommending screening for HCC in high-risk populations (low-level evidence).

CANCER, LUNG

Disease Screening	Organization	Date	Population	Recommendations	Comments	Source
Cancer, Lung	AAFP USPSTF	2008 2004	Asymptomatic persons	Evidence is insufficient to recommend for or against lung CA screening.	1. Counsel all patients against tobacco use, even when age >50 y. Smokers who quit gain ~10 y of increased life expectancy. (*BMJ.* 2004;328)	http://www.aafp.org/online/ en/home/clinical/exam. html http://www.ahrq.gov/clinic/ uspstf/uspslung.htm
	ACCP and ASCO	2013	Asymptomatic persons with >30 pack-year smoking history	Based on good evidence, routine screening for lung CA with chest x-ray (CXR) and sputum cytology is not recommended. Screening with low-dose CT (LDCT) is now recommended following the strict eligibility criteria of the National Lung Screening trial (NLST). This includes ages 50–74 with a 30-pack-year smoking history. People who have not smoked in the last 15 y or who have significant comorbidities are excluded.	2. *Benefits:* Based on fair evidence, screening with sputum cytology or CXR does not reduce mortality from lung CA. *Harms:* Based on solid evidence, screening would lead to false-positive test results and unnecessary invasive procedures. (NCI, 2008)	http://www.chestnet.org/ education/guidelines/ index.php
					3. Spiral CT screening can detect greater number of lung CAs in smokers with a >10-pack-year exposure. (*N Engl J Med.* 2006;355:1763-1771)	*Chest.* 2003;123:835–885
					4. Screening increases the rate of lung CA diagnosis and treatment; it may not reduce the risk of advanced lung CA or death from lung CA. (*JAMA.* 2007;297:995)	*CA Cancer J Clin.* 2004;54:41
	ACS NCCN	2013 2013	Asymptomatic persons with >30-pack-year smoking history	Guidance in shared decision making regarding screening of high-risk persons. Screening with LDCT for 3 consecutive years is recommended for patients meeting the eligibility criteria for the NLST (>30 pack-year smoking history, age 50–74 y, no major medical comorbidities) and the presence of a minimum of a highly skilled support team to evaluate LDCT scans, schedule appropriate follow-ups, and perform lung biopsies safely when indicated.	5. The NCI has reported data from the NLST, a randomized controlled trial comparing LDCT and CXR yearly × 3 with 8-y follow-up. A total of 53,500 men and women age 50–74 y. 30-pack/year smokers were randomized. A 20.3% reduction in deaths from lung CA was reported for the LDCT group (estimated that 10,000–15,000 lives could be saved per year). Problems with false-positives (25% have lung nodules <1 cm that are not cancer) and cost of workup were noted, but benefits have led to a change in guidelines. ACS 2013 guidelines on lung cancer screening recommends adults between the ages of 55 and 74 y (80 y/o for USPSTF). Who meet eligibility criteria of NLST may consider LDCT screening for lung cancer. This should take place in the setting where appropriate resources and expertise are available to minimize morbidity. Patients with a 30-pack-year smoking history but nonsmoking for >15 y are excluded. The ACCP, ACS, NCCN, and ASCO formally recommend LDCT screening for patients who meet the criteria of the NLST study (It is estimated that 8.6 million Americans meet NLST criteria for screening, which would save 12,000 lives annually [*Cancer.* 2013;119:1381-1385]). (*Ann Intern Med.* 2011;155:540. *Ann Intern Med.* 2011;155:537. *N Engl J Med.* 2011;365:395. *JAMA.* 2012;307:2418) *CA Cancer J Clin.* 2013;63:106-117. *CA Cancer J Clin.* 2013;63:87-105. *N Engl J Med.* 2013;368:1980-1991. *N Engl J Med.* 2014;369:910. *N Engl J Med.* 2015;372:2083. *N Engl J Med.* 2015;372:387.	http://www.cancer.org http://www.cancer.gov/nlst

Disease Screening					
	Organization	**Date**	**Population**	**Recommendations**	**Comments**	**Source**

CANCER, ORAL					
Cancer, Oral	AAFP USPSTF	2008 2014	Asymptomatic persons	Evidence is insufficient to recommend for or against routinely screening adults for oral asymptomatic CA.	1. Risk factors: regular alcohol or tobacco use. 2. A randomized controlled trial of visual screening for oral CA (at 3-y intervals) showed decreased oral CA mortality among screened males (but not females) who were tobacco and/or alcohol users over an 8-year period. (*Lancet.* 2005;365:1927)	http://www.aafp.org/online/en/home/clinical/exam.html http://www.ahrq.gov/clinic/uspstf/uspsoral.htm
	AAO-HNS	2011	History of radiation to head, oropharynx, neck, or total body Acute/chronic graft-versus-host disease	Annual oral cavity exam. (*Ann Int Med.* 2014;160:55)	Significant increase in HPV (subtypes 16 and 18)-related squamous cell cancer of the oropharynx (base of tongue and tonsil) in nonsmokers. There is a 20%–30% improvement in cure rate vs. that for smoking-related cancers. (*N Engl J Med.* 2010;363:24) >70% of oropharyngeal squamous cell cancers are HPV positive (*J Clin Onc.* 2013:31:2708. *J Clin Onc.* 2010;28:4142). Prevalence of oral HPV infection in the United States is 6.9% (*JAMA.* 2012:307:693). Studies ongoing to determine if less therapy in HPV-positive patients will result in the same curability with less long- and short-term toxicity. (*J Natl Cancer Inst.* 2008;180:261. *Compr Canc Netw.* 2011;9:665)	http://www.survivorshipguidelines.org

CANCER, OVARIAN

Disease Screening	Organization	Date	Population	Recommendations	Comments	Source
Cancer, Ovarian	USPSTF	2012	Asymptomatic women at average risk[a]	Recommends against routine screening. Beware of symptoms of ovarian CA that can be present in early stage disease (abdominal, pelvic, and back pain; bloating and change in bowel habits; urinary symptoms). (*Ann Intern Med.* 2012;157:900-904. *J Clin Oncol.* 2005;23:7919. *Ann Intern Med.* 2012;156:182)	1. Risk factors: age >60 y; low parity; personal history of endometrial, colon, or breast CA; family history of ovarian CA; and hereditary breast/ovarian CA syndrome. Use of oral contraceptives for 5 y decreases the risk of ovarian CA by 50%. (*JAMA.* 2004;291:2705) 2. *Benefit:* There is inadequate evidence to determine whether routine screening for ovarian CA with serum markers such as CA-125 levels, TVU, or pelvic examinations would result in a decrease in mortality from ovarian CA. *Harm:* Problems have been lack of specificity (positive predictive value) and need for invasive procedures to make a diagnosis. Based on solid evidence, routine screening for ovarian CA would result in many diagnostic laparoscopies and laparotomies for each ovarian CA found. (NCI, 2008) (*JAMA.* 2011;305:2295) 3. Additionally, cancers found by screening have not consistently been found to be lower stage. (*Lancet Oncol.* 2009;10:327) 4. Preliminary results from the Prostate, Lung, Colorectal and Ovarian (PLCO) Cancer Screening Trial: At the time of baseline examination, positive predictive value for invasive cancer was 3.7% for abnormal CA-125 levels, 1% for abnormal TVU results, and 23.5% if both tests showed abnormal results. (*Am J Obstet Gynecol.* 2005;193:1630)	http://www.aafp.org/online/en/home/clinical/exam.html http://www.ahrq.gov/clinic/uspstf/uspsovar.htm
	AAFP USPSTF	2008 2013	Women whose family history is associated with an increased risk for deleterious mutations in *BRCA1* or *BRCA2* genes[b]	Recommends referral for genetic counseling and evaluation for *BRCA* testing. Does not recommend routine screening in this group. Screening with CA-125, TVU, and pelvic exam can be considered, but there is no evidence in this population that screening reduces risk of death from ovarian CA. *A woman with ovarian cancer at any age should be tested for BRCA1 and 2 mutations.* (*USPSTF-publication#12 Dec.* 2013)		http://www.aafp.org/online/en/home/clinical/exam.html http://www.ahrq.gov/clinic/uspstf/uspsbrgen.htm
	ACOG NCCN	2009 2011	High-risk patients with *BRCA1* or 2 mutations or strong family history of ovarian CA	Recommends screening with CA-125 and TVU at age 30–35 y or 5–10 y earlier than earliest onset of ovarian CA in family members. Risk reducing salpingo-oophorectomy should be strongly considered. (*JAMA.* 2010;304:967)		

[a]Lifetime risk of ovarian CA in a woman with no affected relatives is 1 in 70. If 1 first-degree relative has ovarian CA, lifetime risk is 5%. If 2 or more first-degree relatives have ovarian CA, lifetime risk is 7%. Women with two or more family members affected by ovarian cancer have a 3% chance of having a hereditary ovarian cancer syndrome. If *BRCA1* mutation, lifetime risk of ovarian CA is 45%–50%; if *BRCA2* mutation, lifetime risk is 15%–20%. Lynch syndrome = 8%–10% lifetime risk of ovarian CA.

[b]USPSTF recommends against routine referral for genetic counseling or routine BRCA testing of women whose family history is not associated with increased risk for deleterious mutation in *BRCA1* or *BRCA2* genes.

CANCER, PANCREATIC

Disease Screening	Organization	Date	Population	Recommendations	Comments	Source
Cancer, Pancreatic	AAFP USPSTF	2008 2010	Asymptomatic persons	Recommends against routine screening.	1. Cigarette smoking has consistently been associated with increased risk of pancreatic CA. *BRCA2* mutation is associated with a 5% lifetime risk of pancreatic CA. Blood group O with lower risk and diabetes with a 2-fold higher risk of pancreatic CA. (*J Natl Cancer Inst.* 2009;101:424; *J Clin Oncol.* 2009;27:433) 2. USPSTF concluded that the harms of screening for pancreatic CA—the very low prevalence, limited accuracy of available screening tests, invasive nature of diagnostic tests, and poor outcomes of treatment—exceed any potential benefits. Patients with a strong family history (≥2 first-degree relatives with pancreatic CA) should undergo genetic counseling and may benefit from screening with CA 19–9, CT scan, and magnetic resonance cholangiopancreatography (MRCP). (*Nat Rev Gastroenterol Hepatol.* 2012;9:445-453)	http://www.aafp .org/online/en/home/ clinical/exam.html http://www.ahrq .gov/clinic/uspstf/ uspspanc.htm

CANCER, PROSTATE

Disease Screening	Organization	Date	Population	Recommendations	Comments	Source
Cancer, Prostate	ACS	2010	Men age ≥50 y[a]	Offer annual prostate-specific antigen (PSA) and digital rectal exam (DRE) if ≥10-y life expectancy.[b] Discuss risks and benefits of screening strategy.	There are 220,800 new cases of prostate cancer and 27,500 deaths expected in 2015.	http://www.cancer.org
	USPSTF	2012	Asymptomatic men	Do not use PSA-based screening for prostate CA. There is convincing evidence that PSA-based screening results in the detection of many cases of asymptomatic prostate CA and that a substantial percentage of men will have a tumor that will progress so slowly that it would remain asymptomatic for the patient's lifetime. Because of the current inability to distinguish tumors that will remain indolent from those destined to be lethal, many men are subjected to the harms of treatment for a prostate CA that will never become symptomatic. The benefits of PSA-based screening for prostate CA do not outweigh the harms (this recommendation applies to high-risk patients as well—African American/positive family history[c]). There is ongoing significant criticism of the USPSTF prostate screening recommendations. (*JAMA.* 2011;306:2715. *JAMA.* 2011;306:2719. *JAMA.* 2011;306:2721)	1. There is good evidence that PSA can detect early stage prostate CA (2-fold increase in organ-confined disease at presentation with PSA screening), but mixed and inconclusive evidence that early detection improves health outcomes or mortality. 2. Two long-awaited studies add to the confusion. A US study of 76,000 men showed increased prostate CA in screened group, but no reduction in risk of death from prostate CA. A European study of 80,000 men showed a decreased rate of death from prostate CA by 20% but significant overdiagnosis (there was no difference in overall death rate). To prevent 1 death from prostate CA, 1410 men needed to be screened and 48 cases of prostate CA found. Patients older than age 70 y had an increased death rate in the screened group. (*N Engl J Med.* 2009;360:1310, 1320. *N Engl J Med.* 2012;366:981. *N Engl J Med.* 2012;366:1047)	http://www.ahrq.gov/clinic/uspstf/uspsprca.htm *Ann Intern Med.* 2012; 157:120-134 *Ann Intern Med.* 2011;155:762-771
	ACP	2013	Asymptomatic men	Statement of guidance 1. For men between ages 50 and 69 y, discuss limited benefits and substantial harm of screening for prostate CA. Do not do PSA testing unless patient expresses a clear preference for screening. 2. Do not screen PSA in average-risk men younger than 50 or 70 y and older, or in men with a life expectancy of <10 y.	3. *Benefit:* Insufficient evidence to establish whether a decrease in mortality from prostate CA occurs with screening by DRE or serum PSA. *Harm:* Based on solid evidence, screening with PSA and/or DRE detects some prostate CAs that would never have caused important clinical problems. Based on solid evidence, current prostate CA treatments result in permanent side effects in many men, including erectile dysfunction and urinary incontinence. (NCI, 2008) 4. Men with localized, low-grade prostate CAs (Gleason score 2–4) have a minimal risk of dying from prostate CA during 20 years of follow-up (6 deaths per 1000 person-years). (*JAMA.* 2005;293:2095. *N Engl J Med.* 2014;370:932)	*Ann Intern Med.* 2013; 159:761-769 *Ann Intern Med.* 2013; 158:145-153

Disease Screening	Organization	Date	Population	Recommendations	Comments	Source
Cancer, Prostate (continued)	EAU	2010	Asymptomatic men	There is a lack of evidence to support or disregard widely adopted, population-based screening programs for early detection of prostate CA.	5. Radical prostatectomy (vs. watchful waiting) reduces disease-specific and overall mortality in patients with early stage prostate CA (*N Engl J Med.* 2011;364:1708). This benefit was seen only in men age <65 y. Active surveillance for low-risk patients (*J Clin Oncol.* 2010;28:126. *Ann Intern Med.* 2012;156:582) is safe and increasingly used as an alternative to radical prostatectomy. A gene signature profile reflecting virulence and treatment responsiveness in prostate CA is needed. 6. PSA velocity (>0.5–0.75 ng/y rise) is predictive for the presence of prostate CA, especially with a PSA of 4–10. (*Eur Urol.* 2009;56:573) Multi-parametric MRI scanning is emerging as a tool for more accurate detection of early prostate cancer as well as distinguishing indolent from high-grade cancers. (*J Urol.* 2011;185:815. *Nat Rev Clin Oncol.* 2014; 11:346). African American men have double the risk of prostate cancer and a >2-fold risk of prostate cancer–specific death. These patients and those with first-degree relatives <65 y with prostate cancer are at high enough risk to justify PSA screening until a definitive study of this population is available. (*JAMA.* 2014;311:1143).	www.uroweb.org
	UK-NHS NCCN	2007 2013	Asymptomatic men	Informed decision making. —Obtain PSA testing in healthy men age 45–70+. —Men age 45–49 with PSA <0.7 ng/mL, restest in 5 y. —Men age 45–49 with PSA >0.7 ng/mL and those aged 50–59 with PSA >0.9 retest every 1–2 y. —F/U testing should be done every 1–2 y for all men with PSA >1.0. —After age 70 PSA testing should be individualized and indications for biopsy carefully evaluated. —Refer patients. for prostate biopsy if serum PSA rises >0.9 ng/mL in 1 y.	PSA screening is confounded by the morbidity and mortality associated with the treatment of prostate cancer. Molecular profiling that can stratify patients into high-risk and low-risk groups is a critical need for individualized adaptive therapies, which could minimize toxicity from therapy in many patients. See informational leaflet at: http://www.cancerscreening.nhs.uk/prostate/prostate-patient-info-sheet.pdf. This recommendation aims to strike a balance between testing too seldom and testing too often to "maximize benefit and minimize harm."	www.cancerscreening.nhs.uk NCCN Guidelines 2013

[a] Men in high-risk groups (1 or more first-degree relatives diagnosed before age 65 y, African Americans) should begin screening at age 45 y. Men at higher risk because of multiple first-degree relatives affected at an early age could begin testing at age 40 y (http://www.cancer.org/).

[b] Men who ask their doctor to make the decision should be tested. Discouraging testing or not offering testing is inappropriate.

CANCER, SKIN

Disease Screening	Organization	Date	Population	Recommendations	Comments	Source
Cancer, Skin (melanoma)	AAFP USPSTF	2009 2012	Adult general population	Evidence is insufficient to recommend for or against routine screening using a total-body skin examination for early detection of cutaneous melanoma, basal cell carcinoma, or squamous cell skin CA.[a,b] Recommends counseling children, adolescents, and young adults age 10–24 y who have fair skin to minimize exposure to ultraviolet radiation to reduce the risk of skin cancer.	*Benefits:* Evidence is inadequate to determine whether visual exam of the skin in asymptomatic individuals would lead to a reduction in mortality from melanomatous skin CA. *Harms:* Based on fair though unqualified evidence, visual examination of the skin in asymptomatic persons may lead to unavoidable increases in harmful consequences. (NCI, 2008). 28 million people in the United States use UV indoor tanning salons, increasing risk of squamous, basal cell cancer and malignant melanoma (*J Clin Oncol.* 2012;30:1588). No guidelines for patients with familial syndromes (familial atypical mole and melanoma [FAM-M]) syndrome, although systematic surveillance warranted.[c]	http://www.aafp.org/online/en/home/clinical/exam.html http://www.ahrq.gov/clinic/uspstf/uspsskca.htm

[a]Clinicians should remain alert for skin lesions with malignant features when examining patients for other reasons, particularly patients with established risk factors. Risk factors for skin CA include evidence of melanocytic precursors (atypical moles), large numbers of common moles (>50), immunosuppression, any history of radiation, family or personal history of skin CA, substantial cumulative lifetime sun exposure, intermittent intense sun exposure or severe sunburns in childhood, freckles, poor tanning ability, and light skin, hair, and eye color.
[b]Consider educating patients with established risk factors for skin CA (see above) concerning signs and symptoms suggesting skin CA and the possible benefits of periodic self-examination. Alert at-risk patients to significance of asymmetry, border irregularity, color variability, diameter >6 mm, and evolving change in previous stable mole. All suspicious lesions should be biopsied (excisional or punch, not a shave biopsy) (*Ann Intern Med.* 2009;150:188) (USPSTF; ACS; COG).
[c]Consider dermatologic risk assessment if family history of melanoma in ≥2 blood relatives, presence of multiple atypical moles, or presence of numerous actinic keratoses.

CANCER, TESTICULAR

Disease Screening	Organization	Date	Population	Recommendations	Comments	Source
Cancer, Testicular	AAFP USPSTF	2008 2011	Asymptomatic adolescent and adult males[a]	Recommend against routine screening. Be aware of risk factors for testicular CA—previous testis CA (2%–3% risk of second cancer), cryptorchid testis, family history of testis CA, HIV (increased risk of seminoma), Klinefelter syndrome. There is a 3- to 5-fold increase in testis cancer in white men vs other ethnicity.	*Benefits:* Based on fair evidence, screening would not result in appreciable decrease in mortality, in part because therapy at each stage is so effective. *Harms:* Based on fair evidence, screening would result in unnecessary diagnostic procedures. (NCI, 2011)	http://www.aafp.org/online/en/home/clinical/exam.html http://www.ahrq.gov/clinic/uspstf/uspstest.htm
	ACS	2004	Asymptomatic men	Testicular exam by physician as part of routine cancer-related checkup.		http://www.cancer.org
	EAU	2008	High-risk males[a]	Self-physical exam is advisable.		www.uroweb.org

[a]Patients with history of cryptorchidism, orchiopexy, family history of testicular CA, or testicular atrophy should be informed of their increased risk for developing testicular CA and counseled about screening. Such patients may then elect to be screened or to perform testicular self-examination. Adolescent and young adult males should be advised to seek prompt medical attention if they notice a scrotal abnormality. (USPSTF)

CANCER, THYROID

Disease Screening	Organization	Date	Population	Recommendations	Comments	Source
Cancer, Thyroid	USPSTF	2012	Asymptomatic persons	Recommends against the use of ultrasound screening in asymptomatic persons. Be aware of higher-risk patients: radiation administered in infancy and childhood for benign conditions (thymus enlargement, acne) have an increased risk beginning 5 y after radiation and may appear >20 y later; nuclear fallout exposure; history of goiter; family history of thyroid disease; female gender; Asian race. (*Int J Cancer.* 2001;93:745)	Neck palpation for nodules in asymptomatic individuals has sensitivity of 15%–38%, specificity of 93%–100%. Only a small proportion of nodular thyroid glands are neoplastic, resulting in a high false-positive rate. (USPSTF) Fine-needle aspiration (FNA) is the procedure of choice for evaluation of thyroid nodules. (*Otolaryngol Clin North Am.* 2010;43:229–238)	http://www.aafp.org/online/en/home/clinical/exam.html http://www.cancer.org

CAROTID ARTERY STENOSIS					
Disease Screening	Organization	Date	Population	Recommendations	Comments	Source
Carotid Artery Stenosis (CAS) (asymptomatic)	ASN USPSTF AHA/ASA ACCF/ACR/AIUM/ ASE/ASN/IICAVL/ SCAI/SCCT/SIR/ SVM/SVS	2007 2014 2012	Asymptomatic adults	Screening of the general population or a selected population based on age, gender, or any other variable alone is not recommended. Inappropriate to screen asymptomatic adult.	1. The prevalence of internal CAS of ≥70% varies from 0.5% to 8% based on population-based cohort utilizing carotid duplex ultrasound. General population age >65 y estimated prevalence of 1%. No risk stratification tool further distinguishes the importance of CAS. No evidence suggests that screening for asymptomatic CAS reduces fatal or nonfatal strokes.	*J Neuroimaging.* 2007;17:19-47 www.uspreventiveservicestaskforce .org/uspstf/uspsacas.htm USPFT 2007 (AHRQ #08-05102- EF-1; *Stroke.* 2010;42 Appropriate Use Criteria for PVD part 1 *J Am Coll Cardiol.* 2012;50(3):242-276
	ACR–AIUM–SRU	2014		Indications for carotid ultrasound: evaluation of patients with a cervical bruit.	2. Carotid duplex ultrasonography to detect CAS ≥60%: sensitivity, 94%; specificity, 92%. (*Ann Intern Med.* 2007;147(12):860)	http://www.acr.org/~/media/ACR/ Documents/PGTS/guidelines/ US_Extracranial_Cerebro.pdf
	ACC/AHA/ASA/ACR/ SVS	2011		It is reasonable to perform duplex ultrasonography to detect hemodynamically significant carotid stenosis in asymptomatic patients with carotid bruit.	3. If true prevalence of CAS is 1%, number needed to screen to prevent 1 stroke over 5 y = 4368; to prevent 1 disabling stroke over 5 y = 8696. (*Ann Intern Med.* 2007;147(12):860)	Brott TG, Halperin JL, Abbara S, et al. 2011 ASA/ACCF/AHA/ AANN/AANS/ACR/ ASNR/ CNS/SAIP/SCAI/SIR/SNIS/ SVM/SVS guideline on the management of patients with extracranial carotid and vertebral artery disease. *Stroke.* 2011;42(8):e464-e540. http://www.ncbi.nlm.nih.gov/books/ NBK22323O/
	Society of Thoracic Surgeons	2013		Recommends against routine evaluation of carotid artery disease prior to cardiac surgery in the absence of symptoms or other high-risk criteria.		http://www.choosingwisely.org/ wp-content/uploads/2015/02/ STS-Choosing-Wisely-List.pdf
	AAFP	2013		Recommends against screening for carotid artery stenosis in asymptomatic adults.		http://www.choosingwisely.org/ societies/american-academy-of- family-physicians/

Disease Screening	Organization	Date	Population	Recommendations	Comments	Source
CELIAC DISEASE						
Celiac Disease	NICE	2009	Children and adults	Serologic testing to screen for celiac disease should be performed for any of the following signs, symptoms, or associated conditions: chronic diarrhea; failure to thrive; persistent or unexplained gastrointestinal symptoms; prolonged fatigue; recurrent abdominal pain; cramping or distension; unexpected weight loss; unexplained anemia; autoimmune thyroid disease; dermatitis herpetiformis; irritable bowel syndrome; type 1 diabetes; or first-degree relatives with celiac disease.	1. Patients must continue a gluten-containing diet during diagnostic testing. 2. IgA tissue transglutaminase (TTG) is the test of choice. 3. IgA endomysial antibody test is indicated if the TTG test is equivocal. 4. Avoid antigliadin antibody testing. 5. Consider serologic testing for any of the following: Addison disease; amenorrhea; autoimmune hepatitis; autoimmune myocarditis; chronic immune thrombocytopenic purpura (ITP); dental enamel defects; depression; bipolar disorder; Down syndrome; Turner syndrome; epilepsy; lymphoma; metabolic bone disease; chronic constipation; polyneuropathy; sarcoidosis; Sjögren syndrome; or unexplained alopecia.	http://www.nice.org.uk/nicemedia/pdf/CG86FullGuideline.pdf

Disease Screening	Organization	Date	Population	Recommendations	Comments	Source
Chlamydia	CDC ICSI AAFP and USPSTF	2010 2010 2007 2014	Women age ≤25 y who are sexually active	Annual screening.	1. *Chlamydia* is a reportable infection to the Public Health Department in every state. 2. The USPSTF also recommends chlamydia screening in older women who are at increased risk of infection. 3. The USPSTF does not recommend screening sexually active men for chlamydia.	http://www.cdc.gov/mmwr/pdf/rr/rr5912.pdf http://www.icsi.org/preventive_services_for_adults/preventive_services_for_adults_4.html http://www.uspreventiveservicestaskforce.org/Page/Topic/recommendation-summary/chlamydia-and-gonorrhea-screening
	CDC	2010	Women age ≤35 y who are sexually active and in juvenile detention or jail	At intake and then annual screening.		http://www.cdc.gov/mmwr/pdf/rr/rr5912.pdf
	CDC	2010	Young heterosexual men	Insufficient evidence for or against routine screening.		http://www.cdc.gov/mmwr/pdf/rr/rr5912.pdf
	CDC	2010	Homosexual men	Annual testing for men who have had insertive or receptive intercourse in the last year.	1. Urine nucleic amplification acid test (NAAT) for *Chlamydia* for men who have had insertive intercourse. 2. NAAT of rectal swab for men who have had receptive anal intercourse.	http://www.cdc.gov/mmwr/pdf/rr/rr5912.pdf
	AAFP and USPSTF	2007	Pregnant women	Recommends screening for chlamydial infection for all pregnant women 24 y of age and younger and for older women at increased risk. Recommends against routine screening for pregnant women 25 y or older if they are not at high risk.		http://www.uspreventiveservicestaskforce.org/uspstf/uspschlm.htm

CHOLESTEROL AND LIPID DISORDERS

Disease Screening	Organization	Date	Population	Recommendations	Comments	Source
Cholesterol and Lipid Disorders	USPSTF NLA	2007 2011	Infants, children, adolescents, or young adults (age <20 y)	In familial hypercholesterolemia (FH), universal screening at age 9–11 with a fasting lipid panel or nonfasting non-HDL-C. If non-HDL-C ≥145 m/dL, perform fasting lipid panel. Genetic screening for FH is generally not needed for diagnosis or clinical management. Cascade screening: testing lipid levels in all first-degree relatives of diagnosed FH patients. Insufficient evidence to recommend for or against routine population lab screening.[a]	1. Childhood drug treatment of dyslipidemia lowers lipid levels but effect on childhood or adult outcomes pending. 2. Lifestyle approach is recommended starting after age 2 y.	www.uspreventiveservicestask force.org/uspstf/uspschlip.htm *J Clini Lipidol.* 2011;5:S1-S8 doi:10.1016/j.jacl.2011.04.003 *Pediatrics.* 2007;120:e189-e214 *Circulation.* 2007;115:1948-1967 *Pediatrics.* 2008;122:198-208
	AHA	2007		Selective screening age >2 y with a parent age <55 y with coronary artery disease, peripheral artery disease, cerebrovascular disease, or hyperlipidemia should be screened with fasting panel.		
	Pediatrics Integrated Guidelines for CV Heath and Risk Reduction in Children and Adolescents	2008 2011		Selective screening age >2 y if positive family history (FH) of dyslipidemia, presence of dyslipidemia, or the presence of overweight, obesity, hypertension, diabetes, or a smoking history. Universal screening in adolescents regardless of FH between ages 9 and 11 y and again between ages 18 and 21 y.	Fasting lipid profile is recommended. If within normal limits repeat testing in 3–5 y is recommended. Fasting lipid profile or nonfasting non–high-density lipoprotein (HDL) cholesterol level.	http://www.nhlbi.nih gov/guidelines/cvd_ped/ index.htm

CHOLESTEROL AND LIPID DISORDERS

Disease Screening	Organization	Date	Population	Recommendations	Comments	Source
Cholesterol and Lipid Disorders (continued)	ACC/AHA	2013	Asymptomatic adults 40–79 y	Perform 10-year ASCVD Risk Score High-risk categories include 1. Primary elevation of LDL-C ≥ 190 mg/dL. 2. Diabetes (type 1 or 2) with LDL-C 70–189 mg/dL and without clinical ASCVD. 3. Without clinical ASCVD or diabetes with LDL-C 70–189 mg/dL and estimated 10-y ASCVD risk score ≥7.5%	Prior to initiating statin therapy perform: lipid panel, ALT, HgbA1c to R/O DM, baseline CK (if patient's at increased risk for muscle events based on personal or family history of statin intolerance).	*2013 ACC/AHA Guideline on the Treatment of Blood Cholesterol to Reduce Atherosclerotic Cardiovascular Disease Risk in Adults: A Report of the American College of Cardiology/American Heart Association Task Force on Practice Guidelines.* Stone NJ, Robinson J, Lichtenstein AH, et al. *Circulation* published online November 12, 2013 http://circ.ahajournals.org/content/early/2013/11/01/.cir.0000437738.63853.7a.full.pd'+html
	ADA	2013	Adults with diabetes	Measure fasting lipids at least annually in adults with diabetes. Every 2 y for adults with low-risk lipid values (LDL-C < 100 mg/dL, HDL-C >50 mg/dL, TG <150 mg/dL)	No overt CVD: LDL-C goal <100 mg/dL (2.6 mmol/L).	American Diabetes Association. Standards of medical care in diabetes—2013. *Diabetes Care.* 2013;36(suppl 1):S11–S66
	ESC	2012	Adults >40 y old	Perform SCORE risk assessment tool available at: www.heartscore.org Secondary hyperlipidemia should be R/O. LDL-C primary target: goal LDL ≤70 mg/dL in patients with very-high CV risk. LDL ≤100 mg/dL in patients with high CV risk. Non-HDL-C or Apo B should be considered as a second target in combined hyperlipidemias, diabetes, metabolic syndrome, or CKD. HDL is not recommended as a target for treatment.		http://www.escardio.org/guidelines-surveys/esc-guidelines/GuidelinesDocuments/EM_Dyslipidemia_2012.pdf

CHOLESTEROL AND LIPID DISORDERS

Disease Screening	Organization	Date	Population	Recommendations	Comments	Source
Cholesterol and Lipid Disorders (continued)	NLA	2014	Adults >20 y	Fasting lipid profile (LDL-C and TG) or nonfasting lipid panel (non–HDL-C and HDL-C) should be measured at least every 5 y. Also assess ASCVD risk. Non–HDL-C (primary target), Apo-B (secondary target) have more predictive power than LDL-C. Apolipoprotein B (apo B) is considered an optional, secondary target for therapy. More predictive power than LDL-C, but not consistently superior to non–HDL-C. HDL-C is not recommended as a target therapy.	Non–HDL-C values: Desirable <130 mg/dL Above desirable 130–159 Borderline high 160–189 High 190–219 Very high ≥ 220	Jacobson TA, Ito MK, Maki KC, et al. National Lipid Association recommendations for patient-centered management of dyslipidemia: Part 1—executive summary. *J Clin Lipidol.* 2014;8:473-488. http://dx.doi.org/10.1016/j.jacl.2014.07.007
	NCEP III	2004	Adult men and women age >20 y	Check fasting lipoprotein panel (if testing opportunity is nonfasting, use nonfasting total cholesterol [TC] and HDL) every 5 y if in desirable range; otherwise, see management algorithm.[b]	1. There are no recommendations at which age screening should be discontinued. Screening should continue beyond age 65 y if the individual patient would benefit from long-term lipid management. (*Geriatrics.* 2000;55(8):48) 2. Treatment decisions should be based on at least two cholesterol levels. 3. Screen with fasting lipid panel to include TC, low-density lipoprotein-cholesterol (LDL-C), high-density lipoprotein-cholesterol (HDL-C), and triglycerides.	*Circulation.* 2002;106:3143-3421 *Circulation.* 2004;110:227-239 http://www.nhlbi.nih.gov/guidelines/cholesterol/atp3upd04.htm
	USPSTF	2008	Men age >35 y	Grade A recommendation. Optimal screening interval uncertain.		http://www.ahrq.gov/clinic/uspstf/uspschol.htm
			Men age 20–35 y	Only if at increased risk for coronary heart disease (CHD). Grade B recommendation.		
			Women age >45 y	Screen if at increased risk of CHD. Grade A recommendation.		
			Women age 20–45 y	Screen if at increased risk of CHD. Grade B recommendation. No recommendation for or against routine screening in men age 20–35 y or in women age ≥20 y who are not at increased risk of CHD.		

CHOLESTEROL AND LIPID DISORDERS

Disease Screening	Organization	Date	Population	Recommendations	Comments	Source
Cholesterol and Lipid Disorders (continued)	AAFP European Society of Cardiology/ European Atherosclerosis Society	2008 2011	Men age ≥35 y	Strongly recommends routine screening for lipid disorders.		http://www.aafp.org/exam/ http://www.ahrq.gov/clinic/ uspstf/uspschol.htm *Eur Heart J.* 2011:32(4): 1769-1818
			Women age ≥45 y Men age >40 y; women >50 y	Strongly recommends screening only if at increased risk of CHD. [c]		
	Canadian Cardiovascular Society CCS	2013	Men ≥ 40 y Women ≥ 50 y or postmenopausal All patients with any of the following conditions, regardless of age: smoking actively, diabetes, HTN, family hx CVD or HLD, erectile dysfunction, CKD, inflammatory disease, HIV, COPD, clinical evidence of aterosclerosis or AAA, clinical manifestation of HLD, obesity with BMI > 27)	For all, screening should be performed with: history and examination, LDL, HDL, TG, non-HDL, G, eGFR Optional: apoB (instead of standard lipid panel), urine albumin: creatinine ratio (if eGFR > 60, HTN, diabetes) If Framingham Risk Score < 5%, repeat every 4–5 y. If Framingham Risk Score ≥ 5%, repeat every year.		*Can J Cardiol.* 2013:29:151-167

[a]AHA: Low efficacy of targeted screening of children based on family history. Sensitivity and specificity of screening complicated by variability in TC and HDL based on race, gender, and sexual maturation (*Circulation.* 2007;115: 1948-1967).

[b]Classify fasting TC <200 mg/dL as desirable, 200–239 mg/dL as borderline, and ≥240 mg/dL as high. Classify HDL <40 as low and ≥60 as high. Classify LDL <100 as optimal, 100–129 as near or above optimal, 130–159 as borderline high, 160–189 as high, and ≥190 as very high. If TC <200 mg/dL and HDL ≥40 mg/dL, then repeat in 5 years; if nonfasting TC ≥200 mg/dL or HDL <40 mg/dL, then check fasting lipids and risk-stratify based on low-density lipoprotein (LDL) (see Management Algorithm). It remains unclear how much additional information is provided by advanced lipoprotein testing over the standard lipid panel (*Circulation.* 2009;119:819-2404).

[c]Hypertension, smoking, diabetes, FH of CHD before age 50 y (male relatives) or age 60 y (female relatives), FH suggestive of familial hyperlipidemia.

CHOLESTEROL GUIDELINES			
Source	Recommended Lipoprotein Measurements for Risk Assessment	Recommended Lipoprotein Targets of Therapy	Recommended Risk Assessment Algorithm
National Cholesterol Education Program Adult Treatment Panel III[7,8]	Fasting lipid panel Calculation of non-HDL-C when TG > 200 mg/dl	Primary target: LDL-C Secondary target: non-HDL-C	Identify number of CHD risk factors Framingham 10-y absolute CHD risk
International Atherosclerosis Society[16]	Fasting lipid panel with calculation of non-HDL-C	Non-HDL-C LDL-C is considered alternative target of therapy	Lifetimes risk of total ASCVD morbidity/mortality (by Framingham, CV Lifetime Risk pooling Project, or QRISK)
European Society of Cardiology/European Atherosclerosis Society[22]	Fasting lipid panel with calculation of non-HDL-C and TC/HDL-C ratio apoB or apoB/apoA1 ration are considered alternative risk markers	Primary target: LDC-C Secondary targets: non-HDL or apoB in patients with cardiometabolic risk	10-y risk total fatal ASCVD risk by the Systematic Coronary Risk Evaluation (SCORE) system
Canadian Cardiovascular Society[27]	Fasting lipid panel with calculation of non-HDL-C apoB considered alternative marker of risk	Primary target: LDL-C Secondary targets: non-HDL-C and apoB	10-y risk of total ASCVD events by the Framingham Risk Score
American Association of Clinical Endocrinologists[31]	Fasting lipid panel Calculation of non-HDL-C more accurate risk assessment if TG in between 200–500 mg/dl, diabetes, insulin resistance, or established CAD	Primary targets : LDC-C Secondary targets: non-HDL-in patients with cardiometabolic risk or established CAD apoB recommended to assess success of LDL-C-lowering therapy	Men: Framingham Risk Score 10-y risk of coronary event Women: Reynolds Risk Score (10-y risk of coronary event, stroke, or other major heart disease)
American Diabetes Association/ American Heart Association Statement on Cardiometabolic Risk[38]	Stronger risk discrimination provided by non-HDL-C, apoB, LDL-P	Strong recommendation for apoB and non-HDL-C as secondary targets	30-year/lifetime global ASCVD risk
American Diabetes Association: Standards of Medical Care in Diabetes[39]	Fasting lipid panel	LDL-C	Not applicable in setting of diabetes (CHD risk equivalent)
Kidney Disease: Improving Global Outcomes: Clinical Practice Guideline for Lipid Management in Chronic Kidney Disease[41]	Fasting lipid panel to screen for more severe forms of dyslipidemia and secondary causes of dyslipidemia	None: therapy guided by absolute risk of coronary event based on age, Stage of CKD or eGFR	CKD considered CHD risk equivalent Treatment with evidence-based statins/statin doses based on age, Stage of CKD or eGFR
Secondary Prevention of Atherosclerotic Cardiovascular Disease in Older Adults: A Scientific Statement from the American Heart Association[36]	Fasting lipid panel Calculation of non-HDL-C when TG >200 mg/dL	Primary target: LDL-C Secondary target: non-HDL-C	N/A
National Lipid Association: Familial Hypercholesterolemia[40]	Fasting lipid panel	LDL-C	Not applicable due to extremely high lifetime risk
Expert Panel on Integrated Guidelines for Cardiovascular Health and Risk Reduction in Children and Adolescents[34,35]	Fasting lipid panel with calculation of non-HDL-C	Primary target: LDL-C Secondary target: non-HDL-C	No risk algorithm, treatment based on number of ASCVD risk factors

CHOLESTEROL GUIDELINES			
Source	Recommended Lipoprotein Measurements for Risk Assessment	Recommended Lipoprotein Targets of Therapy	Recommended Risk Assessment Algorithm
AHA Women's Cardiovascular Disease Prevention Guidelines[17]	Fasting lipid panel Consider hs-CRP in women >60 y and CHD risk >10%	LDL-C	Updated Framingham risk profile (coronary, cerebrovascular, and peripheral arterial disease and heart failure events) Reynolds Risk Score (10-y risk of coronary event, stroke, or other major heart disease)
2013 American College of Cardiology/American Heart Association: Blood Cholesterol Guidelines for ASCVD Prevention[50]	Fasting lipid panel to screen for more severe forms of dyslipidemia and secondary causes of dyslipidemia	LDL-C measured for assessment of therapeutic response and compliance Therapy guided by indentification of 40 categories of patients who benefit from high or moderate-dose statin therapy	CV Risk Calculator based on Pooled Risk Equations (10-y risk of total ASCVD events) Lifetime risk provided for individuals 20–59 y of age
CENTRAL ILLUSTRATION Comparison of Clinical Guidelines for the Management of Risks Related to LDL in ASCVD			

apoA1, apolipoprotein A1; apoB, apolipoprotein B; ASCVD, atherosclerotic cardiovascular disease; CAD, coronary artery disease; CHD, coronary heart disease; CKD, chronic kidney disease; CV, cardiovascular; eGFR, estimated glomerular fitration rate; HDL-C, high-density lipoprotein cholestrol; hs-CRP, high-sensitivity C-reactive protein; LDL-C, low-density lipoprotein cholesterol; LDL-P, low-density lipoprotein paritcle, TC, total cholesterol; TG, triglycerides

Source: Morris et al. "Review of clinical practice Guidelines for the management of LDL-related risk. *JACC* Vol. 64, No.2, 2014, page 198

CHRONIC OBSTRUCTIVE PULMONARY DISEASE

Disease Screening	Organization	Date	Population	Recommendations	Comments	Source
Chronic Obstructive Pulmonary Disease (COPD)	AAFP USPSTF	2008	Adults	Recommends *against* screening asymptomatic adults for COPD using spirometry.		http://www.guidelines.gov/content.aspx?id=38619
Coronary Artery Disease	AAFP USPSTF	2012 2004	Adults at low risk of CHD events[a]	Recommends against routine screening in men and women with resting electrocardiogram (ECG), exercise treadmill test (ETT), or electron-beam CT for coronary calcium at low risk for CHD risk.[b]	USPSTF recommends against screening asymptomatic individuals because of the high false-positive results, the low mortality with asymptomatic disease, and the iatrogenic diagnostic and treatment risks.	http://www.aafp.org/online/en/home/clinical/exam.html *Circulation.* 2005;111:682-696 http://www.ahrq.gov/clinic/uspstf/uspsacad.htm *Ann Intern Med.* 2004;140:569 *Circulation.* 2005;112:771-776

CORONARY ARTERY DISEASE

Disease Screening	Organization	Date	Population	Recommendations	Comments	Source
Coronary Artery Disease (continued)	ACC/AHA ESC	2013 2012	All asymptomatic adults age ≥20 years Risk Score Assessment in asymptomatic adults	ASCVD Risk Score has replaced the FRS in the United States for patients ages 40–79. Assess 10-y ASCVD risk score every 4–6 y (see page 192, Chapter 3). Framingham Risk Score (FRS), including blood pressure (BP) and cholesterol level, should be obtained in asymptomatic adults ≥ age 20. The SCORE Risk Score remains the screening choice in Europe. No benefit in genetic testing advanced lipid testing, natriuretic peptide testing, high-sensitivity C-reactive protein (CRP), ankle-brachial index, carotid intima-medial thickness, coronary artery score on electron-beam CT, homocysteine level, lipoprotein (a) level, CT angiogram, MRI, or stress echocardiography regardless of CHD risk.	10-year ASCVD risk calculator (The Pooled Cohort Equation) can be found at: http://tools.acc.org/ASCVD-Risk-Estimator/	*Circulation.* 2007;115:402-426 *J Am Coll Cardiol.* 2010;56(25):2182-2199 http://www.uspreventiveservicestaskforce.org/uspstf/uspscoronaryhd.htm *Eur Heart J.* 2007;28(19): 2375-2414 *Eur Heart J.* 2012;33:1635-1701 *J Am Coll Cardiol.* 2007;49:378-402 http://circ.ahajournals.org/content/early/2013/11/11/01.cir.0000437741.48606.98.full.pdf
			Adults at intermediate risk of CHD events	May be reasonable to consider use of coronary artery calcium and high-sensitivity CRP (hsCRP) measurements in patients at intermediate risk according to Framingham Score.[b] hsCRP is not recommended in low- or high-risk individuals.		
	AAFP	2012	Adults at high risk of CHD events[a]	Insufficient evidence to recommend for or against routine screening with ECG, ETT.		*Arch Intern Med.* 2011;171(11): 977-982
	AHA	2007		In addition, there is insufficient evidence to recommend routine MRI.		http://www.aafp.org/patient-care/clinical-recommendations/all/coronary-heart-disease.html http://www.ahrq.gov/clinic/uspstf/uspsacad.htm *Ann Intern Med.* 2009;151:474-482
	USPSTF	2012				*Eur Heart J.* 2012;33:1635-1701
	USPSTF	2009	Men and Women with no History of CHD	Insufficient evidence to assess the balance of benefits and harms of using the nontraditional risk factors to prevent CHD events. (hs-CRP, ankle-brachial index [ABI], leukocyte count, fasting blood glucose level, periodontal disease, carotid intima-media thickness, coronary artery calcification [CAC] score on electron-beam computed tomography, homocysteine level, and lipoprotein[a] level)		http://www.uspreventiveservicestaskforce.org/Page/Topic/recommendation-summary/coronary-heart-disease-screening-using-non-traditional-risk-factors

CORONARY ARTERY DISEASE

Disease Screening	Organization	Date	Population	Recommendations	Comments	Source
Coronary Artery Disease (continued)	ACCF/AHA	2010	Women	Cardiac risk stratification by the Framingham Risk Score should be used. High risk in women should be considered when the risk is ≥10% rather than ≥20%. An alternative 10-y risk score to consider is the Reynolds Risk Score, although it requires measurement of hsCRP.		AHA Guidelines. *J Am Coll Cardiol.* 2011;57(12):1404-1423
	CCS	2013	Adults with stable CAD	Risk assessment by Framingham Risk Score should be completed every 3–5 y for men age 40–75 y and women age 50–75 y. Frequency of measurement should increase if history of premature cardiovascular disease (CVD) is present. Calculate and discuss a patient's "cardiovascular age" to improve the likelihood that the patient will reach lipid targets and that poorly controlled hypertension will be treated.		*Can J Cardiol.* 2013;29:151-167
	AAFP	2009		All patients with acute myocardial infarction (MI) to be screened for depression at regular intervals during and posthospitalization.		*Ann Fam Med.* 2009;7(1):71-79
	AHA/APA	2008		Routine screening for depression in patients with CHD.		*Circulation.* 2008;118:1768-1775
	American College of Physicians	2012		Recommends against screening with exercise electrocardiogram testing in asymptomatic individuals with low risk for CHD.		http://www.choosingwisely.org/societies/american-college-of-physicians/
	AAFP	2013		Recommends against annual ECGs or any other cardiac screening for asymptomatic low-risk patients.		http://www.choosingwisely.org/societies/american-academy-of-family-physicians/
	American Society of Echocardiography	2013		Recommends against stress echocardiograms being performed on asymptomatic patients with low risk for CAD.		http://www.choosingwisely.org/societies/american-society-of-echocardiography/
	ACC	2014		1. Against stress cardiac imaging or advanced non-invasive imaging in the initial evaluation of patients without cardiac symptoms, unless high-risk markers are present. 2. Against annual stress cardiac imaging or advanced non-invasive imaging as part of routine follow-up in asymptomatic patients.		http://www.choosingwisely.org/societies/american-college-of-cardiology/

[a] Increased risk for CHD events: older age, male gender, high BP, smoking, elevated lipid levels, diabetes, obesity, sedentary lifestyle. Risk assessment tool for estimating 10-year risk of developing CHD events available online, or see Appendices VI and VII. http://cvdrisk.nhlbi.nih.gov/calculator.asp

[b] AHA scientific statement (2006): Asymptomatic persons should be assessed for CHD risk. Individuals found to be low risk (<10% 10-y risk) or at high risk (>20% 10-y risk) do not benefit from coronary calcium assessment. High-risk individuals are already candidates for intensive risk-reducing therapies. In clinically selected, intermediate-risk patients, it may be reasonable to use electron-beam CT or multidetector computed tomography (MDCT) to refine clinical risk prediction and select patients for more aggressive target values for lipid-lowering therapies (*Circulation.* 2006;114:1761-1791).

DEMENTIA						

Disease Screening	Organization	Date	Population	Recommendations	Comments	Source
Dementia	ICSI	2010	Adults	Insufficient evidence to recommend for or against routine dementia screening.		http://www.icsi.org/preventive_services_for_adults/ preventive_services_for_adults_4.html
	USPSTF	2014	Elderly adults over 65 y			http://www.guideline.gov/content.aspx?id=48059

DEPRESSION

Disease Screening	Organization	Date	Population	Recommendations	Comments	Source
Depression	USPSTF	2009	Children age 7–11 y	Insufficient evidence to recommend for or against routine screening.		http://www.uspreventiveservicestaskforce.org/uspstf09/depression/chdeprart.pdf
	USPSTF	2009	Adolescents	Screen all adolescents age 12–18 y for major depressive disorder (MDD) when systems are in place to ensure accurate diagnosis, appropriate psychotherapy, and adequate follow-up.	1. Screen in primary care clinics with the Patient Health Questionnaire for Adolescents (PHQ-A) (73% sensitivity; 94% specificity) or the Beck Depression Inventory-Primary Care (BDI-PC) (91% sensitivity; 91% specificity). See Appendix I. 2. Treatment of adolescents with selective serotonin reuptake inhibitors (SSRIs), psychotherapy, or combined therapy decreases MDD symptoms. 3. SSRI may increase suicidality in some adolescents, emphasizing the need for close follow-up.	

	USPSTF
	ICSI
		2009
		2010
			Adults	Recommend screening adults for depression when staff-assisted support systems are in place for accurate diagnosis, effective treatment, and follow-up.	1. Asking two simple questions may be as accurate as formal screening tools:
					  a. "Over the past 2 wk, have you felt down, depressed, or hopeless?"
					  b. "Over the past 2 wk, have you felt little or no interest or pleasure in doing things?"
					2. Optimal screening interval is unknown.
						http://www.uspreventiveservicestaskforce.org/uspstf09/adultdepression/addeprs.pdf
						http://www.icsi.org/preventive_services_for_adults/preventive_services_for_adults_4.html

DEVELOPMENTAL DYSPLASIA OF THE HIP

Disease Screening	Organization	Date	Population	Recommendations	Comments	Source
Developmental Dysplasia of the Hip (DDH)	ICSI AAFP	2010 2010	Infants	Evidence is insufficient to recommend routine screening for DDH in infants as a means to prevent adverse outcomes.	There is evidence that screening leads to earlier identification; however, 60%–80% of the hips of newborns identified as abnormal or suspicious for DDH by physical examination, and >90% of those identified by ultrasound in the newborn period, resolve spontaneously, requiring no intervention.	http://www.icsi.org/preventive_services_for_children_guideline_/preventive_services_for_children_and_adolescent_2531.html
	USPSTF	2006	Infants	Same recommendation as above.	The USPSTF was unable to assess the balance of benefits and harms of screening for DDH, but was concerned about the potential harms associated with treatment, both surgical and nonsurgical, of infants identified by routine screening.	http://www.guideline.gov/content.aspx?id=38619
	AAOS	2014	Infants up to 6 mo	1. Recommend against universal ultrasound screening of newborns. 2. Ultrasound recommended for infants before 6 mo for a history of breech presentation, family history, or history of clinical hip instability. 3. Limited evidence supports brace treatment for hips in infants with a positive instability examination.		http://www.guideline.gov/content.aspx?id=48516

GESTATIONAL DIABETES

Disease Screening	Organization	Date	Population	Recommendations	Comments	Source
Diabetes Mellitus, Gestational (GDM)	USPSTF	2014	Pregnant women after 24 wk of gestation	Recommends screening for gestational diabetes mellitus in asymptomatic pregnant women.	Insufficient evidence to support screening for gestational diabetes prior to 24 gestational weeks.	http://www.uspreventiveservicestaskforce.org/Page/Topic/recommendation-summary/gestational-diabetes-mellitus-screening
	ACOG	2013		1-hour glucose screening test with 50-g anhydrous glucose load should be performed between 24 and 28 gestational weeks with a cutoff value of either 135 or 140 mg/dL. A 3-h glucose tolerance test should be performed if the 1-h glucose screening test is abnormal. • May use either the Carpenter and Coustan criteria or the National Diabetes Data Group criteria. Screen women with GDM 6–12 wk postpartum for overt diabetes.		http://www.guideline.gov/content.aspx?id=47014

DIABETES, TYPE 2

Disease Screening	Organization	Date	Population	Recommendations	Comments	Source
Diabetes Mellitus (DM), Type 2	ADA	2012	Pregnant women	1. Screen for undiagnosed DM type 2 at first prenatal visit if age ≥45 y or if risk factors for DM are present.[a] 2. For all other women, screen at 24–28 wk with a 75-g 2-h oral glucose tolerance test (OGTT) in the morning after an overnight fast of at least 8 h.	1. Preexisting diabetes if: a. Fasting glucose ≥126 mg/dL b. 2-h glucose ≥200 mg/dL after 75-g glucose load c. Random glucose ≥200 mg/dL with classic hyperglycemic symptoms d. Hemoglobin A1c ≥6.5% 2. Criteria for GDM by 75-g 2-h OGTT if any of the following are abnormal: a. Fasting ≥92 mg/dL (5.1 mmol/L) b. 1 h ≥180 mg/dL (10.0 mmol/L) c. 2 h ≥153 mg/dL (8.5 mmol/L)	http://care.diabetesjournals.org/content/35/Supplement_1/S11.full
	ADA	2011	Children at start of puberty or age ≥10 y	Screen all children at risk for DM type 2.[b]		
	ADA	2011	Adults	Screen asymptomatic adults age ≥45 y or if risk factors for DM are present.[a]	1. Australian Carbohydrate Intolerance Study in Pregnant Women (ACHOIS): Treatment of a screening-detected population with mild gestational diabetes reduced serious neonatal and maternal outcomes. (*Ann Intern Med.* 2008;148(10):766) 2. Fasting plasma glucose ≥126 mg/dL or a casual plasma glucose ≥200 mg/dL meets threshold for diabetes diagnosis, if confirmed on a subsequent day. *and precludes the need for glucose challenge.* (ADA)	http://www.guideline.gov/content.aspx?id=38619 http://www.ahrq.gov/clinic/pocketgd1011/pocketgd1011.pdf
	AAFP USPSTF	2010 2010	Hypertensive adults	Screen asymptomatic adults with sustained BP (either treated or untreated) >135/80 mm Hg.		
	AAFP USPSTF	2010 2010	Adults	Evidence is insufficient to recommend for or against routinely screening asymptomatic adults with a BP <135/80 mm Hg.	Screen at least every 3 years in asymptomatic adults.	

[a]DM risk factors: overweight (BMI ≥25 kg/m²) *and* an additional risk factor: physical inactivity; first-degree relative with DM; high-risk ethnicity (eg, African American, Latino, Native American, Asian American, Pacific Islander); history of GDM; prior baby with birth weight >9 lb; hypertension (HTN) on therapy or with BP ≥140/90 mm Hg; HDL–C level <35 mg/dL (0.90 mmol/L) and/or a triglyceride level >250 mg/dL (2.82 mmol/L); polycystic ovary syndrome; history of impaired glucose tolerance or HgbA1c ≥5.7%; *Acanthosis nigricans*; or cardiovascular disease.

[b]Test asymptomatic children if BMI >85% for age/gender, weight for height >85th percentile, or weight >120% of ideal for height *plus any two* of the following: FH of DM in first- or second-degree relative; high-risk ethnic group (eg, Native American, African American, Latino, Asian American, or Pacific Islander); *Acanthosis nigricans*; HTN; dyslipidemia; polycystic ovary syndrome; small-for-gestational-age birth weight; maternal history of DM or GDM during the child's gestation.

FALLS IN THE ELDERLY

Disease Screening	Organization	Date	Population	Recommendations	Comments	Source
Falls in the Elderly	NICE	2004	All older persons	Ask at least yearly about falls.[a,c]	1. Individuals are at increased risk if they report at least 2 falls in the previous year, or 1 fall with injury. 2. Calcium and vitamin D supplementation reduces falls by 45% over 3 y in women, but no effect is seen in men. (*Arch Intern Med.* 2006;166:424) 3. A fall prevention clinic appears to reduce the number of falls among the elderly. (*Am J Phys Med Rehabil.* 2006;85:882) 4. See also page 102 for fall prevention and Appendix II. 5. Of US adults age ≥65 y, 15.9% fell in the preceding 3 months; of these, 31.3% sustained an injury that resulted in a doctor visit or restricted activity for at least 1 d. (*MMWR Morb Mortal Wkly Rep.* 2008;57(9):225)	http://www.nice.org.uk
	AAOS	2001				*J Am Geriatr Soc.* 2001;49:664–672
	AGS	2001				http://www .americangeriatrics.org/ health_care_professionals/ clinical_practice/clinical_ guidelines_ recommendations/ prevention_of_falls_ summary_of_ recommendations
	British Geriatrics Society	2001				
	CTF	2005	All persons admitted to long-term care facilities	Recommend programs that target the broad range of environmental and resident-specific risk factors to prevent falls and hip fractures.[d]		http://canadiantaskforce .ca/guidelines/ all-guidelines/2005- prevention-of-falls-in-long- term-care-facilities/

[a]All who report a single fall should be observed as they stand up from a chair without using their arms, walk several paces, and return (see Appendix II). Those demonstrating no difficulty or unsteadiness need no further assessment. Those who have difficulty or demonstrate unsteadiness, have ≥1 fall, or present for medical attention after a fall should have a fall evaluation (see Fall Prevention, page 128).
[b]Risk factors: Intrinsic: lower-extremity weakness, poor grip strength, balance disorders, functional and cognitive impairment, visual deficits. Extrinsic: polypharmacy (≥4 prescription medications), environment (poor lighting, loose carpets, lack of bathroom safety equipment).
[c]Free "Tip Sheet" for patients from AGS (http://www.healthinaging.org/public_education/falls_tips.php).
[d]Postfall assessments may detect previously unrecognized health concerns.

FAMILY VIOLENCE AND ABUSE					
Disease Screening	Organization	Date	Population	Recommendations	Comments	Source
Family Violence and Abuse	AAFP	2010	Children, women, and older adults	Insufficient evidence to recommend for or against routine screening of parents or guardians for the physical abuse or neglect of children, of women for intimate partner violence, or of older adults or their caregivers for elder abuse.	1. Recent studies show that screening for intimate partner violence in emergency departments and pediatric clinics shows high prevalence (10%–20%) and does not increase harm. (*Ann Emerg Med.* 2008;51:433. *Pediatrics.* 2008;121:e85)	http://www.uspreventive servicestaskforce.org/ uspstf/uspsfamv.htm http://www.guideline.gov/ content.aspx?id=38619
Elder Abuse and Neglect	USPSTF	2013	Elderly people and vulnerable adults	Insufficient evidence to recommend for or against routine screening all elderly people or vulnerable adults for abuse and neglect.	2. In screening for intimate partner violence, women prefer self-completed approaches (written or computer-based) over face-to-face questioning. (*JAMA.* 2006;296:530) 3. All providers should be aware of physical and behavioral signs and symptoms associated with abuse and neglect, including burns, bruises, and repeated suspect trauma.	www.guidelines.gov/content. aspx?id=39425
Intimate Partner Violence	USPSTF	2013	Women age 14–46 y	Recommends that clinicians screen women of childbearing age for intimate partner violence and provide or refer women who screen positive to intervention services.	It is thought that nearly 31% of women and 26% of men report experiencing intimate partner violence at some time during their lives	www.guidelines.gov/content. aspx?id=39425

Disease Screening	Organization	Date	Population	Recommendations	Comments	Source
GLAUCOMA						
Glaucoma	AAFP	2005	Adults	Insufficient evidence to recommend for or against screening adults for glaucoma.		http://www.guidelines.gov/content.aspx?id=38619 http://www.uspreventiveservicestaskforce.org/uspstf/uspsglau.htm
	USPSTF	2013	Adults	The available evidence is insufficient to recommend for or against routine screening of adults for primary open-angle glaucoma.		http://www.guideline.gov/content.aspx?id=46922

GONORRHEA

Disease Screening	Organization	Date	Population	Recommendations	Comments	Source
Gonorrhea	CDC	2010	Sexually active women	Annually screen all women at risk for gonorrhea.[a]	Gonorrhea is a reportable illness to state Public Health Departments.	http://www.cdc.gov/mmwr/pdf/rr/rr5912.pdf
	USPSTF	2014	Sexually active women age 24 y or younger and older women at high risk			http://www.uspreventiveservicestaskforce.org/Page/Topic/recommendation-summary/chlamydia-and-gonorrhea-screening
	CDC	2010	Women age ≤35 y who are sexually active and in juvenile detention or jail	Screen at intake and then annual screenings.		http://www.cdc.gov/mmwr/pdf/rr/rr5912.pdf
	CDC	2010	Homosexual men	Annual testing for men who have had insertive or receptive intercourse in the past year.		http://www.cdc.gov/mmwr/pdf/rr/rr5912.pdf

[a]Women age <25 y are at highest risk for gonorrhea infection. Other risk factors that place women at increased risk include a previous gonorrhea infection, the presence of other sexually transmitted diseases (STDs), new or multiple sex partners, inconsistent condom use, commercial sex work, and drug use.

GROUP B STREPTOCOCCAL DISEASE

Disease Screening	Organization	Date	Population	Recommendations	Comments	Source
Group B Streptococcal (GBS) Disease	CDC	2010	Pregnant women	Universal screening of all women at 35–37 gestational weeks for GBS colonization with a vaginal–rectal swab.	Women who are colonized with GBS should receive intrapartum antibiotic prophylaxis to prevent neonatal GBS sepsis.	http://www.cdc.gov/mmwr/ preview/mmwrhtml/rr5910a1 .htm?s_cid=rr5910a1_w

GROWTH ABNORMALITIES, INFANT

Disease Screening	Organization	Date	Population	Recommendations	Comments	Source
Growth Abnormalities, Infant	CDC	2010	Children 0–59 mo	Use the 2006 World Health Organization (WHO) international growth charts for children age <24 mo.	1. The Centers for Disease Control and Prevention (CDC) and American Academy of Pediatricians (AAP) recommend the WHO as opposed to the CDC growth charts for children age <24 mo. 2. The CDC growth charts should still be used for children age 2–19 y. 3. This recommendation recognizes that breastfeeding is the recommended standard of infant feeding, and therefore the standard against which all other infants are compared.	http://www.cdc.gov/ mmwr/preview/ mmwrhtml/rr5909a1. htm

HEARING IMPAIRMENT

Disease Screening	Organization	Date	Population	Recommendations	Comments	Source
Hearing Impairment	AAFP USPSTF	2010 2008	Newborns	Routine screening of all newborn infants for hearing loss.	1. Screening involves either a 1-step or a 2-step process. 2. The 2-step process includes otoacoustic emissions (OAEs) followed by auditory brainstem response (ABR) in those who fail the OAE test. 3. The 1-step process uses either OAE or ABR testing.	http://www.guideline.gov/content.aspx?id=38619 http://www.uspreventive servicestaskforce.org/uspstf08/newbornhear/newbhears.htm
	ICSI	2010	Newborns	Universal screening of infants for congenital hearing loss should be performed during the first month of life.		http://www.icsi.org/preventive_services_for_children_guideline_/preventive_services_for_children_and_adolescents_2531.html
	AAFP ICSI USPSTF	2010 2010 2011	Adults age >50 y	Question older adults periodically about hearing impairment, counsel about availability of hearing aid devices, and make referrals for abnormalities when appropriate. See also Appendix II: Functional Assessment Screening in the Elderly.	1. Of adults age >50 y 20%–40%, and >80% of adults age ≥80 y, have some degree of hearing loss. 2. Additional research is required to determine if hearing loss screening can lead to improved health outcomes. 3. No harm from hearing loss screening. 4. No harm related to hearing aid use.	http://www.guideline.gov/content.aspx?id=38619 http://www.icsi.org/preventive_services_for_adults/preventive_services_for_adults_4.html http://www.uspreventive servicestaskforce.org/uspstf11/adulthearing/adulthearart.pdf

HEMOCHROMATOSIS

Disease Screening	Organization	Date	Population	Recommendations	Comments	Source
Hemochromatosis (Hereditary)	AASLD	2011	Adults	Screen people with iron studies and a serum *HFE* mutation analysis if they have first-degree relatives with *HFE*-related hemochromatosis (*Blood.* 2008;111:3373)		http://www.aasld.org/practiceguidelines/Practice%20Guideline%20Archive/Diagnosis%20 and%20Management%20of%20Hemochromatosis.pdf
	AAFP USPSTF	2008 2006	Asymptomatic adults	Recommends against routine genetic screening for hemochromatosis in asymptomatic adults. Patients with a family history should be counseled with further testing based on clinical considerations. (*Arch Intern Med.* 2006;166:269. *Blood.* 2008 111 3373)	1. There is fair evidence that clinically significant disease caused by hereditary hemochromatosis is uncommon in the general population. Male homozygotes for C282Y gene mutation have a 2-fold increase in the incidence of iron overload-related symptoms, compared with females. 2. There is poor evidence that early therapeutic phlebotomy improves morbidity and mortality in screening-detected vs clinically detected individuals.	http://www.aafp.org/online/en/home/clinical/exam.html http://www.ahrq.gov/clinic/uspstf/uspshemoch.htm

HEMOCHROMATOSIS

Disease Screening	Organization	Date	Population	Recommendations	Comments	Source
Hemochromatosis (Hereditary) (continued)	ACP	2005	Adults	Insufficient evidence to recommend for or against screening.[a] In case-finding for hereditary hemochromatosis, serum ferritin and transferrin saturation tests should be performed.	1. If testing is performed, cutoff values for serum ferritin levels >200 µg/L in women and >300 µg/L in men and transferrin saturation >45% may be used as criteria for case-finding, but there is no general agreement about diagnostic criteria. 2. For clinicians who choose to screen, one-time screening of non-Hispanic white men with serum ferritin level and transferrin saturation has highest yield.	*Ann Intern Med.* 2005;143:517-521 http://www.acponline.org/ clinical/guidelines/ *N Engl J Med.* 2004;350:2383

[a]Discuss the risks, benefits, and limitations of genetic testing in patients with a positive FH of hereditary hemochromatosis, or those with elevated serum ferritin levels or transferrin saturation.

HEMOGLOBINOPATHIES					
Disease Screening	Organization	Date	Population	Recommendations	Comments	Source
Hemoglobinopathies	AAFP USPSTF	2010 2007	Newborns	Recommend screening all newborns for hemoglobinopathies (including sickle cell disease).	Newborn screen tests for phenylketonuria (PKU), hemoglobinopathies, and hypothyroidism.	http://www.guideline.gov/content .aspx?id=38619 http://www.uspreventive servicestaskforce.org/uspstf07/ sicklecell/sicklers.htm

HEPATITIS B VIRUS INFECTION

Disease Screening	Organization	Date	Population	Recommendations	Comments	Source
Hepatitis B Virus Infection	NICE	2013	Adults	• Offer transient elastography as the initial test of liver cirrhosis for all adults with HBV infection. • Liver ultrasound and α-fetoprotein every 6 mo for HBV infection with cirrhosis to screen for hepatocellular carcinoma.		http://www.guideline.gov/content.aspx?id=46933

HEPATITIS B VIRUS INFECTION, CHRONIC

Disease Screening	Organization	Date	Population	Recommendations	Comments	Source
Hepatitis B Virus (HBV) Infection, Chronic	USPSTF ACOG AAP AAFP CDC	2009 2007 2006 2010 2010	Pregnant women	Screen all women with HBsAg at their first prenatal visit.	1. Breastfeeding is not contraindicated in women with chronic HBV infection if the infant has received hepatitis B immunoglobulin (HBIG)-passive prophylaxis and vaccine-active prophylaxis. 2. All pregnant women who are HBsAg-positive should be reported to the local Health Department to ensure proper follow-up. 3. Immunoassays for HBsAg have sensitivity and specificity >98% (*MMWR.* 1993;42:707).	http://www.annals.org/content/150/12/I-36.full http://www.guideline.gov/content.aspx?id=38619 http://www.cdc.gov/mmwr/pdf/rr/rr5912.pdf
	NIH AASLD	2009 2009	Adults and children	1. Recommend routine screening for HBV infection of newly arrived immigrants from countries where the HBV prevalence rate is >2%.[a] 2. Screen all patients with chronically elevated alanine transaminase (ALT), homosexual men, persons with multiple sexual partners, injection-drug users, jail inmates, dialysis patients, household contacts of persons with chronic HBV infection, and persons infected with either hepatitis C virus (HCV) or HIV.		http://www.guidelines.gov/content.aspx?id=14240 http://www.guidelines.gov/content.aspx?id=15475
	USPSTF	2014	Nonpregnant adults and adolescents	USPSTF recommends screening for HBV infection in persons at high risk of infection.		http://www.uspreventiveservicestaskforce.org/Page/Topic/recommendation-summary/hepatitis-b-virus-infection-screening-2014

[a]Immigrants from Asia, Africa, South Pacific, Middle East (except Israel), Eastern Europe (except Hungary), the Caribbean, Malta, Spain, Guatemala, and Honduras.

HEPATITIS C VIRUS INFECTION, CHRONIC

Disease Screening	Organization	Date	Population	Recommendations	Comments	Source
Hepatitis C Virus (HCV) Infection, Chronic	ACOG CDC	2007 2010	Pregnant women at increased risk[a]	Perform routine counseling and testing at the first prenatal visit.	1. Route of delivery has not been shown to influence rate of vertical transmission of HCV infection. Cesarean section should be reserved for obstetric indications only. 2. Breast-feeding is not contraindicated in women with chronic HCV infection.	http://www.guidelines.gov/content.aspx?id=12627 http://www.cdc.gov/mmwr/pdf/rr/rr5912.pdf
	AASLD USPSTF USPSTF WHO	2009 2013 2013 2014	Persons at increased risk for HCV infection[a] Adults born between 1945 and 1965	Recommend HCV antibody testing by enzyme immunoassay in all high-risk adults. One-time HCV antibody testing for HCV screening in all adults born between 1945 and 1965.	1. HCV RNA testing should be performed for: a. Positive HCV antibody test result in a patient b. When antiviral treatment is being considered c. Unexplained liver disease in an immunocompromised patient with a negative HCV antibody test result d. Suspicion of acute HCV infection 2. HCV genotype should be determined in all HCV-infected persons prior to interferon treatment. 3. Seroconversion may take up to 3 months. 4. Of persons with acute hepatitis C, 15%–25% resolve their infection; of the remaining, 10%–20% develop cirrhosis within 20–30 y after infection, and 1%–5% develop hepatocellular carcinoma.	http://www.bccdc.ca/NR/rdonlyes/9F6B2AE8-D8A9-4DCB-A83D-710045A62B3A/0/AASLO_guidelines_HEP_C_2009.pdf http://www.uspreventiveservicestaskforce.org/uspstf/uspshepc.htm http://www.guideline.gov/content.aspx?id=48895
	AAFP	2010	General asymptomatic adults	Recommends against routine screening for HCV infection in adults who are not at increased risk.[a]	5. Patients testing positive for HCV antibody should receive a nucleic acid test to confirm active infection. A quantitative HCV RNA test and genotype test can provide useful prognostic information prior to initiating antiviral therapy. (JAMA. 2007;297:724)	http://www.guidelines.gov/content.aspx?id=34005

[a] HCV risk factors: HIV infection; sexual partners of HCV-infected persons; persons seeking evaluation or care for STDs, including HIV; history of injection-drug use; persons who have ever been on hemodialysis; intranasal drug use; history of blood or blood component transfusion or organ transplant prior to 1992; hemophilia; multiple tattoos; children born to HCV-infected mothers; and health care providers who have sustained a needlestick injury.

HERPES SIMPLEX VIRUS, GENITAL

Disease Screening	Organization	Date	Population	Recommendations	Comments	Source
Herpes Simplex Virus (HSV), Genital	AAFP CDC	2010 2010	Adolescents and adults	Recommends against routine serologic screening for HSV.		http://www.guideline.gov/content.aspx?id=38619 http://www.cdc.gov/mmwr/pdf/rr/rr5912.pdf
	AAFP CDC	2010 2010	Pregnant women	Recommends against routine serologic screening for HSV to prevent neonatal HSV infection.	1. In women with a history of genital herpes, routine serial cultures for HSV are not indicated in the absence of active lesions. 2. Women who develop primary HSV infection during pregnancy have the highest risk for transmitting HSV infection to their infants.	http://www.guideline.gov/content.aspx?id=38619 http://www.cdc.gov/mmwr/pdf/rr/rr5912.pdf

HUMAN IMMUNODEFICIENCY VIRUS

Disease Screening	Organization	Date	Population	Recommendations	Comments	Source
Human Immunodeficiency Virus (HIV)	AAFP USPSTF	2010 2005	Pregnant women	Clinicians should screen all pregnant women for HIV.	Rapid HIV antibody testing during labor identified 34 HIV-positive women among 4849 women with no prior HIV testing documented (prevalence: 7 in 1000). Eighty-four percent of women consented to testing. Sensitivity was 100%, specificity was 99.9%, positive predictive value was 90%. (*JAMA.* 2004;292:219).	http://www.guideline.gov/content.aspx?id=38619 http://www.ahrq.gov/clinic/uspstf/uspshivi.htm
	CDC	2010	Pregnant women	Include HIV testing in panel of routine prenatal screening tests. Retest high-risk women at 36 wk' gestation. Rapid HIV testing of women in labor who have not received prenatal HIV testing.		http://www.cdc.gov/mmwr/pdf/rr/rr5912.pdf
	CDC	2010	Adolescents and adults who seek evaluation and treatment for STDs	HIV screening should be offered to all people who seek evaluation for STDs and all adolescents who are sexually active or who engage in injection drug use.	1. HIV testing should be voluntary and must have a verbal consent to test. Patients may "opt out" of testing. 2. Educate and counsel all high-risk patients regarding HIV testing, transmission, risk-reduction behaviors, and implications of infection.	http://www.cdc.gov/mmwr/pdf/rr/rr5912.pdf
	AAFP	2010	Adolescents and adults at increased risk[a]	Strongly recommends screening.	1. If acute HIV is suspected, also use plasma RNA test. 2. False-positive results with electroimmunoassay (EIA): nonspecific reactions in persons with immunologic disturbances (eg, systemic lupus erythematosus or rheumatoid arthritis), multiple transfusions, recent influenza, or rabies vaccination. 3. Confirmatory testing is necessary using Western blot or indirect immunofluorescence assay. 4. Awareness of HIV positively reduces secondary HIV transmission risk and high-risk behavior and viral load if on highly active antiretroviral therapy (HAART). (CDC, 2006)	http://www.guideline.gov/content.aspx?id=38619
	AAFP USPSTF	2010 2005	Adolescents and adults who are not at increased risk[a]	Insufficient evidence to recommend for or against routine screening.		http://www.guideline.gov/content.aspx?id=38619 http://www.uspreventiveservicestaskforce.org/uspstf/uspshivi.htm
	USPSTF	2013	Adolescents and adults age 15–65 y	Screen people age 15–65 y for HIV infection.	Consider screening younger adolescents or older adults who are at increased risk.	http://www.guideline.gov/content.aspx?id=45148
			Pregnant women	All pregnant women should be screened for HIV infection.		

[a]Risk factors for HIV: men who have had sex with men after 1975; multiple sexual partners; history of intravenous drug use; prostitution; history of sex with an HIV-infected person; history of sexually transmitted disease; history of blood transfusion between 1978 and 1985; or persons requesting an HIV test.

HYPERTENSION, CHILDREN AND ADOLESCENTS

Disease Screening	Organization	Date	Population	Recommendations	Comments	Source
Hypertension (HTN), Children and Adolescents	AAFP Pediatrics	2013 2004 2011	Age 3–20 y[a]	Children age ≥3 years should have BP measured as part of routine evaluation.	1. Hypertension: average systolic blood pressure (SBP) or diastolic blood pressure (DBP) ≥95th percentile for gender, age, and height on ≥3 occasions. See Appendices. 2. Prehypertension: average SBP or DBP 90th–95th percentile. 3. Adolescents with BP ≥120/80 mm Hg are prehypertensive. 4. Evaluation of hypertensive children: assess for additional risk factors. Follow-up BP: if normal, repeat in 1 y; if prehypertensive, repeat BP in 6 mo; if stage 1, repeat in 2 wk; if symptomatic or stage 2, refer or repeat in 1 wk. 5. Indications for antihypertensive drug therapy in children: symptomatic HTN, secondary HTN, target-organ damage, diabetes, persistent HTN despite nonpharmacologic measures.	http://www.aafp.org/patient-care/clinical-recommendations/all/hypertension.html *Pediatrics.* 2004;114:555-576 http://www.nhlbi.nih.gov/guidelines/cvd_ped/index.htm http://www.nhlbi.nih.gov/health/public/heart/hbp/bp_child_pocket/bp_child_pocket.pdf *Am Fam Physician.* 2006;73(9):1558-1568
	NHLBI	2004	Age 3–20 y[a]		6. Accumulating evidence suggests that ambulatory BP monitoring is a more accurate method for diagnosis of HTN in children and allows better assessment for therapy.	http://www.nhlbi.nih.gov/ *Contemp Pediatr.* 2008;
	Bright Futures	2008	Age 3–21 y[a]	Annual screening.	7. Screening for hypertension in children and adolescents hasn't been proven to reduce adverse cardiovascular outcomes in adults.	http://www.brightfutures.org *Hypertension.* 2008;52:433-451 *Pediatrics.* 2013;131(3):490-525 www.uspreventiveservicestaskforce.org/uspstf/uspshypechld.htm
	USPSTF	2013			The USPSTF concludes that the current evidence is insufficient to assess the balance of benefits and harms of screening for primary hypertension in asymptomatic children and adolescents to prevent subsequent cardiovascular disease in childhood or adulthood.	http://www.uspreventiveservicestaskforce.org/Page/Topic/recommendation-summary/blood-pressure-in-children-and-adolescents-hypertension-screening

[a]In children age <3 y, conditions that warrant BP measurement: prematurity, very low birth weight, or neonatal complications; congenital heart disease; recurrent urinary tract infections (UTIs), hematuria, or proteinuria; renal disease or urologic malformations; FH of congenital renal disease; solid-organ transplant; malignancy or bone marrow transplant; drugs known to raise BP; systemic illnesses; increased intracranial pressure.

HYPERTENSION, ADULTS

Disease Screening	Organization	Date	Population	Recommendations	Comments	Source
Hypertension (HTN), Adults	USPSTF AAFP USPSTF CHEP ESH	2009 2008 2007 2015 2007	Adults age >18 y	1. Screen for HTN. 2. HTN >140/90 mm Hg. 3. Diagnosis after two or more BP readings obtained at least two visits over several weeks. 4. All adults should have their BP assessed at all appropriate clinical visits. 5. Home BP monitoring (HBPM) is an important toll in self-monitoring and self-management. 6. Annual F/U of patients with high-normal BP (2-y risk of developing HTN is 40%).	8. Electronic (oscillometric) measurement methods are preferred to manual measurements. Routine auscultatory OBPMs are 9/6 mm Hg higher than standardized research BPs (primarily using oscillometric devices)CHEP 2015. 9. Out-of-office measurement should be performed to confirm the initial diagnosis of hypertension. 10. ABPM has better predictive ability than OBPM and is the recommended out-of-office measurement method. 11. HBPM has better predictive ability than OBPM and is recommended if ABPM is not tolerated, not readily available or due to patient preference. HBPM and ABPM identify white coat hypertension (as well as diagnose masked hypertension).	Am Fam Physician. 2009;79(12):1087–1088 http://www.aafp.org/online/en/home/clinical/exam.html http://www.ahrq.gov/clinic/uspstf/uspshype.htm http://www.hypertension.ca/en/chep J Hypertens. 2007;25:1105 http://www.escardio.org/ knowledge/ guidelines/ Guidelines_list.htm?hit=quick
	ESC	2013		In cases of severe BP elevation, especially if associated with end-organ damage, the diagnosis can be based on measurements taken at a single visit. In asymptomatic subjects with hypertension but free of CVD, chronic kidney disease (CKD), and diabetes, total cardiovascular risk stratification using the SCORE model is recommended as a minimal requirement.	12. The first reading should be discardedand the latter two averaged. 13. Assess global cardiovascular risk in all hypertensive patients. Informing patients of their global risk ("vascular age") improves the effectiveness of risk factor modification.	Hypertens. 2007;25:1105 http://www.escardio.org/ knowledge/guidelines/ Guidelines_list.htm?hit=quick Eur Heart J. 2013;34:2159–2219
	JNC VII (NHLBI)	2003	Age >18 y	Normal: recheck in 2 y (see Comments). Pre-HTN: Recheck in 1 y. Stage 1 HTN: Confirm within 2 mo. Stage 2 HTN: Evaluate or refer to source of care within 1 mo (evaluate and treat immediately if BP >180/110 mm Hg).	1. Pre-HTN: SBP 120–139 mm Hg or DBP 80–89 mm Hg. 2. Stage 1 HTN: SBP 140–159 mm Hg or DBP 90–99 mm Hg. 3. Stage 2 HTN: SBP ≥160 mm Hg or DBP ≥100 mm Hg (based on average of ≥2 measurements on ≥2 separate office visits).[a] 4. Perform physical examination and routine labs.[b] 5. Pursue secondary causes of HTN.[b] 6. Treatment goals are for BP <140/90 mm Hg, unless the patient has diabetes or renal disease (<130/80 mm Hg). See page 266, Chapter 3 for JNC 8 Management Algorithm. 7. Ambulatory BP monitoring is a better (and independent) predictor of cardiovascular outcomes compared with office visit monitoring and is covered by Medicare when evaluating white-coat HTN. (N Engl J Med. 2006;354:2368)	JAMA. 2003;289:2560 Hypertension. 2003;42:1206 J Am Coll Cardiol. 2011;57(20):2037–2110
	ACCF/AHA	2011	Age >65 y	Identification and treatment of systolic and diastolic HTN in the very elderly is beneficial in reduction in all-cause mortality and stroke death.	Increased frequency of systolic HTN compared with younger patients. HTN is more likely associated with end-organ damage and more often associated with other risk factors.	

OBPM, Office BP Measurement; HBPM, Home BP Measurement; ABPM, Ambulatory BP Measurement
[a]Physical examination should include: measurements of height, weight, and waist circumference; funduscopic exam (retinopathy); carotid auscultation (bruit); jugular venous pulsation; thyroid gland (enlargement); cardiac auscultation (left ventricular heave, S3 or S4, murmurs, clicks); chest auscultation (rales, evidence of chronic obstructive pulmonary disease); abdominal exam (bruits, masses, pulsations); examination of lower extremities (diminished arterial pulsations, bruits, edema); and neurologic examination (focal findings). Routine labs include urinalysis, complete blood count, electrolytes (potassium, calcium), creatinine, glucose, fasting lipids, and 12-lead electrocardiogram.
[b]Pursue secondary causes of HTN when evaluation is suggestive (clues in parentheses) of (1) pheochromocytoma (labile or paroxysmal HTN accompanied by sweats, headaches, and palpitations); (2) renovascular disease (abdominal bruits); (3) autosomal dominant polycystic kidney disease (abdominal or flank masses); (4) Cushing syndrome (truncal obesity with purple striae); (5) primary hyperaldosteronism (hypokalemia); (6) hyperparathyroidism (hypercalcemia); (7) renal parenchymal disease (elevated serum creatinine, abnormal urinalysis); (8) poor response to drug therapy; (9) well-controlled HTN with an abrupt increase in BP; (10) SBP >180 mm Hg or DBP >110 mm Hg; or (11) sudden onset of HTN.

ILLICIT DRUG USE

Disease Screening	Organization	Date	Population	Recommendations	Comments	Source
Illicit Drug Use	AAFP USPSTF ICSI	2010 2008 2010	Adults, adolescents, and pregnant women	Insufficient evidence to recommend for or against routine screening for illicit drug use.		http://www.guideline.gov/content .aspx?id=38619 http://www.uspreventive servicestaskforce.org/uspstf08/druguse/ drugrs.htm http://www.icsi.org/preventive_services_for_ adults/preventive_services_for_adults_4.html

KIDNEY DISEASE, CHRONIC

Disease Screening	Organization	Date	Population	Recommendations	Comments	Source
Kidney Disease, Chronic (CKD)	NICE	2008	Adults	1. Monitor glomerular filtration rate (GFR) at least annually in people prescribed drugs known to be nephrotoxic.[a] 2. Screen renal function in people at risk for CKD.[b]		http://www.nice.org.uk/nicemedia/live/12069/42117/42117.pdf

[a]Examples: calcineurin inhibitors, lithium, or nonsteroidal anti-inflammatory drugs (NSAIDs).
[b]DM, HTN, CVD, structural renal disease, nephrolithiasis, benign prostatic hyperplasia (BPH), multisystem diseases with potential kidney involvement (eg, systemic lupus erythematosus [SLE]), FH of stage 5 CKD or hereditary kidney disease, or personal history of hematuria or proteinuria.

Disease Screening	Organization	Date	Population	Recommendations	Comments	Source

Lead Poisoning	AAFP	2010	Children age 1–5 y	1. Insufficient evidence to recommend for or against routine screening in asymptomatic children at increased risk.
				2. Recommends against screening in asymptomatic children at average risk.
					1. Risk assessment should be performed during prenatal visits and continue until age 6 y.
					2. CDC personal risk questionnaire:
					  a. Does your child live in or regularly visit a house (or other facility, eg, daycare) that was built before 1950?
					  b. Does your child live in or regularly visit a house built before 1978 with recent or ongoing renovations or remodeling (within the last 6 mo)?
					  c. Does your child have a sibling or playmate who has or did have lead poisoning? (http://www.cdc.gov/nceh/lead/publications/screening.htm)
						http://www.guidelines.gov/content.aspx?id=36873

	AAFP	2010	Pregnant women	Recommends against screening in asymptomatic pregnant women.		http://www.guidelines.gov/content.aspx?id=36873
	CDC	2010	Pregnant women	Routine blood lead testing of pregnant women is recommended in clinical settings that serve populations with specific risk factors for lead exposure.[a]		http://www.cdc.gov/nceh/lead/publications/LeadandPregnancy2010.pdf
	CDC	2009	Children age 1–5 y	Recommend blood lead screening in Medicaid-eligible children at increased risk for lead exposure.[b]	Screen at ages 1 and 2 y, or by age 3 y if a high-risk child has never been screened.	http://www.cdc.gov/mmwr/preview/mmwrhtml/rr5809a1.htm

[a]Important risk factors for lead exposure in pregnant women include recent immigration, pica practices, occupational exposure, nutritional status, culturally specific practices such as the use of traditional remedies or imported cosmetics, and the use of traditional lead-glazed pottery for cooking and storing food.

[b]Child suspected by parent, health care provider, or Health Department to be at risk for lead exposure; sibling or playmate with elevated blood lead level; recent immigrant, refugee, or foreign adoptee; child's parent or caregiver works with lead; household member uses traditional folk or ethnic remedies or cosmetics or who routinely eats food imported informally from abroad; residence near a source of high lead levels.

MOTOR VEHICLE SAFETY

Disease Screening	Organization	Date	Population	Recommendations	Comments	Source
Motor Vehicle Safety	ICSI	2010	Children and adolescents	Recommend that all health care providers ask about 1. Car seats 2. Booster seats 3. Seat belt use 4. Helmet use while riding motorcycles	One study demonstrated a 21% reduction in mortality with the use of child restraint systems vs seat belts in children age 2–6 y involved in motor vehicle collisions. (*Arch Pediatr Adolesc Med.* 2006;160: 617-621)	http://www.icsi.org/preventive_services_for_children_guideline_/preventive_services_for_children_and_adolescents_2531.html

NEWBORN SCREENING

Disease Screening	Organization	Date	Population	Recommendations	Comments	Source
Newborn Screening	ICSI	2010	Newborns	All newborns should receive a newborn metabolic screening test prior to hospital discharge.	The newborn screen should be performed after 24 h of age. Infants who receive their newborn screen before 24 h of age should have it repeated before 2 wk of age.	http://www.icsi.org/preventive_services_for_children_guideline/preventive_services_for_children_and_acolescents_2531.html

OBESITY

Disease Screening	Organization	Date	Population	Recommendations	Comments	Source
Obesity	AAFP USPSTF	2010 2010	Children age ≥6 y	The AAFP recommends that clinicians screen children age 6 y and older for obesity.	Obese children should be offered intensive counseling and behavioral interventions to promote improvement in weight status.	http://www.guideline.gov/content.aspx?id=38619 http://www.uspreventive servicestaskforce.org/uspstf/uspschobes.htm
	ICSI	2010	Children age ≥2 y	Height, weight, and body mass index (BMI) should be recorded annually starting at age 2 y.	1. Children with a BMI ≥25 are 5 times more likely to be overweight as adults when compared with their normal-weight counterparts. 2. Overweight children should be counseled about wholesome eating, 30–60 min of daily physical activity, and avoiding soft drinks.	http://www.icsi.org/preventive_services_for_children_guideline_/preventive_services_for_children_and_adolescents_2531.html
	AAFP	2012	Adults age >18 y	Recommends screening all adults and offering intensive counseling and behavioral interventions to promote sustained weight loss in obese adults with BMI ≥30 kg/m².	Intensive counseling involves more than one session per month for at least 3 mo.	http://www.guideline.gov/content.aspx?id=38619 http://www.uspreventive servicestaskforce.org/uspstf/uspsobes.htm
	ICSI	2010	Adults age >18 y	Height, weight, and BMI should be measured at least annually.	Intensive intervention to promote weight loss should be offered to all obese adults (BMI ≥30 or waist circumference ≥40 in [men] or ≥35 in [women]).	http://www.icsi.org/preventive_services_for_adults/preventive_services_for_adults_4.html
	VA/DoD	2006	Adults	1. Height, weight, and BMI should be measured at least annually. 2. Waist circumference should be measured at least annually.	1. Intensive intervention to promote weight loss should be offered to a. Obese adults (BMI ≥30 or waist circumference ≥40 in [men] or ≥35 in [women]) b. Overweight adults (BMI 25–29.9) with an obesity-associated condition[a]	http://www.healthquality.va.gov/obesity/obe06_final1.pdf

[a]HTN, DM type 2, dyslipidemia, obstructive sleep apnea, degenerative joint disease, or metabolic syndrome.

OSTEOPOROSIS					
Disease Screening	Organization	Date	Population	Recommendations	Comments	Source
Osteoporosis	USPSTF ACPM	2011 2009	Women age ≥65 y or younger women whose fracture risk is ≥ that of a 65-y-old white woman	Routine screening for women using either dual-energy x-ray absorptiometry (DXA) of the hip and lumbar spine, or quantitative ultrasonography of the calcaneus.	1. The optimal screening interval is unclear. 2. Screening should not be performed more frequently than every 2 y. 3. Ten-year risk for osteoporotic fractures can be calculated for individuals by using the FRAX tool (http://www.shef.ac.uk/FRAX/). 4. Quantitative ultrasonography of the calcaneus predicts fractures of the femoral neck, hip, and spine as effectively as does DXA. 5. The criteria for treatment of osteoporosis rely on DXA measurements.	http://www.uspreventiveservicestask force.org/uspstf10/osteoporosis/ osteors.htm http://www.guideline.gov/content. aspx?id=15270
	AAFP	2010	Women age ≥65 y or age ≥60 y at an increased risk for osteoporotic fracture	Routine screening for osteoporosis.		http://www.guideline.gov/content. aspx?id=38619
	USPSTF	2011	Older men	Insufficient evidence to recommend for or against routine osteopcrosis screening.		http://www.uspreventive servicestaskforce.org/uspstf10/ osteoporosis/osteors.htm
	ICSI	2010	Women age ≥65 y	Routine screening for osteoporosis.		http://www.icsi.org/preventive_ services_for_adults/preventive_ services_for_adults_4.html
	NOF ACPM	2008 2009	Men age ≥70 y	Recommends routine screening via bone mineral density (BMD).	Repeat every 3–5 y if "normal" baseline score; if high risk, then every 1–2 y.	http://www.guideline.gov/content. aspx?id=15270

PELVIC EXAMINATIONS

Disease Screening	Organization	Date	Population	Recommendations	Comments	Source
Pelvic Examinations	ACP	2014	Asymptomatic, nonpregnant women	Recommend against routine screening pelvic examinations.		http://www.guideline.gov/content.aspx?id=48334

PHENYLKETONURIA

Disease Screening	Organization	Date	Population	Recommendations	Comments	Source
Phenylketonuria (PKU)	AAFP USPSTF	2010 2007	Newborns	Recommend screening all newborns for PKU.	Newborn screen tests for PKU, hemoglobinopathies, and hypothyroidism.	http://www.guideline.gov/content.aspx?id=38619 http://www.uspreventiveservicestaskforce.org/uspstf07/sicklecell/sicklers.htm

RH (D) INCOMPATIBILITY

Disease Screening	Organization	Date	Population	Recommendations	Comments	Source
Rh (D) Incompatibility	AAFP USPSTF	2010 2007	Pregnant women	1. Recommend blood typing and Rh (D) antibody testing for all pregnant women at their first prenatal visit. 2. Repeat Rh (D) antibody testing for all unsensitized Rh (D)-negative women at 24–28 wk gestation.	Rh (D) antibody testing at 24–28 wk can be skipped if the biologic father is known to be Rh (D)-negative.	http://www.guideline.gov/content.aspx?id=38619 http://www.uspreventiveservicestaskforce.org/3rduspstf/rh/rhrs.htm

SCOLIOSIS

Disease Screening	Organization	Date	Population	Recommendations	Comments	Source
Scoliosis	AAFP USPSTF	2010 2004	Adolescents	Recommend against routine screening of asymptomatic adolescents for idiopathic scoliosis.		http://www.guideline.gov/content .aspx?id=38619 http://www.uspreventive servicestaskforce.org/3rduspstf/ scoliosis/scoliors.htm

SPEECH AND LANGUAGE DELAY

Disease Screening	Organization	Date	Population	Recommendations	Comments	Source
Speech and Language Delay	AAFP	2008	Preschool children	Evidence is insufficient to recommend for or against routine use of brief, formal screening instruments in primary care to detect speech and language delay in children up to age 5 y.	1. Fair evidence suggests that interventions can improve the results of short-term assessments of speech and language skills; however, no studies have assessed long-term consequences. 2. In a study of 9000 toddlers in the Netherlands, 2-time screening for language delays reduced the number of children who required special education (2.7% vs 3.7%) and reduced deficient language performance (8.8% vs 9.7%) at age 8 y. (*Pediatrics.* 2007;120:1317) 3. Studies have not fully addressed the potential harms of screening or interventions for speech and language delays, such as labeling, parental anxiety, or unnecessary evaluation and intervention.	http://www.aafp.org/online/en/home/clinical/exam.html
	USPSTF	2006				http://www.ahrq.gov/clinic/uspstf/uspschdv.htm

SYPHILIS					

Disease Screening	Organization	Date	Population	Recommendations	Comments	Source
Syphilis	CDC AAFP USPSTF	2010 2010 2009	Pregnant women	Strongly recommends routine screening of all pregnant women at the first prenatal visit.	1. A nontreponemal test (Venereal Disease Research Laboratory [VDRL] or rapid plasma reagent [RPR] test) should be used for initial screening. 2. All reactive nontreponemal tests should be confirmed with a fluorescent treponemal antibody absorption (FTA-ABS) test. 3. Women at high risk for syphilis or who are previously untested should be tested again at 28 gestational weeks. Consider testing a third time at the time of delivery. 4. Syphilis is a reportable disease in every state.	http://www.cdc.gov/mmwr/pdf/rr/rr5912.pdf http://www.guideline.gov/content.aspx?id=38619 http://www.uspreventiveservicestaskforce.org/uspstf/uspssyphpg.htm
	AAFP CDC USPSTF	2010 2010 2004	Persons at increased risk[a]	Recommends screening high-risk persons.		http://www.guideline.gov/content.aspx?id=38619 http://www.cdc.gov/mmwr/pdf/rr/rr5912.pdf

[a]High risk includes commercial sex workers, persons who exchange sex for money or drugs, persons with other STDs (including HIV), sexually active homosexual men, and sexual contacts of persons with syphilis, gonorrhea, *Chlamydia*, or HIV infection.

THYROID DISEASE

Disease Screening	Organization	Date	Population	Recommendations	Comments	Source
Thyroid Disease	AAFP ICSI	2010 2010	Adults	Insufficient evidence to recommend for or against routine screening for thyroid disease.	Individuals with symptoms and signs potentially attributable to thyroid dysfunction and those with risk factors for its development may require TSH testing. Higher risk individuals are those with an autoimmune disorder, pernicious anemia, history of neck radiation, first-degree relative with a thyroid disorder, and those with psychiatric disorders.	http://www.guideline.gov/content .aspx?id=38619 http://www.icsi.org/preventive_services_ for_adults/preventive_services_for_ adults_4.html https://www.aace.com/files/final-file-hypo-guidelines.pdf
	ATA	2012	Adults	ATA recommends screening men and women older than age 35 y for hypothyroidism every 5 y.		
	AACE	2012	Adults	AACE recommends screening older adults with a thyroid-stimulating hormone (TSH) measurement.		
	ICSI AAFP and USPSTF	2010 2008	Newborns	Recommends screening for congenital hypothyroidism in newborns.		http://www.icsi.org/preventive_services_ for_children_guideline_/preventive_ services_for_children_and_ adolescents_2531.html http://www.guidelines.gov/content. aspx?id=38619 http://www.uspreventiveservicestaskforce. org/uspstf/uspscghy.htm

THYROID DISEASE, PREGNANCY AND POSTPARTUM

Disease Screening	Organization	Date	Population	Recommendations	Comments	Source
Thyroid Disease, Pregnancy and Postpartum	ATA	2011	Women who are pregnant or immediately postpartum	TSH levels should be obtained in first trimester for: • History of thyroid dysfunction or prior thyroid surgery • Age >30 y • Symptoms of thyroid dysfunction • Goiter • Thrombopoietin (TPO) antibody+ • Autoimmune disorder • History of miscarriage • History of preterm delivery • History of head or neck radiation • Family history of thyroid disease • Morbid obesity • Use of amiodarone or lithium use • Infertility • Lives in an area of severe iodine deficiency		http://thyroidguidelines.net/sites/thyroidguidelines.net/files/file/thy.2011.0087.pdf

Disease Screening	Organization	Date	Population	Recommendations	Comments	Source
Tobacco Use	AAFP USPSTF ICSI	2010 2009 2010	Adults	Recommends screening all adults for tobacco use and provide tobacco cessation interventions for those who use tobacco products.	The "5-A" framework is helpful for smoking cessation counseling: a. Ask about tobacco use. b. Advise to quit through clear, individualized messages. c. Assess willingness to quit. d. Assist in quitting. e. Arrange follow-up and support sessions.	http://www.guideline.gov/content. aspx?id=38619 http://www.uspreventiveservicestaskforce. org/uspstf/uspstbac2.htm http://www.icsi.org/preventive_services_ for_adults/preventive_services_for_ adults_4.html
	AAFP USPSTF ICSI	2010 2009 2010	Pregnant women	Recommends screening all pregnant women for tobacco use and provide pregnancy-directed counseling and literature for those who smoke.		http://www.guideline.gov/content. aspx?id=38619 http://www.uspreventiveservicestaskforce. org/uspstf/uspstbac2.htm http://www.icsi.org/preventive_services_ for_adults/preventive_services_for_ adults_4.html
	AAFP	2010	Children and adolescents	Evidence is insufficient to recommend for or against routine screening.	The avoidance of tobacco products by children and adolescents is desirable. It is uncertain whether advice and counseling by health care professionals in this area is effective.	http://www.guideline.gov/content. aspx?id=38619
	ICSI	2010	Children and adolescents age ≥10 y	Screen for tobacco use and reassess at every opportunity.	Provide ongoing cessation services to all tobacco users at every opportunity.	http://www.icsi.org/preventive_services_ for_children_guideline_/preventive_ services_for_children_and_ adolescents_2531.html

TOBACCO USE

TUBERCULOSIS, LATENT

Disease Screening	Organization	Date	Population	Recommendations	Comments	Source
Tuberculosis, Latent	CDC	2010	Persons at increased risk of developing tuberculosis (TB)	Screening by tuberculin skin test (TST) or interferon-gamma release assay (IGRA) is recommended. Frequency of testing is based on likelihood of further exposure to TB and level of confidence in the accuracy of the results.	1. Typically, a TST is used to screen for latent TB. 2. IGRA is preferred if: a. Testing persons who have a low likelihood of returning to have their TST read b. Testing persons who have received a bacille Calmette- Guérin (BCG) vaccination	http://www.cdc.gov/ mmwr/pdf/rr/rr5905 .pdf

VISUAL IMPAIRMENT, GLAUCOMA, OR CATARACT

Disease Screening	Organization	Date	Population	Recommendations	Comments	Source
Visual Impairment, Glaucoma, or Cataract	USPSTF AAFP	2009 2010	Older adults	Insufficient evidence to recommend for or against visual acuity screening or glaucoma screening in older adults.		http://www.uspreventiveservicestaskforce.org/uspstf09/visualscr/viseldrs.htm http://www.guideline.gov/content.aspx?id=38619
	ICSI	2010	Older adults	Objective vision testing (Snellen chart) recommended for adults age ≥65 y.		http://www.icsi.org/preventive_services_for_adults/preventive_services_for_adults_4.html
	AAO	2011	Adults	Avoid routine genetic testing for genetically complex disorders like age-related macular degeneration and late-onset primary open-angle glaucoma.	Genotyping of such individuals should be confined to research studies until more definitive data are available.	http://one.aao.org/CE/PracticeGuidelines/ClinicalStatements_Content.aspx?cid=f84ff8ef-9772-42ea-a168-8e096ac24d00#section7
	ICSI	2010	Children ≤4 y	Vision screening recommended for children age ≤4 y.	Screen for amblyopia, strabismus, or decreased visual acuity.	http://www.icsi.org/preventive_services_for_children_guideline_/preventive_services_for_children_and_adolescents_2531.html
	USPSTF USPSTF	2011 2011	Children 3–5 y Children <3 y	Vision screening for all children 3–5 y at least once to detect amblyopia. Insufficient evidence for vision screening in children <3 y of age.	May screen with a visual acuity test, a stereoacuity test, a cover–uncover test, and the Hirschberg light reflex test.	http://www.uspreventiveservicestaskforce.org/uspstf11/vischildren/vischildrs.htm

VITAMIN D DEFICIENCY

Disease Screening	Organization	Date	Population	Recommendations	Comments	Source
Vitamin D Deficiency	USPSTF	2015	Nonpregnant adults aged 18 y or older	Insufficient evidence to screen for vitamin D deficiency in asymptomatic adults.		http://www.guideline.gov/content.aspx?id=48961

					ASTHMA	
Disease Prevention	Organization	Date	Population	Recommendations	Comments	Source
Asthma	Global Initiative for Asthma (GINA)	2012	Children	• Pregnant women and parents of young children should be advised not to smoke.	• Level of Evidence B. • Passive smoking increases the risk of allergic sensitization in children.	http://www.ginasthma.org/local/uploads/files/GINA_Pocket_2014_Jun11.pdf

			Adults and children over 5 y	• Reducing exposure to asthma "triggers" can reduce asthma exacerbations and improve asthma control.
				  ○ Mattress encasing for mite control
				  ○ Eliminate suitable environments for cockroaches
				  ○ Eliminate passive smoke exposure
				  ○ Reduce aggravating occupational exposures
						http://www.ginasthma.org/local/uploads/files/GINA_Pocket2013_May 15.pdf

Back Pain, Low	AAFP USPSTF	2004	Adults	• Insufficient evidence for or against the use of interventions to prevent low back pain in adults in primary care settings.	• Insufficient evidence to support back strengthening exercises, mechanical supports, or increased physical activity to prevent low back pain.	http://www.guidelines.gov/content.aspx?id=38619http://www.uspreventiveservicestaskforce.org/3rduspstf/lowback/lowbackrs.htm

PRIMARY PREVENTION OF CANCER (CA): NCI EVIDENCE SUMMARY 2015

CA Type[a,b]	Minimize Risk Factor Exposure	Strength of Evidence That Modifying or Avoiding Risk Factor Will Reduce CA	Therapeutic	Strength of Evidence
Breast[a,b]	Hormone replacement therapy —Approximately 26% increased incidence of invasive breast cancer (CA) with combination hormone replacement therapy (HRT) (estrogen and progesterone) —Estrogen alone with mixed evidence—unlikely to increase risk significantly (decreases risk in African Americans)	Solid	TAMOXIFEN (postmenopausal and high-risk premenopausal women) —Treatment with tamoxifen for 5 y reduced breast CA risk by 40%–50% USPSTF reemphasizes discussion with women at increased risk of breast cancer to strongly consider chemoprevention with selective estrogen receptor modulators (SERMs) and aromatase inhibitors (AIs) (*Ann Intern Med.* 2013;159:698-718) —Meta-analysis shows RR = 2.4 (95% confidence interval [CI], 1.5–4.0) for endometrial CA and 1.9 (95% CI, 1.4–2.6) for venous thromboembolic events	Solid
	Ionizing radiation to chest and mediastinum —Increased risk occurs approximately 10 y after exposure. Risk depends on dose and age at exposure (woman with radiation from age 15 to 30 at highest risk)	Solid	RALOXIFENE (postmenopausal women) —Similar effect as tamoxifen in reduction of invasive breast CA but does not reduce the incidence of noninvasive tumors—studied only in postmenopausal women —Similar risks as tamoxifen for venous thrombosis, but no risk of endometrial CA or cataracts (*Lancet.* 2013;381:1827)	Solid
	Obesity —In Women's Health Initiative (WHI), relative risk (RR) = 2.85 for breast CA for women >82.2 kg compared with women <58.7 kg	Solid	AROMATASE INHIBITORS —Anastrozole reduces the incidence of new primary breast CAs by 50% compared with tamoxifen; similar results have been reported with letrozole and exemestane treatment (*Lancet.* 2014; 383:1041) 100 needed to treat to prevent 1 breast cancer —There is a 65% reduction in the risk of breast CA occurrence in postmenopausal women treated with exemestane for 5 y (*N Engl J Med.* 2011; 364:2381)	Fair
	Alcohol —RR for intake of 4 alcoholic drinks/d is 1.32 —RR increases approximately 7% for each drink per day	Solid	—Harmful effects of aromatase inhibitors include decreased bone mineral density and increased risk of fracture, hot flashes, increased falls, decreased cognitive function, fibromyalgia, and carpal tunnel syndrome —Fracture rate for women being treated with anastrozole was 5.9% compared with 3.7% for those being treated with tamoxifen	Fair
	Factors of unproven or disproven association —Abortions —Environmental factors —Diet and vitamins *epidemiologic studies suggest vitamin D may decrease risk of breast CA—more studies needed. (*N Engl J Med.* 2011;364:1385) (*Medicine.* 2013;92:123) —Active and passive cigarette smoking —Use of statin drugs —Use of low-dose daily aspirin *Population based studies have shown reduction in breast CA risk but more data needed. (*J Clin Oncol.* 2010;25:1467. *Lancet Oncol.* 2012;13:518) —Use of biphosphonates		PROPHYLACTIC BILATERAL MASTECTOMY (high-risk women) —Reduces risk as much as 90% —Approximately 6% of women were dissatisfied with their decision; regrets about mastectomy were less among women who opted not to have reconstruction PROPHYLACTIC SALPINGO-OOPHORECTOMY among *BRCA*-positive women —Breast CA incidence decreased as much as 50% —Nearly all women experience some sleep disturbances, mood changes, hot flashes, and bone demineralization, but the severity of these symptoms varies greatly EXERCISE —Exercising >4 h/wk results in average risk reduction of 30%–40% The effect may be greatest for premenopausal women of normal or low body weight BREAST-FEEDING —The RR of breast CA is decreased 4.3% for every 12 mo of breast-feeding, in addition to 7% for each birth PREGNANCY before age 20 y —Approximately 50% decrease in breast CA compared with nulliparous women or those who give birth after age 35 y DENSE BREASTS —Women have increased risk of Breast CA proportionate to breast density. Relative risk 1.79 for 50% density and 4.64 for women with > 75% breast density. (*Cancer Epidemiol Biomarkers Prev.* 2006;15:1159) No known method to reduce breast density	

PRIMARY PREVENTION OF CANCER (CA): NCI EVIDENCE SUMMARY 2015 (CONTINUED)

CA Type	Minimize Risk Factor Exposure	Strength of Evidence That Modifying or Avoiding Risk Factor Will Reduce CA	Therapeutic	Strength of Evidence
Cervical	Human papillomavirus (HPV) infection[c]		HPV-16/HPV-18 vaccination[d]	Solid
	—Abstinence from sexual activity; condom and/or spermicide use (RR, 0.4)	Solid	—Reduces incident and persistent infections with efficacy of 91.6% (95% CI, 64.5–98.0) and 100% (95% CI, 45–100), respectively; duration of efficacy is not yet known; impact on long-term cervical CA rates also unknown but likely to be significant (*Lancet.* 2009; 374:1975)	Solid
	Cigarette smoke (active or passive)			
	—HPV vaccination ideally at age 9–13—also given to females age 13–26 if no previous vaccination	Solid	—Also will likely decrease risk of other HPV-driven malignancies	Fair
	—Increases risk of high-grade cervical intraepithelial neoplasia (CIN) or invasive CA 2- to 3-fold among HPV-infected women		Screening with PAP smears	
	High parity		—Estimates from population studies suggest that screening may decrease CA incidence and mortality by <80%. Adding screening for HPV after age 30 y increases sensitivity and reduces frequency of screening to every 5 y if both are negative	Solid
	—HPV-infected women with seven or more full-term pregnancies have a 4-fold increased risk of squamous cell CA of the cervix compared with nulliparous women	Solid	HPV screening only without a PAP smear is being studied in developing countries	
	Long-term use of oral contraceptives (>5 y)			
	—Increases risk by 3-fold	Solid		
	—Longer use related to higher risk			
Colorectal[b,c]	Excessive alcohol use, RR is 1.41 for >45 g/d (>4.5 drinks/d)	Solid	ASPIRIN AND NSAID USE	Solid
	Cigarette smoking—RR for current smokers vs never smokers, 1.18	Solid	—Based on solid evidence, nonsteroidal antinflammatory drugs (NSAIDs) reduce the risk of adenomas, but how much this reduces the risk of CRC is uncertain. Harms include upper gastrointestinal (UGI) bleeding (4–5/1000 people/y), chronic kidney disease (CKD), and cardiovascular (CV) events[f]	
	Obesity—RR for woman with a body mass index (BMI) >29 is 1.45. Similar increase seen in colorectal CA (CRC) mortality	Solid	—Based on solid evidence, daily aspirin use for at least 5 y reduces CRC incidence and mortality (37%), with an absolute risk reduction from 3.1% to 1.9%. Harm of low-dose aspirin use includes approximately 10–30 extra cases of UGI complications per 1000 users over a 1-y period. Risk increases with age. Benefit shown in other GI cancers as well (*Lancet.* 2011;377:31) (*JAMA.* 2015;313:1133)	
	Regular physical activity—a meta-analysis of 52 studies showed a 24% reduction in incidence of CRC	Solid	POSTMENOPAUSAL COMBINATION HORMONE REPLACEMENT (not estrogen alone)	Solid
	B6 (Pyridoxal 5′-phosphate) levels are inversely associated with risk of colon CA. B6 found in cereals, meat, fish, vegetables, bananas, and avocado. (*JAMA.* 2010;303:1077)		—Based on solid evidence (WHI), 44% reduction in CRC incidence among HRT users	
			—Based on solid evidence (WHI), combination HRT users have a 26% increased invasive breast CA risk, a 29% increase in coronary heart disease (CHD) events, and a 41% increase in stroke rates. These risks obviate use of HRT for CRC prevention. Estrogen-only HRT does not impact on the incidence of or survival of CRC	
			POLYP REMOVAL	
			—Based on fair evidence, removal of adenomatous polyps reduces the risk of CRC, especially polyps >1 cm (*Ann Intern Med.* 2011;154:22) (*Gastrointest Endosc.* 2014;80:471.)	
			—Based on fair evidence, complications of polyp removal include perforation of the colon and bleeding estimated at 7–9 events per 1000 procedures	
			Low-fat, high-fiber diet does not reduce the risk of CRC to a significant degree	

PRIMARY PREVENTION OF CANCER (CA): NCI EVIDENCE SUMMARY 2015 (CONTINUED)

CA Type	Minimize Risk Factor Exposure	Strength of Evidence That Modifying or Avoiding Risk Factor Will Reduce CA	Therapeutic	Strength of Evidence
Colorectal[b,c] (continued)			Increased consumption of fruits and vegetables and reduction in red meat intake may decrease risk of colorectal CA. (*JAMA.* 2005;293:172) INTERVENTIONS WITHOUT BENEFIT Statins do not reduce the incidence or mortality of CRC Data are inadequate to show a reduction in the risk of CRC from calcium or vitamin D supplementation. Fair data that calcium intake >1000 mg/day will increase risk of myocardial infarction (MI). (*BMJ.* 2010;341:3691)	
Endometrial	Unopposed estrogen —Use in postmenopausal women (>5 y of use = 10-fold higher risk) —Obesity—risk increases 1.59-fold for each 5 kg/m² change in body mass —Lack of exercise—regular exercise (2 h/wk) with 38%–48% decrease in risk —Tamoxifen—used for >2 y has a 2.3- to 7.5-fold increased risk of endometrial CA (usually stage I— 95% cure rate with surgery). Nulliparous women have a 35% increased risk of endometrial CA	Solid Solid Solid Solid	Insufficient evidence to assess benefits and harms of regular use of multivitamins to prevent cancer (*Ann Intern Med.* 2013;159:824 Oral contraception (estrogen and progesterone containing) —Use of oral contraceptions for 4 y reduces the risk of endometrial CA by 56%; 8 y, by 67%; and 12 y, by 72% but will increase risk of breast cancer by 26% and pulmonary embolus by 113% INCREASING PARITY AND LACTATION —35% reduction vs nulliparous women-increasing length of breastfeeding with decreasing risk WEIGHT LOSS —Insufficient evidence to conclude weight loss is associated with a decreased incidence of endometrial cancer	Fair Fair Inadequate Solid
Esophagus	Avoidance of tobacco abuse and alcohol would decrease risk of squamous cell CA The combination use of alcohol and smoking is associated with a 3- to 7-fold increased risk of esophageal cancer (account for 90% squamous cell esophageal CA). Diet high in cruciferous vegetables will decrease risk of esophageal CA ASA or NSAID use decreases the risk of developing or dying from esophageal CA by 43% (*Gastroenterology.* 2003;124:47–56)	Solid Fair	Randomized controlled trial has shown that radiofrequency ablation of Barrett's esophagus (BE) with moderate or severe dysplasia may lead to eradication of dysplasia and reduced risk of progression to malignancy (*NEJM.* 2009;360:2277–2288) Longstanding GERD associated with BE Uncertain if elimination of GERD by surgical or medical therapy will reduce the risk of esophageal adenocarcinoma No trials in the United States have shown any benefit from the use of chemoprevention with the use of vitamins and minerals.	Fair Uncertain
Gastric	*Helicobacter pylori* eradication with decreased risk of gastric cancer from 1.7% to 1.1% Excessive salt intake Deficient consumption of fruits/vegetables Avoid salted, smoked, or poorly preserved foods Smoking cessation – relative risk = 1.6 (*Tumor.* 2009;95:13)	Solid Fair Fair	Anti-*H. pylori* therapy may reduce risk but effect on mortality unclear. Dietary interventions—eating more fruits, vegetables and less processed foods reduces risk of gastric cancer by 10%–15%. Smoking cessation will reduce risk by 20%–30%. Patients with hereditary susceptibility (HNPCC, e-cadherin mutation, Li Fraumeni syndrome), pernicious anemia, atrophic gastritis, or gastric polyps should be followed carefully for dysplasia or early cancer.	Inadequate Inadequate

PRIMARY PREVENTION OF CANCER (CA): NCI EVIDENCE SUMMARY 2015 (CONTINUED)

CA Type	Minimize Risk Factor Exposure	Strength of Evidence That Modifying or Avoiding Risk Factor Will Reduce CA	Therapeutic	Strength of Evidence
Liver	Avoidance of cirrhosis (hepatitis B and C, excessive alcohol use, hepatic steatosis in diabetes mellitus, hemochromatosis)	Fair	Hepatitis B virus (HBV) vaccination (newborns of mothers infected with HBV) —HBV vaccination of newborns of Taiwanese mothers reduced the incidence of hepatocellular carcinoma (HCC) from 0.7 to 0.36 per 100,000 children after about 10 y —New effective anti-viral therapy for hepatitis C will likely decrease the risk for HCC in near future (N Engl J Med. 2013;368:1907).	Solid
Lung	Cigarette smoking (20-fold increased risk) and second-hand exposure to tobacco smoke (20% increased risk) both medication and counseling better than either alone in increasing cessation rates.	Solid	No evidence that vitamin E/tocopherol, retinoids, vitamin C, or beta-carotene in any dose reduces the risk of lung CA (Ann Inter Med. 2013; 159:824.)	
	Beta-carotene, pharmacologic doses, actually increases the risk of lung CA, especially in high-intensity smokers	Solid	Minimize indoor exposure to radon, especially if smoker. Avoid occupational exposures (asbestos, arsenic, nickel, chromium)	
	Radon gas exposure, severe air pollution (Am J Respir Crit Care Med. 2006;173:667.)	Solid	Stopping tobacco use will lower risk of lung and other cancers but at 15 y there is still a 2 to 3 times increased risk of lung cancer.	
	Avoid occupational exposures (asbestos, arsenic, nickel, and chromium) Air pollution—40% increased risk of lung CA with highest pollution exposure			
Oral	Tobacco cessation (in any form, including smokeless) Alcohol and dietary factors—double the risk for people who drink 3–4 drinks/d vs nondrinkers	Solid	Oropharyngeal squamous cell CAs (tonsil and base of tongue) are related to HPV infection (types 16 and 18) in 70% of patients—related to sexual practices, number of partners, and may be prevented by HPV vaccine. HPV (+), non-smokers with improved cure rate by 25%–30%. (N Engl J Med. 2010;363:82. N Engl J Med. 2010;363:24) Inadequate evidence to suggest change in diet will reduce risk of oral cancer	
	Oral HPV infection—found in 6.9% of general population and found in 70%–75% of patients with oropharyngeal squamous cell cancer Lip cancer—avoid chronic sun exposure	Inadequate		
Ovarian	POSTMENOPAUSAL USE OF HRT (estrogen replacement only) with a 3.2-fold increased risk after >20 y of use	Fair	ORAL CONTRACEPTIVES —5%–10% reduction in ovarian CA per year of use, up to 80% maximum risk reduction. —Increased risk of deep venous thrombosis (DVT) with oral contraceptive pill (OCP) use of about 3 events per 10,000 women per year; increased breast CA risk among long-term OCP users of about 1 extra case per 100,000 women per year	Solid
	OBESITY —Elevated BMI including during adolescence associated with increased mortality from ovarian CA (J Natl Cancer Inst. 2003;95:1244) TALC EXPOSURE and use of fertility drugs with inadequate data to show increased risk of ovarian CA If a woman is newly diagnosed with ovarian cancer she should be tested for BRCA 1 or 2 at any age—if positive, family members should be tested for that specific gene mutation.	Fair	PROPHYLACTIC SALPINGO-OOPHORECTOMY—in high-risk women (eg, BRCA1 or BRCA2) —Ninety percent reduction in ovarian CA risk and 50% reduction in breast cancer with bilateral salpingo-oophorectomy —When prior to menopause, approximately 50% of women experience vasomotor symptoms; 4.5-fold increased RR of heart disease especially in women <40 y old.	Solid

PRIMARY PREVENTION OF CANCER (CA): NCI EVIDENCE SUMMARY 2015 (CONTINUED)

CA Type	Minimize Risk Factor Exposure	Strength of Evidence That Modifying or Avoiding Risk Factor Will Reduce CA	Therapeutic	Strength of Evidence
Prostate	Family history of prostate CA in men age <60 y defines risk. One first-degree relative with prostate CA increases the risk 3-fold, 2 first-degree relatives increase the risk 5-fold—incidence of prostate CA in African Americans increased by 2-fold, occurs at a younger age and is more virulent with increased death rate. —High dietary fat intake does not increase risk for prostate CA but is associated with aggressive cancers and shorter survivals	Cannot be modified	Finasteride —Decreased 7-y prostate CA incidence from 25% (placebo) to 18% (finasteride), but no change in mortality. —Trial participants report reduced ejaculate volume (47% → 60%); increased erectile dysfunction (62% → 67%); increased loss of libido (60% → 65%); increased gynecomastia (3% → 4.5%) Dutasteride —Absolute risk reduction of 22.8% —No difference in prostate CA-specific or overall mortality. Increase in more aggressive CA (Gleason 7–10) in dutasteride group (*N Engl Med.* 2013;369:603.) Vitamin E/alfa-tocopherol—inadequate data—one study showed a 17% increase in prostate CA with vitamin E alone (*JAMA.* 2011:306:1549) Selenium—no study shows benefit in reducing risk of prostate CA Lycopene—largest trials to date show no benefit (*Am J Epidemiol.* 2010;172:566)	Solid
Skin	Avoid sunburns and tanning booths[g]	Fair	Sunscreen, protective clothing, limited time in the sun, avoid blistering sunburn in adolescence and young adults (squamous cell, basal cell carcinoma of the skin and malignant melanoma)	Inadequate

[a]National Surgical Adjuvant Breast and Bowel Project (NS ABP) Study of Tamoxifen and Raloxifene (STAR) trial: raloxifene is as effective as tamoxifen in reducing the risk of invasive breast CA among postmenopausal women with at least a 5-y predicted breast CA risk of 1.66% based on the Gail model (http://bcra.nci.nih.gov/brc). Raloxifene does not reduce the risk of noninvasive CA and is not associated with endometrial CA.

[b]Women's Health Initiative (WHI): alternate-day use of low-dose aspirin (100 mg) for an average of 10 y of treatment does not lower the risk of total, breast, colorectal, or other site-specific CAs. There was a trend toward reduction in risk for lung CA (*JAMA.* 2005;294:47–55).

[c]Methods to minimize risk of HPV infection include abstinence from sexual activity and the use of barrier contraceptives and/or spermicidal gel during sexual intercourse.

[d]On June 8, 2006, the U.S. Food and Drug Administration (FDA) announced approval of Gardasil, the first vaccine developed to prevent cervical CA, precancerous genital lesions, and genital warts caused by HPV types 6,11,16, and 18. The vaccine is approved for use in females age 9–26 y (http://www.fda.gov). A bivalent vaccine, Cervarix, is also FDA approved with activity against HPV subtypes 16 and 18 (*N Engl J Med.* 2006;354:1109-1112).

[e]Cereal fiber supplementation and diets low in fat and high in fiber, fruits, and vegetables do no reduce the rate of adenoma recurrence over a 3-to 4-y period.

[f]There is solid evidence that NSAIDs reduce the risk of adenomas, but the extent to which this translates into a reduction in CRC is uncertain.

[g]Twenty-eight million Americans/year use indoor tanning salons—increased risk of squamous cell and basal cell cancers greater than melanoma.

Source: http://www.cancer.gov/cancertopics/pdq/prevention.

CATHETER-RELATED BLOODSTREAM INFECTIONS

Disease Prevention	Organization	Date	Population	Recommendations	Comments	Source
Catheter-Related Bloodstream Infections	IDSA	2011	Adults and children requiring intravascular catheters	1. Educate staff regarding proper procedures for insertion and maintenance of intravascular catheters. 2. The arm is preferred over the leg for catheter insertion. 3. Use a central venous catheter (CVC) when the duration of IV therapy is likely to exceed 6 d. 4. Avoid the femoral vein for central venous access in adult patients. 5. Subclavian vein is preferred over femoral or internal jugular vein to minimize infection risk for nontunneled CVC. 6. Use ultrasound guidance to place CVCs to minimize mechanical complications. 7. Promptly remove a CVC that is no longer essential. 8. Wash hands before and after catheter insertion, replacement, accessing, or dressing an intravascular catheter. 9. Use maximal sterile barrier precau→tions including a cap, mask, sterile gown, sterile gloves, and a sterile full-body drape for the insertion of CVCs. 10. Chlorhexidine skin antisepsis preferred over povidone-iodine. 11. Avoid antibiotic ointments on insertion sites.	Clean gloves should be worn when changing the catheter dressings.	http://www.cdc.gov/hicpac/BSI/01-BSI-guidelines-2011.html

	COLITIS, *CLOSTRIDIUM DIFFICILE*				
Disease Prevention	Organization	Date	Population	Recommendations	Comments	Source
Colitis, *Clostridium difficile*	Cochrane Database of systematic reviews	2013	Adults and children taking antibiotics	• Recommend probiotics for prevention of *C. difficile-associated* diarrhea (CDAD) after a course of antibiotics.	• Probiotics lower the incidence of CDAD by about 65% after a course of antibiotics.	http://onlinelibrary.wiley.com/doi/10.1002/14651858.CD006095.pub3/abstract
	ACG	2013	Adults and children	• Hospital-based infection control programs can decrease the spread of CDI. • Recommend antibiotic stewardship programs. • Contact precautions should be maintained until the patient no longer has diarrhea. • Patients with CDI should be treated in a private room. • Hand hygiene and barrier precautions, including gloves and gowns, should be used by all health care workers and visitors entering the room of any patient with known or suspected CDI. • Single-use disposable equipment should be used for prevention of CDI transmission. Nondisposable medical equipment should be dedicated to the patient's room and other equipment should be thoroughly cleaned after use in a patient with CDI. • Disinfection of environmental surfaces is recommended using an Environmental Protective Agency (EPA)–registered disinfectant with *C. difficile* sporicidal label claim or 5000 p.p.m. Chlorine-containing cleaning agents in areas of potential contamination by *C. difficile.* • Although there is moderate evidence that two probiotics (*Lactobacillus rhamnosus* GG and *Saccharomyces boulardii*) decrease the incidence of antibiotic associated diarrhea, there is insufficient evidence that probiotics prevent *C. difficile* infection.		http://www.guideline.gov/content.aspx?id=45139

CONCUSSION

Disease Prevention	Organization	Date	Population	Recommendations	Comments	Source
Concussion	AAN	2013	Children and young adults	• School-based professionals should be educated by licensed healthcare professionals to understand the risks of a concussion. • Licensed health care professionals should educate athletes about concussion risks. • Athletes with a concussion should be prohibited from returning to play or practice in contact sports until a licensed healthcare provider has cleared them to return. • Licensed healthcare providers should recommend retirement for any athlete with repeated concussions who has chronic, persistent neurologic or cognitive deficits.		http://www.guideline.gov/content.aspx?id=43947

DENTAL CARIES					

Disease Prevention	Organization	Date	Population	Recommendations	Comments	Source
Dental Caries	AAFP	2010	Children and adolescents	Recommends fluoride supplementation to prevent dental caries for infants and children age 6 mo through 15 y residing in areas with inadequate fluoride in the water supply (<0.6 ppm).		http://www.guideline.gov/ content.aspx?id=38619
	USPSTF	2014	Infants and children up to age 5 y	1. Recommends application of fluoride varnish to the primary teeth of all infants and children starting at the age of primary teeth eruption. 2. Recommends oral fluoride supplementation starting at age 6 mo for children whose water supply is fluoride deficient.		http://www.uspreventive- servicestaskforce.org/ Page/Document/ UpdateSummaryFinal/ dental-caries-in- children-from-birth- through-age-5-years- screening

DIABETES MELLITUS (DM), TYPE 2

Disease Prevention	Organization	Date	Population	Recommendations	Comments	Source

Diabetes Mellitus (DM), Type 2	ADA	2013	Persons with impaired glucose tolerance (IGT)[a]	1. Recommend initiation of an effective ongoing program targeting weight loss. Program should emphasize moderate activity most days of the week.
				2. Consider initiation of metformin for patients at highest risk for developing diabetes (eg, HgbA1c 5.7%–6.4%, BMI 35 kg/m^2 or greater, those age 60 y or younger, and those with prior gestational diabetes mellitus [GDM]).
					1. Goal of program is weight loss of at least 7% of body weight and to encourage at least 30 min of moderate activity a minimum of 5 d/wk.
					2. Program should include follow-up counseling. Recommend annual screening for the development of type 2 DM.
					3. Recommendations for disease prevention:
					  a. Annual influenza vaccine
					  b. Pneumococcal polysaccharide vaccine if 2 y or older with one-time revaccination when over 64 y
					  c. Hepatitis B vaccine series if unvaccinated and 19–59 y of age
					  d. Aspirin 81 mg daily for primary prevention if 10-y risk of significant CAD is at least 10% (by Framingham Risk Score); includes most men over 50 y and most women over 60 y
						http://care.diabetesjournals.org/content/36/Supplement_1/S11.full

[a]IGT if fasting glucose 110–125 mg/dL, 2-h glucose after 75-g anhydrous glucose load 140–199 mg/dL, or HgbA1c 5.7%–6.4%.

DOMESTIC VIOLENCE

Disease Prevention	Organization	Date	Population	Recommendations	Comments	Source
Domestic Violence	WHO	2010	Adolescents and adult women	Recommend school-based programs that emphasize preventing dating violence.	Interventions of possible, but not proven, efficacy include: 1. School-based programs that teach children to recognize and avoid sexually abusive situations 2. Empowerment and relationship skills training for women 3. Programs that change social and cultural gender norms	http://www.who.int/violence_injury_prevention/publications/violence/9789241564007_eng.pdf

Disease Prevention	Organization	Date	Population	Recommendations	Comments	Source
DRIVING RISK						
Driving Risk	AAN	2010	Adults with dementia	Assess patients with dementia for the following characteristics that place them at increased risk for unsafe driving: 1. Caregiver's assessment that the patient's driving ability is marginal or unsafe 2. History of traffic citations 3. History of motor vehicle collisions 4. Reduced driving mileage 5. Self-reported situational avoidance 6. Mini-Mental Status Exam score <24 7. Aggressive or impulsive personality		http://www.guidelines.gov/content .aspx?id=15853

ENDOCARDITIS

Disease Prevention	Organization	Date	Population	Recommendations	Comments	Source
Endocarditis	AHA ESC	2007 2009	Endocarditis is more likely a result of random exposure to bacteremia rather than associated with procedures. Certain persons are at highest risk for adverse sequelae from endocarditis.[a]	1. Give antibiotic prophylaxis[b] before certain dental[c] procedures, as well as before certain other procedures, only to those patients at highest risk.[d] 2. Antibiotic prophylaxis is no longer indicated for native valvular heart disease unless previous endocarditis is present.	1. Emphasis is on providing prophylaxis to patients at greatest risk of endocarditis. 2. General consensus suggests few cases of infective endocarditis can be prevented by preprocedure prophylaxis with antibiotics.	*Circulation.* 2007;116:1736 *Eur Heart J.* 2009;30:2369-2413 *Circulation.* 2008;52:676-685

[a]Patients with prosthetic valves; previous endocarditis; selected patients with congenital heart disease (unrepaired cyanotic congenital heart disease; completely repaired cyanotic congenital heart defect with prosthetic material or device during first 6 mo after procedure; repaired cyanotic CHD with residual defects at or near-repair site); and cardiac transplant recipients who develop valvulopathy.

[b]Standard prophylaxis regimen: amoxicillin (adults 2.0 g; children 50 mg/kg orally 1 h before procedure). If unable to take oral medications, give ampicillin (adults 2.0 g IM or IV; children 50 mg/kg IM or IV within 30 min of procedure). If penicillin-allergic, give clindamycin (adults 600 mg; children 20 mg/kg orally 1 h before procedure) or azithromycin or clarithromycin (adults 500 mg; children 15 mg/kg orally 1 h before procedure). If penicillin-allergic and unable to take oral medications, give clindamycin (adults 600 mg; children 20 mg/kg IV within 30 min before procedure). If allergy to penicillin is not anaphylaxis, angioedema, or urticaria, options for nonoral treatment also include cefazolin (1 g IM or IV for adults, 50 mg/kg IM or IV for children); and for penicillin-allergic, oral therapy includes cephalexin 2 g PO for adults or 50 mg/kg PO for children (IM, intramuscular; IV, intravenous; PO, by mouth, orally).

[c]All dental procedures that involve manipulation of gingival tissue or the periapical region of teeth or perforation of oral mucosa only in high-risk patients.

[d]Antibiotic prophylaxis is recommended for procedures in the respiratory tract or infected skin, skin structures, or musculoskeletal tissue in high-risk patients. Antibiotic prophylaxis for genitourinary (GU) or gastrointestinal (GI) procedures is indicated with ongoing infection.

FALLS IN THE ELDERLY

Disease Prevention	Organization	Date	Population	Recommendations	Comments	Source
Falls in the Elderly	USPSTF Cochrane Database of Systematic Reviews	2012	Older adults	1. Recommends vitamin D supplementation (800 international units [IU] orally daily). 2. Recommends home-hazard modification (eg, adding nonslip tape to rugs and steps, provision of grab bars, etc.) for all homes of persons age >65 y. 3. Recommends exercise or physical therapy interventions targeting gait and balance training. 4. Insufficient evidence to recommend a multifactorial assessment and management approach for all elderly persons (65 y and older). 5. Recommends vitamin D supplementation to elderly patients in care facilities. This reduces the rate of falls by 37%.	1. 30%–40% of all community-dwelling persons age >65 y fall at least once a year. 2. Falls are the leading cause of fatal and nonfatal injuries among persons age >65 y. 3. A review and modification of chronic medications, including psychotropic medications, is important although not proven to reduce falls.	http://www.uspreventiveservice staskforce.org/uspstf/uspsfalls. htm http://onlinelibrary.wiley.com/doi/10.1002/14651858. CD005465.pub3/abstract

FRACTURES

Disease Prevention	Organization	Date	Population	Recommendations	Comments	Source
Fractures	USPSTF	2013	Noninstitutionalized postmenopausal women	• Recommends against daily supplementation with ≤400 IU Vitamin D and ≤1000 mg calcium for primary prevention of fractures.	Insufficient evidence for vitamin D and calcium supplementation in anyone for the primary prevention of fractures.	http://www.guideline.gov/content.aspx?id=43793

GONORRHEA, OPHTHALMIA NEONATORUM

Disease Prevention	Organization	Date	Population	Recommendations	Comments	Source
Gonorrhea, Ophthalmia Neonatorum	AAFP USPSTF	2010 2005	Newborns	Recommend prophylactic ocular topical medication against gonococcal ophthalmia neonatorum for all newborns.		http://www.guideline.gov/content.aspx?id=38619 http://www.uspreventiveservices taskforce.org/uspstf/uspsgono.htm

Gout	American College of Rheumatology (ACR)	2012	Adults	• Recommend a urate-lowering diet and lifestyle measures for patients with gout to prevent exacerbations.
				• Urate-lowering medications are indicated for gout with Stage 2–5 CKD or recurrent gout attacks and hyperuricemia (uric acid >6 mg/dL.)
				   ○ Allopurinol
				   ○ Febuxostat
				   ○ Probenecid
				   ○ Goal uric acid level <6 mg/dL
					• Minimize or avoid alcohol and purine-rich meat and seafood.
					• Limit consumption of high-fructose corn syrup-sweetened soft drinks and energy drinks.
					• Increase low-fat dairy products and vegetable intake.
						http://www.guidelines.gov/content.aspx?id=38624

	American College of Rheumatology (ACR)	2012	Adults	• Anti-inflammatory prophylaxis of acute gout attacks indicated for the greater of 6 or 3 mo after uric acid level <6 mg/dL
				   ○ Colchicine 0.6 mg daily-bid
				   ○ Less preferable option is naproxen 250 mg bid
					• Low-dose prednisone is an alternative if neither colchicine nor NSAIDS may be used.	http://www.guidelines.gov/content.aspx?id=38625

GROUP B STREPTOCOCCAL INFECTION

Disease Prevention	Organization	Date	Population	Recommendations	Comments	Source
Group B Streptococcal (GBS) Infection	CDC	2010	Pregnant women	1. Intrapartum antibiotic prophylaxis (IAP) to prevent early onset invasive GBS disease in newborns is indicated for high-risk pregnancies.[a] 2. IAP is **not** indicated for GBS colonization or GBS bacteriuria **during a previous pregnancy,** negative vaginal-rectal GBS culture, or if a cesarean delivery is performed with intact membranes and before the onset of labor (regardless of GBS screening culture status).	1. Penicillin G is the agent of choice for IAP. 2. Ampicillin is an acceptable alternative to penicillin G. 3. Cefazolin may be used if the patient has a penicillin allergy that does not cause anaphylaxis, angioedema, urticaria, or respiratory distress. 4. Clindamycin or erythromycin may be used if the patient has a penicillin allergy that causes anaphylaxis, angioedema, urticaria, or respiratory distress.	http://www.cdc.gov/mmwr/preview/mmwrhtml/rr5910a1.htm?s_cid=rr5910a1_w

[a]Indications for IAP: previous infant with invasive GBS disease; history of GBS bacteriuria during current pregnancy; positive GBS vaginal-rectal screening culture within 5 wk of delivery; unknown GBS status with any of the following: preterm labor at <37 gestational weeks, amniotic membrane rupture ≥18 h, intrapartum fever ≥100.4°F (≥38°C; intrapartum nucleic acid amplification test positive for GBS.

HORMONE REPLACEMENT THERAPY

Disease Prevention	Organization	Date	Population	Recommendations	Comments	Source
Hormone Replacement Therapy	AAFP USPSTF	2012	Postmenopausal women	• Recommends against the use of combined estrogen and progestin for the prevention of chronic conditions (eg, osteoporosis).		http://www.guidelines.gov/content.aspx?id=38619
	AAFP USPSTF	2012	Postmenopausal women who have had a hysterectomy	• Recommends against the use of estrogen for the prevention of chronic conditions (eg, osteoporosis).	• This recommendation does not apply to women under the age of 50 who have undergone a surgical menopause and require estrogen for hot flashes and vasomotor symptoms.	http://www.uspreventiveservicestaskforce.org/uspstf12/menohrt/menohrtfinalrs.htm
Human Immunodeficiency Virus (HIV), Opportunistic Infections	CDC	2009	HIV-infected adults and adolescents	See table below (from the clinical practice guidelines at http://www.cdc.gov/mmwr/preview/mmwrhtml/rr5804a1.htm).		http://www.cdc.gov/mmwr/preview/mmwrhtml/rr5804a1.htm
	CDC	2009	HIV-infected children	See table below (from the clinical practice guidelines at http://www.cdc.gov/mmwr/preview/mmwrhtml/rr5811a1.htm).		http://www.cdc.gov/mmwr/preview/mmwrhtml/rr5811a1.htm

PROPHYLAXIS TO PREVENT FIRST EPISODE OF OPPORTUNISTIC DISEASE AMONG HIV-INFECTED ADULTS

Pathogen	Indication	First Choice	Alternative
Pneumocystis carinii Pneumonia (PCP)	CD4+ count <200 cells/μL (AII) or oropharyngeal candidiasis (AII) CD4+ <14% or history of AIDS-defining illness (BII) CD4+ count >200 but <250 cells/μL if monitoring CD4+ count every 1–3 mo is not possible (BIII)	Trimethoprim-sulfamethoxazole (TMP-SMX), 1 DS PO daily (AII): or 1SS daily (AII)	• TMP-SMX 1DSPOTIW (BI); or • Dapsone 100 mg PO daily or 50 mg PO bid (BI); or • Dapsone 50 mg PO daily + pyrimethamine 50 PO weekly + leucovorin 25 mg PO weekly (BI); or • Aerosolized pentamidine 300 mg via Respirgard III nebulized every month (BI); or • Atovaquone 1500 mg PO daily (BI); or • Atovaquone 1500 mg + pyrimethamine 25 mg + leucovorin 10 mg PO daily (CIII)
Toxoplasma gondii encephalitis	*Toxoplasma* IgG-positive patients with CD4+ count <100 cells/μL (AII) Seronegative patients receiving PCP prophylaxis not active against toxoplasmosis should have toxoplasma serology retested if CD4+ count declines to <100 cells/μL (CIII) Prophylaxis should be initiated if seroconversion occurred (AII)	TMP-SMX 1 DS PO daily (AII)	• TMP-SMX 1DSOTIW (BIII); or • TMP-SMX 1 SS PO daily (BIII); • Dapsone 50 mg PO daily + pyrimethamine 50 mg PO weekly + leucovorin 25 mg PO weekly (BI); or • (Dapsone 200 mg + pyrimethamine 75 mg + leucovorin 25 mg) PO weekly (BIII); • (Atovaquone 1500 mg ± pyrimethamine 25 mg + leucovorin 10 mg) PO daily (CIII)
Mycobacterium tuberculosis infection (TB) (treatment of latent TB infection [LTBI])	(+) diagnostic test for LTBI, no evidence of active TB, and no prior history of treatment for active or latent TB (AII) (−) diagnostic test for LTBI and no evidence of active TB, but close contact with a person with infectious pulmonary TB (AII) A history of untreated or inadequately treated healed TB (ie, old fibrotic lesions) regardless of diagnostic tests for LTBI and no evidence of active TB (AII)	Isoniazid (INH) 300 mg PO daily (AII) or 900 mg PO biw (BII) for 9 mo—both plus pyridoxine 50 mg PO daily (BIII); or For persons exposed to drug-resistant TB, selection of drugs after consultation with public health authorities (AII)	• Rifampin (RIF) 600 mg PO daily × 4 mo (BIII); or • Rifabutin (RFB) (dose adjusted based on concomitant antiretroviral therapy [ART]) × 4 mo (BIII)
Disseminated *Mycobacterium avium* complex (MAC) disease	CD4+ count <50 cells/μL—after ruling out active MAC infection (AI)	Azithromycin 1200 mg PO once weekly (AI); or Clarithromycin 500 mg PO bid (AI); or Az thromycin 600 mg PO twice weekly (BIII)	• RFB 300 mg PO daily (BI) (dosage adjustment based on drug–drug interactions with ART); rule out active TB before starting RFB
Streptococcus pneumoniae infection	CD4+ count >200 cells/μL and no receipt of pneumococcal vaccine in the last 5 y (AII) CD4+ count <200 cells/μL—vaccination can be offered (CIII) In patients who received polysaccharide pneumococcal vaccination (PPV) when CD4+ count <200 cells/μL but has increased to >200 cells/μL in response to ART (CIII)	23-valent PPV 0.5 mL IM × 1 (BII) Revaccination every 5 y may be considered (CIII)	
Influenza A and B virus infection	All HIV-infected patients (AII)	Inactivated influenza vaccine 0.5 mL IM annually (AIII)	

PROPHYLAXIS TO PREVENT FIRST EPISODE OF OPPORTUNISTIC DISEASE AMONG HIV-INFECTED ADULTS (CONTINUED)

Pathogen	Indication	First Choice	Alternative
Histoplasma capsulatum infection	CD4+ count >150 cells/μL and at high risk because of occupational exposure or live in a community with a hyperendemic rate of histoplasmosis (>10 cases/100 patient-y) (CI)	Itraconazole 200 mg PO daily (CI)	
Coccidioidomycosis	Positive IgM or IgG serologic test in a patient from a disease-endemic area, and CD4+ count <250 cells/μL (CIII)	Fluconazole 400 mg PO daily (CIII); Itraconazole 200 mg PO bid (CIII)	
Varicella-zoster virus (VZV) infection	*Preexposure prevention:* Patient with CD4+ count >200 cells/μL, who have no history of varicella or herpes zoster, or who are seronegative for VZV (CIII). Note: Routine VZV serologic testing in HIV-infected adults is not recommended. *Postexposure-close contact with a person who has active varicella or herpes zoster:* For susceptible patients (those who have no history of vaccination or infection with either condition, or are known to be VZV seronegative [AIII])	*Preexposure prevention:* Primary varicella vaccination (Varivax), 2 doses (0.5 mL SQ) administered 3 mo apart (CIII). If vaccination results in disease because of vaccine virus, treatment with acyclovir is recommended (AIII). *Postexposure therapy:* Varicella-zoster immune globulin (VZIG) 125 IU per 10 kg (maximum of 625 IU) IM, administered within 96 h after exposure to a person with active varicella or herpes zoster (AIII). Note: As of June 2007, VZIG can be obtained only under a treatment IND (1-800-843-7477, FFF Enterprises)	• VZV-susceptible household contacts of susceptible HIV-infected persons should be vaccinated to prevent potential transmission of VZV to their HIV-infected contacts (BIII). *Alternative postexposure therapy:* • Postexposure varicella vaccine (Varivax) 0.5 mL SQ × 2 doses, 3 mo apart if CD4+ count >200 cells/μL (CIII); or • Preemptive acyclovir 800 mg PO 5×/d for 5 d (CIII) • These two alternatives have not been studied in the HIV population
Human papillomavirus (HPV) infection	Women age 15–26 y (CIII)	HPV quadrivalent vaccine 0.5 mL IM months 0, 2, and 6 (CIII)	
Hepatitis A virus (HAV) infection	HAV-susceptible patients with chronic liver disease, or who are injection-drug users, or men who have sex with men (AII). Certain specialists might delay vaccination until CD4+ count >200 cells/μL (CIII)	Hepatitis A vaccine 1 mL IM × 2 doses—at 0 and 6–12 mo (AII). IgG antibody response should be assessed 1 mo after vaccination; nonresponders should be revaccinated (BIII)	
Hepatitis B virus (HBV) infection	All HIV patients without evidence of prior exposure to HBV should be vaccinated with HBV vaccine, including patients with CD4+ count <200 cells/μL (AII). *Patients with isolated anti-HBc:* (BIII) (consider screening for HBV DNA before vaccination to rule out occult chronic HBV infection)	Hepatitis B vaccine IM (Engerix-B 20 μg/mL or Recombivax HB 10 μg/mL) at 0, 1, and 6 mo (AII). Anti-HBs should be obtained 1 mo after receipt of the vaccine series (BIII)	Some experts recommend vaccinating with 40-μg doses of either vaccine (CIII)

PROPHYLAXIS TO PREVENT FIRST EPISODE OF OPPORTUNISTIC DISEASE AMONG HIV-INFECTED ADULTS (CONTINUED)

Pathogen	Indication	First Choice	Alternative
	Vaccine nonresponders: Defined as anti-HBs <10 IU/mL 1 mo after a vaccination series. For patients with low CD4$^+$ count at the time of first vaccination series, certain specialists might delay revaccination until after a sustained increase in CD4$^+$ count with ART.	Revaccinate with a second vaccine series (BIII)	Some experts recommend revaccinating with 40 µg doses of either vaccine (CIII)
Malaria	Travel to disease-endemic area	Recommendations are the same for HIV-infected and noninfected patients. One of the following three drugs is usually recommended, depending on location: atovaquone/proguanil, doxycycline, or mefloquine. Refer to the following Web site for the most recent recommendations based on region and drug susceptibility. http://www.cdc.gov/malaria/ (AII)	

BID, twice daily; DS, double strength; IM, intramuscular; PO, by mouth; SS, single strength; SQ, subcutaneous; TIW, three times weekly.

PROPHYLAXIS TO PREVENT FIRST EPISODE OF OPPORTUNISTIC INFECTIONS AMONG HIV-EXPOSED AND HIV-INFECTED INFANTS AND CHILDREN, UNITED STATES[a,b]

Pathogen	Indication	Preventive Regimen	
		First Choice	**Alternative**
		STRONGLY RECOMMENDED AS STANDARD OF CARE	
Pneumocystis pneumoniae[c]	HIV-infected or HIV-indeterminate infants age 1–12 mo; HIV-infected children age 1–5 y with CD4 count of <500 cells/mm³ or CD4 percentage of <15%; HIV-infected children age 6–12 y with CD4 count of <200 cells/mm³ or CD4 percentage of <15%	• TMP-SMX 150/750 mg/m²body surface area per day (max: 320/1600 mg) orally divided into 2 doses daily and administered 3 times weekly on consecutive days (AI) • Acceptable alternative dosage schedules for the same dose (AI): single dose orally 3 times weekly on consecutive days; 2 divided doses orally daily; or 2 divided doses orally 3 times weekly on alternate days	• Dapsone: children age >1 mo, 2 mg/kg body weight (max 100 mg) orally daily; or 4 mg/kg body weight (max 200 mg) orally weekly (BI) • Atovaquone: children age 1–3 mo and >24 mo, 30 mg/kg body weight orally daily; children age 4–24 mo, 45 mg/kg body weight orally daily (BI) • Aerosolized pentamidine: children age >5 y, 300 mg every month by Respirgard II (Marquest, Englewood, CO) nebulizer (BI) • Doxycycline 100 mg orally daily for children >8 y (2.2 mg/kg/d)

Malaria	Travel to area in which malaria is endemic	• Recommendations are the same for HIV-infected and HIV-uninfected children. Refer to http://www.cdc. gov/malaria/ for the most recent recommendations based on region and drug susceptibility
		• Mefloquine 5 mg/kg body weight orally 1 time weekly (max 250 mg)
		• Atovaquone/proguanil (Malarone) 1 time daily
		  11–20 kg = 1 pediatric tablet (62.5 mg/25 mg)
		  21–30 kg = 2 pediatric tablets (125 mg/50 mg)
		  31–40 kg = 3 pediatric tablets (187.5 mg/75 mg)
		  >40 kg = 1 adult tablet (250 mg/100 mg)
			• Chloroquine base 5 mg/kg base orally up to 300 mg weekly for sensitive regions only (7.5 mg/kg chloroquine phosphate)

Mycobacterium tuberculosis Isoniazid-sensitive	Tuberculin skin test (TST) reaction >5 mm or prior positive TST result without treatment, regardless of current TST result TST result and previous treatment, close contact with any person who has Contagious TB. TB disease must be excluded before start of treatment	• Isoniazid 10–15 mg/kg body weight (max 300 mg) orally daily for 9 mo (AII); or 20–30 mg/kg body weight (max 900 mg) orally 2 times weekly for 9 mo (BII)	• Rifampin 10–20 mg/kg body weight (max 600 mg) orally daily for 4–6 mo (BIII)
Isoniazid-resistant	Same as previous pathogen; increased probability of exposure to isoniazid-resistant TB	• Rifampin 10–20 mg/kg body weight (max 600 mg) orally daily for 4–6 mo (BIII)	• Uncertain
Multidrug-resistant (isoniazid and rifampin)	Same as previous pathogen; increased probability of exposure to multidrug-resistant TB	• Choice of drugs requires consultation with public health authorities and depends on susceptibility of isolate from source patient	
Mycobacterium avium complex[d]	For children age >6 y with CD4 count of <50 cells/mm³; age 2–5 y with CD4 count of <75 cells/mm³; age 1–2 y with CD4 count of <500 cells/mm³; age <1 y with CD4 count of <750 cells/mm³	• Clarithromycin 7.5 mg/kg body weight (max 500 mg) orally 2 times daily (AII), or azithromycin 20 mg/kg body weight (max 1200 mg) orally weekly (AII)	• Azithromycin 5 mg/kg body weight (max 250 mg) orally daily (AII); children age >6 y, rifabutin 300 mg orally daily (BI)

PROPHYLAXIS TO PREVENT FIRST EPISODE OF OPPORTUNISTIC INFECTIONS AMONG HIV-EXPOSED AND HIV-INFECTED INFANTS AND CHILDREN, UNITED STATES[a,b] (CONTINUED)

Pathogen	Indication	Preventive Regimen	
		First Choice	**Alternative**
		STRONGLY RECOMMENDED AS STANDARD OF CARE	
Varicella-zoster virus[c]	Substantial exposure to varicella or shingles with no history of varicella or zoster or seronegative status for VZV by a sensitive, specific antibody assay or lack of evidence for age-appropriate vaccination	• VZIG 125 IU per 10 kg (max 625 IU) IM, administered within 96 h after exposure[e] (AIII)	• If VZIG is not available or >96 h have passed since exposure, some experts recommend prophylaxis with acyclovir 20 mg/kg body weight (max 800 mg) per dose orally 4 times a day for 5–7 d. Another alternative to VZIG is intravenous immune globulin (IVIG), 400 mg/kg, administered once. IVIG should be administered within 96 h after exposure (CIII)
Vaccine-preventable pathogens	Standard recommendations for HIV-exposed and HIV-infected children	Routine vaccinations	
Toxoplasma gondii[g]	Immunoglobulin G (IgG) antibody to *Toxoplasma* and severe immunosuppression: HIV-infected children age <6 y with CD4 <15%; HIV-infected children age >6 y with CD4 <100 cells/mm³ (BIII)	• TMP-SMX, 150/750 mg/m² body surface area daily orally in 2 divided doses (BIII) • Acceptable alternative dosage schedules for same dosage (AI): single dose orally 3 times weekly on consecutive days; 2 divided doses orally daily; or 2 divided doses orally 3 times weekly on alternate days	• Dapsone (children age >1 mo) 2 mg/kg body weight or 15 mg/m² body surface area (max 25 mg) orally daily; *plus* pyrimethamine 1 mg/kg body weight (max 25 mg) orally daily; *plus* leucovorin 5 mg orally every 3 d (BI) • Atovaquone (children age 1–3 mo and >24 mo, 30 mg/kg body weight orally daily; children age 4–24 mo, 45 mg/kg body weight orally daily) with or without pyrimethamine 1 mg/kg body weight or 15 mg/m² body surface area (max 25 mg) orally daily; *plus* leucovorin 5 mg orally every 3 d (CIII)
Invasive bacterial infections	Hypogammaglobulinemia (ie, IgG <400 mg/dL)	• IVIG (400 mg/kg body weight every 2–4 wk) (AI)	
Cytomegalovirus (CMV)	CMV antibody positivity and severe immunosuppression (CD4 <50 cells/mm³)	• Valganciclovir 900 mg orally 1 time daily with food for older children who can receive adult dosing (CIII)	

[a]Abbreviations: CMV, cytomegalovirus; FDA, Food and Drug Administration; HIV, human immunodeficiency virus; IgG, immunoglobulin G; IM, intramuscularly; IVIG, intravenous immune globulin; PCP, *Pneumocystis pneumoniae*; TB, tuberculosis; TMP-SMX, trimethoprim-sulfamethoxazole; TST, tuberculin skin test; VZV, varicella-zoster virus.

[b]Information in these guidelines might not represent FDA approval or FDA-approved labeling for products or indications. Specifically, the terms "safe" and "effective" might not be synonymous with the FDA-defined legal standards for product approval. Letters and roman numerals in parentheses after regimens indicate the strength of the recommendation and the quality of the evidence supporting it.

[c]Daily trimethoprim-sulfamethoxazole (TMP-SMX) reduces the frequency of certain bacterial infections. TMP-SMX, dapsone-pyrimethamine, and possibly atovaquone (with or without pyrimethamine) protect against toxoplasmosis; however, data have not been prospectively collected. Compared with weekly dapsone, daily dapsone is associated with lower incidence of PCP but higher hematologic toxicity and mortality. Patients receiving therapy for toxoplasmosis with sulfadiazine-pyrimethamine are protected against PCP and do not need TMP-SMX.

[d]Substantial drug interactions can occur between rifamycins (ie, rifampin and rifabutin) and protease inhibitors and nonnucleoside reverse transcriptase inhibitors. A specialist should be consulted.

[e]Children routinely being administered IVIG should receive VZIG if the last dose of IVIG was administered >21 d before exposure.

[f]As of 2007, VZIG can be obtained only under a treatment Investigational New Drug protocol.

[g]Protection against toxoplasmosis is provided by the preferred *anti-Pneumocystis* regimens and possibly by atovaquone.

HYPERTENSION (HTN)

Disease Prevention	Organization	Date	Population	Recommendations	Comments	Source
Hypertension (HTN)	CHEP[c] JNC 8 ICSI 14th Edition ESC	2015 2014 2012 2013	Persons at risk for developing HTN[a]	Recommend weight loss, reduced sodium intake, moderate alcohol consumption, increased physical activity, potassium supplementation, and modification of eating patterns.[b]	1. A 5 mm Hg reduction in systolic blood pressure in the population would result in a 14% overall reduction in mortality from stroke, a 9% reduction in mortality from CHD, and a 7% decrease in all-cause mortality. 2. Weight loss of as little as 10 lb (4.5 kg) reduces blood pressure and/or prevents HTN in a large proportion of overweight patients.	https://www.hypertension.ca/en/chep *JAMA.*doi:10.1001/jama.2013.284427 Luehr D, Woolley T, Burke R, et al. Institute for Clinical Systems Improvement. *Hypertension Diagnosis and Treatment.* http://bit.ly/Hypertension1112. Updated November 2012. *Eur Heart J* 2013;34:2159-2219
	CHEP	2014		Above the normal replacement levels, supplementation of K, Ca, and Mg is not recommended for the prevention or treatment of HTN.		https://www.hypertension.ca/en/chep
	ACCF/AHA	2011	Patients age >65 y	Lifestyle management is effective in all ages.		*J Am Coll Cardiol.* 2011;57(20): 2037-2114
		2008	Patients age >80 y	A higher target systolic blood pressure (SBP) and diastolic blood pressure (DBP) at >140/70 mm Hg.		*N Engl J Med* 2008;358:1887-1898

[a]Family history of HTN; African American (black race) ancestry; overweight or obesity; sedentary lifestyle; excess intake of dietary sodium; insufficient intake of fruits, vegetables, and potassium; excess consumption of alcohol.
[b]See Lifestyle Modifications for Primary Prevention of Hypertension on page 113 and refer to *JAM Coll Cardiol* 2011;57:2037-2110.
[c]Canadian Hypertension Education Program

LIFESTYLE MODIFICATIONS FOR PRIMARY PREVENTION OF HYPERTENSION

- Maintain a healthy body weight for adults (BMI, 18.5–24.9 kg/m²; waist circumference <102 cm for men and <88 cm for women).
- Reduce dietary sodium intake to no more than 100 mmol/d (approximately 6 g of sodium chloride or 2.4 g of sodium/d).
- Per CHEP 2015: adequate intake 2000 mg daily (all >19 y old) (80% in processed foods; 10% at the table or in cooking).
- 2000 mg sodium (Na) = 87 mmol sodium (Na)= 5 g of salt (NaCl) ~1 teaspoon of table salt
- Engage in regular aerobic physical activity, such as brisk walking, jogging, cycling, or swimming (30–60 min per session, 4–7 d/wk), in addition to the routine activities of daily living. Higher intensities of exercise are not more effective. Weight training exercise does not adversely influence BP.
- Limit alcohol consumption to no more than two drinks (eg, 24 oz [720 mL] of beer, 10 oz [300 mL] of wine, or 3 oz [90 mL] of 100-proof whiskey) per day in most men and to no more than one drink per day in women and lighter-weight persons.
- Maintain adequate intake of dietary potassium (>90 mmol [3500 mg]/d).
- Above the normal replacement levels, supplementation of potassium, calcium, and magnesium is not recommended for prevention or treatment of hypertension.Daily K dietary intake > 80 mmol
- Daily K dietary intake > 80 mmol
- Consume a diet that is rich in fruits and vegetables and in low-fat dairy products with a reduced content of saturated and total fat (Dietary Approaches to Stop Hypertension [DASH] eating plan).
- Advice in combination with pharmacotherapy (varenicline, bupropion, nicotine replacement therapy) should be offered to all smokers with a goal of smoking cessation.
- Stress management should be considered as an intervention in hypertensive patients in whom stress may be contributing to BP elevation.

Sources: CHEP 2015 http://www.hypertension.ca. *Hypertension.* 2003;42:1206-1252. ASH 2009 *J Clin Hypertens (Greenwich).* 2009;11: 358-368.
Eckel RH, Jakicic JM, Ard JD, et al. 2013 ACC/AHA Guideline on lifestyle management to reduce CV risk: a report of the American College of Cardiology/American Heart Association Task Force on Practice Guidelines. http://circ.ahajournals.org/content/early/2013/11/11/01. cir.0000437740.48606.d1

IMMUNIZATIONS

Disease Prevention	Organization	Date	Population	Recommendations	Comments	Source
Immunizations, Adults	CDC	2013	Adults	Recommend immunizing adults according to the Centers for Disease Control and Prevention (CDC) recommendations unless contraindicated (see Appendix IX).		http://www.cdc.gov/vaccines/schedules/hcp/imz/adult.html
Immunizations, Infants and Children	CDC	2013	Infants and children age 0–18 y	Recommend immunizing infants and children according to the CDC recommendations unless contraindicated (see Appendix IX).		http://www.cdc.gov/vaccines/schedules/hcp/imz/child-adolescent.html http://www.cdc.gov/vaccines/schedules/hcp/imz/catchup.html

INFECTIONS						

Disease Prevention	Organization	Date	Population	Recommendations	Comments	Source
Intravascular device-related infections	CDC	2011	Adults and children with intravascular devices	• Educate health care staff on the proper procedures for insertion and maintenance of intravascular devices. • Ensure appropriate nursing staffing levels in ICUs. • Recommend upper extremity sites for adults. • Avoid using the femoral vein in adults. • Subclavian vein is preferred over the internal jugular or femoral veins in adults. • Evaluate the catheter insertion site daily. • Remove peripheral catheters if the site develops signs of infection, phlebitis, or infiltration. • Promptly remove any central venous catheter that is no longer needed. • Hand hygiene should be performed before and after accessing central venous catheter. • Maximal sterile barrier precautions should be followed when inserting a central line. • Prepare the skin with an antiseptic solution prior to vascular device placement. • Use 2% chlorhexidine daily wash to lower incidence of central line-associated bloodstreams infections. • Replace dressings used on short-term CVC sites at least every 7 d for transparent dressings or if dressings become damp, loosened, or soiled. • Recommend antimicrobial-impregnated central venous catheters. • Recommend against routinely replace CVCs, PICCs, hemodialysis catheters, or pulmonary artery catheters to prevent catheter-related infections. • In adults, use of the radial, brachial, or dorsalis pedis sites is preferred over the femoral or axillary sites of insertion to reduce the risk of infection.		www.guideline.gov/content.aspx?id=34426
Surgical site infections (SSI)	Cochrane Database of Systematic Reviews	2014	Women undergoing cesarean sections	Recommend a vaginal preparation with povidone-iodine solution immediately prior to cesarean delivery.	A vaginal prep prior to cesarean section reduces the incidence of postpartum endometritis. This benefit was especially true for women in active labor or with rupture membranes	http://www.cochrane.org/CD007892/PREG_vaginal-cleansing-before-cesarean-delivery-to-reduce-post-cesarean-infections
				Recommend administration of prophylactic IV antibiotics preoperatively within 60 min of skin incision as opposed to administration after cord clamping.	The incidence of maternal infectious morbidity is decreased (RR 0.54) when prophylactic antibiotics are administered preoperatively as opposed to after cord clamping	http://www.cochrane.org/CD009516/PREG_when-should-antibiotics-be-given-to-prevent-infectious-complications-after-cesarean-birth

INFLUENZA, CHEMOPROPHYLAXIS

Disease Prevention	Organization	Date	Population	Recommendations	Comments	Source

Influenza, Chemoprophylaxis	IDSA
	CDC
		2009
		2011
			Children and adults	1. Consider antiviral chemoprophylaxis for adults and children age >1 y at high risk of influenza complications (see the Influenza, Vaccination section) when any of the following conditions are present:
				  a. Influenza vaccination is contraindicated.[a]
				  b. Unvaccinated adults or children when influenza activity has been detected in the community. Vaccinate simultaneously.
				  c. Unvaccinated adults and children in close contact with people diagnosed with influenza.
				  d. Residents of extended-care facilities with an influenza outbreak.
					1. Influenza vaccination is the best way to prevent influenza.
					2. Antiviral chemoprophylaxis is not a substitute for influenza vaccination.
					3. Duration of chemoprophylaxis is 2 wk postvaccination in most persons but is indicated for 6 wk in children who were not previously vaccinated or who require 2 vaccine doses.
					4. Chemoprophylaxis for 10 d in a household in which a family member has influenza.
					5. Agents for chemoprophylaxis of influenza A (H1N1) and B: zanamivir or oseltamivir.
						http://www.guidelines.gov/content.aspx?id=14173
						http://www.cdc.gov/mmwr/preview/mmwrhtml/rr6001a1.htm?s_cid=rr6001a1_w

[a]Contraindications for influenza vaccination: anaphylactic hypersensitivity to eggs, acute febrile illness, history of Guillain-Barré syndrome within 6 wk of a previous influenza vaccination.

INFLUENZA, VACCINATION					
Disease Prevention	Organization	Date	Population	Recommendations	Comments	Source

Influenza, Vaccination	CDC	2013	All persons age >6 mo	1. All persons age >6 mo should receive the seasonal influenza vaccine annually.
				2. All children age 6 mo to 8 y should receive 2 doses of the 2013–2014 seasonal influenza vaccine (>4 wk apart) if:
				    a. Vaccination status is unknown.
				    b. Persons have never received the influenza vaccine before.
				    c. Those who did not receive the 2009 H1N1 vaccine.
				3. A quadrivalent live attenuated influenza vaccine (Flumist quadrivalent) is available for all healthy, nonpregnant people ages 2–49 y.
					1. Highest-risk groups for influenza complications are:
					    – Pregnant women
					    – Children age 6 mo to 5 y
					    – Adults age >50 y
					    – Persons with chronic medical conditions[a]
					    – Residents of extended-care facilities
					    – Morbidly obese (BMI >40) persons
					    – Health care personnel
					    – Household contacts of persons with high-risk medical conditions or caregivers of children age <5 y or adults age >50 y
					    – Children and adolescents receiving long-term aspirin therapy.
					    – American Indians or Alaska Natives
						http://www.cdc.gov/mmwr/preview/mmwrhtml/rr6207a1.htm

[a]Chronic heart, lung, renal, liver, hematologic, cancer, neuromuscular, or seizure disorders, severe cognitive dysfunction, diabetes, HIV infection, or immunosuppression.

Disease Prevention	Organization	Date	Population	Recommendations	Comments	Source
Influenza, Prevention	AAP	2011	Children and adolescents >6mo	Annual trivalent seasonal influenza immunization for all children and adolescents >6mo.	High-risk children include infants born prematurely, children with chronic heart disease, lung disease, kidney disease, neurologic disorders, diabetes, HIV infection, immunosuppression, sickle cell anemia, or chronic metabolic disorders.	http://pediatrics. aappublications.org/ content/128/4/813.full

		2013	Children 6 mo of age and older	• Recommend annual seasonal influenza vaccine for all children 6 mo of age and older.
				  ○ Children 9 y and older need only 1 dose.
				  ○ Children 6 mo through 8 y of age receiving the seasonal influenza vaccine for the first time should receive a second dose this season at least 4 wk after the first dose.
				  ○ Children 6 mo through 8 y of age who received seasonal influenza vaccine before the 2013–2014 influenza season
				  ○ Need only 1 dose of vaccine, if they previously received 2 or more doses of seasonal vaccine since July 1, 2010
				  ○ Healthy children 2 y and older can receive either inactivated influenza vaccine (IIV) or live-attenuated influenza vaccine (LAIV)
				• For children at high risk of complications from influenza for whom influenza vaccine is contraindicated
				• For children at high risk during the 2 wk after influenza immunization
				• For family members or HCP who are unimmunized and are likely to have ongoing, close exposure to
				  ○ Unimmunized children at high risk; or
				  ○ Unimmunized infants and toddlers who are younger than 24 mo
				• Indications for chemoprophylaxis with oseltamivir:
				  ○ For control of influenza outbreaks for unimmunized staff and children in a closed institutional setting with children at high risk (eg, extended-care facilities)
				  ○ As a supplement to immunization among children at high risk, including children who are immunocompromised and may not respond to vaccine
				  ○ As postexposure prophylaxis for family members and close contacts of an infected person if those people are at high risk of complications from influenza
				  ○ For children at high risk and their family members and close contacts, as well as HCP, when circulating strains of influenza virus in the community are not matched with seasonal influenza vaccine strains, on the basis of current data from the CDC and local health departments
					Highest-risk groups are:
					• All children, including infants born preterm, who are 6 mo of age and older with conditions that increase the risk of complications from influenza (eg, children with chronic medical conditions, such as asthma, diabetes mellitus, hemodynamically significant cardiac disease, immunosuppression, or neurologic and neurodevelopmental disorders).
					• Children of American Indian/Alaskan Native heritage.
					• All household contacts and out-of-home care providers of:
					  ○ Children with high-risk conditions; and
					  ○ Children younger than 5 y, especially infants younger than 6 mo
					• All health care personnel (HCP).
					• All women who are pregnant, are considering pregnancy, have recently delivered, or are breast-feeding during the influenza season.
					• Chemoprophylaxis is not a substitute for vaccination.
						http://www.guideline.gov/ content.aspx?id=47372

KIDNEY INJURY, ACUTE

Disease Prevention	Organization	Date	Population	Recommendations	Comments	Source

Kidney Injury, Acute	NICE
	VA/DoD
		2013
		2014
			Adults and children	• Recommend volume expansion to at risk adults who will receive intravenous iodinated contrast.
				  ○ CKD with eGFR <40 mL/min
				  ○ CHF
				  ○ Renal transplant
				  ○ 75 y or over
				• Consult a pharmacist to assist with drug dosing in adults or children at risk for AKI.
					Inconsistent evidence for N-acetylcysteine use to prevent contrast-induced nephropathy	http://www.guideline.gov/content.aspx?id=47080
						http://www.guideline.gov/content.aspx?id=48951

MOTOR VEHICLE INJURY

Disease Prevention	Organization	Date	Population	Recommendations	Comments	Source
Motor Vehicle Injury	ICSI	2010	Infants, children, and adolescents	1. Providers should ask the family about the use of car seats, booster seats, and seat belts. 2. Ask children and adolescents about helmet use in recreational activities.	1. Head injury rates are reduced by approximately 75% in motorcyclists who wear helmets compared with those who do not. 2. Properly used child restraint systems can reduce mortality up to 21% compared with seat belt usage in children age 2–6 y.	https://www.icsi.org/_asset/x1mmv1/PrevServKids.pdf

Disease Prevention	Organization	Date	Population	Recommendations	Comments	Source
MYOCARDIAL INFARCTION (MI)						
Myocardial Infarction (MI)	*In a report showing a 50% reduction in the population's CHD mortality rate, 81% was attributable to primary prevention of CHD through tobacco cessation and lipid- and blood pressure-lowering activities. Only 19% of CHD mortality reduction occurred in patients with existing CHD (secondary prevention).*					*BMJ.* 2005;331(7517):614
	FDA ASPC (American Society for Preventive Cardiology) USPSTF ESC	2014 2011 2009 2012	Asymptomatic adults Establish risk factors by the Framingham Heart Study in all men and women Aspirin therapy in adults	Data do not support the use of Aspirin for primary prevention of a heart attack or stroke. Aspirin is associated with "serious risks," including increased risk of intracerebral and GI bleeding. 1. Recommends aspirin (ASA) usage for MI prevention in men age 45–79 y when the potential benefit outweighs the risk. 2. Recommends against ASA usage for MI prevention in men age <45 y. 3. Recommends ASA usage for MI prevention in women age 55–79 y when the potential benefit outweighs the risk. 4. Insufficient evidence to recommend ASA usage for CV disease prevention in men and women age >80 y.	1. Meta-analysis concludes ASA prophylaxis reduces ischemic stroke risk in women (−17%) and MI events in men (−32%). No mortality benefit is seen in either group. Risk of bleeding is increased in both groups to a similar degree as the event rate reduction. *Initiation of therapy based on a case by case basis. (JAMA.* 2006;295:306-313; *Arch Intern Med.* 2012;172:209-216)	http://www.fda.gov/downloads/ForConsumers/ConsumerUpdates/UCM395477.pdf *Clin Cardiol.* 2011;34:6562 http://www.uspreventive servicestaskforce.org/uspstf/uspsasmi.htm http://eurheartj.oxfordjournals.org.
	ADA	2014	Aspirin therapy in diabetics type 1 or 2	Consider ASA (75–162 mg/d) if at increased CV risk (10-y > 10% based on Framingham risk score (see Appendix VI, pages 396–397), and in men age >50 y or women age >60 y with one additional risk factor.		*Diabetes Care.* 2014;37(1):S14-S80
	CHEP	2015	Hypertensive patients	Recommends low-dose ASA for vascular protection, in hypertensive patients ≥ 50 y; caution should be exercised if BP is not controlled.		h tps://www.hypertension.ca/en/chep

MYOCARDIAL INFARCTION (MI)

Disease Prevention	Organization	Date	Population	Recommendations	Comments	Source
Myocardial Infarction (MI) (continued)	AHA/ACC ESC AHA/ACCF	2013 2012 2011	Dietary therapy in all children and adults	*Dietary guidelines:* (1) Balance calorie intake and physical activity to achieve or maintain a healthy body weight. (2) Consume a diet rich in vegetables and fruit. (3) Choose whole grain, high-fiber foods. (4) Consume fish, especially oily fish, at least twice a week. (5) Limit intake of saturated fats to <7% energy, trans fats to <1% energy, and cholesterol to <300 mg/d by: • Choosing lean meats and vegetable alternatives • Selecting fat-free (skim), 1% fat, and low-fat dairy products • Minimizing intake of partially hydrogenated fats. (6) Minimize intake of beverages and foods with added sugars. (7) Choose and prepare foods with little or no salt. (8) If you consume alcohol, do so in moderation. (9) Follow these recommendations for food consumed/prepared inside *and* outside of the home. (7) Recommended diets: DASH, USDA Food Pattern, or AHA Diet *Avoid use of and exposure to tobacco products.*		Eckel RH, Jakicic JM, Ard JD, et al. 2013 ACC/AHA Guideline on lifestyle management to reduce CV risk: a report of the American College of Cardiology/American Heart Association Task Force on Practice Guidelines. http://circ.ahajournals.org/content early/2013/11/11/01. cir.0000437740.48606.d1
	CCS	2013		The Mediterranean, Portfolio, or DASH diets are recommended to improve lipid profiles or decrease cardiovascular disease (CVD) risk.		*Can J Cardiol.* 2013;29:151-167
	AHA/ASA	2012	History of CVA	Large-vessel ischemic stroke is a CHD risk. Small-vessel disease, may be considered CHD risk equivalent.		*Stroke.* 2012;43:199 8-2027
	ACC/AHA	2013		10-y ASCVD risk score (updated ATP III guidelines) three high-risk groups identified, based on ASCVD score and LDL-C levels. Lifestyle management and drug therapy recommended in all three categories. Statin drugs remain the treatment of choice based upon outcome data. See pages 192–193. For therapy see Chapter 3. (Pages 192–196)	1. Short-term reduction in low-density lipoprotein (LDL) using dietary counseling by dietitians is superior to that achieved by physicians. *(Am J Med.* 2000;109:549) 2. Statin therapy can safely reduce the 5-y incidence of major CVD events (coronary revascularization, stroke) by about one-fifth per mmol/L reduction in LDL cholesterol. *(Lancet.* 2005;366(9493): 1267-1278)	2013 ACC/AHA Guideline on the Treatment of Blood Cholesterol to Reduce Atherosclerotic Cardiovascular Disease Risk in Adults: A Report of the American College of Cardiology/American Heart Association Task Force on Practice Guidelines. Neil J Stone, Jennifer Robinson, Alice H. Lichtenstein, et al. Circulation published online November 12, 2013. http://circ.ahajournals.org/content/early/2013/11/11/01. cir.0000437738.63853.7a.full. pdf+html

MYOCARDIAL INFARCTION (MI)

Disease Prevention	Organization	Date	Population	Recommendations	Comments	Source
Myocardial Infarction (MI) (continued)	Cochrane	2011		Statin therapy should be employed in primary prevention only in high-risk patients (Framingham risk >20%). Restraint should be exercised in patients at low or intermediate 10-y risk (<10%; 10%–20%). If low or intermediate 10-year risk, calculate *lifetime risk* to better assess benefit of statin therapy.		*Cochrane Database Syst Rev.* 2011;(1):CD004816 *Am J Med.* 2012;125: 440-446 *Circulation.* 2006;113: 791-798 *N Engl J Med.* 2012;366:321-329
	ACP	2004		Statins should be used for primary prevention of macrovascular complications if patient has type 2 DM and other CV risk factors (age >55 y, left ventricular hypertrophy, previous cerebrovascular disease, peripheral arterial disease, smoking, or HTN).		*N Engl J Med.* 2012;366:321-329 *Ann Intern Med.* 2004;140:644-649
	FDA Warning CCS	2012 2013		Statins may cause nonserious reversible cognitive side effects as well as increased blood sugar and HbA1c levels.	No longer required to monitor liver enzymes.	
	JNC 8	2013	HTN	See page 266 for JNC 8 treatment algorithms.		*JAMA.* doi:10.1001/jama.2013. 284427
	AHA/ACCF/ACP AHA/ACC/ASH	2012 2007 2015		Goal: blood pressure (BP) <140/90 mm Hg for population with stable CAD. BP target < 140/90 mm Hg is reasonable for the secondary prevention of CV events in patients with HTN and CAD. Class IIa, LOE: 3 BP target < 130/80 mm Hg may be appropriate in some individuals with CAD, previous MI, stroke or TIA, or CAD risk equivalents (carotid artery disease, PAD, abdominal aortic aneurysm). Class IIb, LOE: B In patients with an elevated DBP and CAD with evidence of myocardial ischemia, BP should be lowered slowly, and caution is advised in inducing decreases in DBP < 60 mm Hg in any patients with DM or who is > 60 y. In older hypertensive patients with wide pulse pressures, lowering SBP may cause very low DBP values < 60 mm Hg. This should alert clinicians to assess carefully any untoward signs or symptoms, especially those resulting from myocardial ischemia. Class IIa, LOE C. If ventricular dysfunction is present, lowering the goal to 120/80 mm Hg may be considered.		*Circulation.* 2007;115:2761-2788 *Circulation.* 2012;26:3097-3137 Rosencorff C, Lackland DT, Allison M, et al. Treatment of HTN in patients with CAD. *JACC.* 2015;65(18):1998-2038.
	ESC/ECH	2013		<130/80 mm Hg goal in diabetics and other high-risk patients has not been supported by trials. No benefit and possible harm is suggested with SEP <130 mm Hg. Elderly patients' SBP goal is <160 mm Hg.		*J Hypertens* 2013;31:1281-1357

				MYOCARDIAL INFARCTION (MI)		
Disease Prevention	Organization	Date	Population	Recommendations	Comments	Source
Myocardial Infarction (MI) (continued)	CCS	2013		An increased risk of new-onset type 2 diabetes might apply to statin therapy. A recent review of the existing data suggest that potential mechanisms include increased insulin levels, reduced insulin sensitivity, and selection bias. However, the overall data strongly suggest that the reduction in CVD events outweighs the minor effect on glucose homeostasis.		*Can J Cardiol.* 2013;29:151–167
	Society of General Internal Medicine	2015		Statin use was associated with an increased likelihood of new diagnoses of DM, diabetic complications, and overweight/obesity in healthy people taking statin for primary prevention.		Mansi I, Frei CR, Wang CP, et al. Statins and new-onset diabetes mellitus and diabetic complications: a retrospective cohort study of US healthy adults. *J Gen Intern Med.* 2015. DOI:10.007/s11606-015-3335-1
	ADA	2014	Diabetes mellitus	Goals: Normal fasting glucose (≤130 mg/dL) and HbA1c (<7.5%), BP <140/80 mm Hg; low-density-lipoprotein cholesterol (LDL–C) <100 mg/dL (or <70 for high risk), high-density-lipoprotein cholesterol (HDL–C) >50 mg/dL and triglycerides <150 mg/dL.	1. Intensive glucose lowering should be avoided in patients with a history of hypoglycemic spells, advanced microvascular or macrovascular complications, long-standing DM, or if extensive comorbid conditions are present. 2. DM with BP readings of 130–139/80–89 mm Hg that persist after lifestyle and behavioral therapy should be treated with angiotensin-converting enzyme (ACE) inhibitor or angiotensin receptor blocker (ARB) agents. Multiple agents are often needed. *Administer at least one agent at bedtime.* No advantage of combining ACE inhibitor and ARB in HTN Rx (ONTARGET Trial). (*N Engl J Med.* 2008;358:1547-1559)	*Diabetes Care.* 2014;37 (1) *Circulation.* 2006;114: 82-96 *N Engl J Med.* 2008;358:1547-1559 *N Engl J Med.* 2008;358:2545-2559 *N Engl J Med.* 2008;358:2560-2572
	AHA ADA	2006 2012	Smoking	Advise all patients not to smoke.		
	ESC	2012		Avoid passive smoking.	New evidence on the health effects of passive smoking strengthens the recommendation on passive smoking. Smoking bans in public places, by law, lead to a decrease in incidence of myocardial infarction.	*Eur Heart J.* 2012;33:1635-1701

MYOCARDIAL INFARCTION (MI)

Disease Prevention	Organization	Date	Population	Recommendations	Comments	Source
Myocardial Infarction (MI) (continued)	AHA	2011	Women	Standard CVD lifestyle recommendations, *plus*: Waist circumference <35 in. Omega-3 fatty acids if high-risk (EPA 1800 mg/d).[a] BP <120/80 mm Hg. Lipids: LDL-C <100 mg/dL, HDL-C >50 mg/dL, triglycerides <150 mg/dL. ASA (75–325 mg/d) indicated only in high-risk women.[a] In women age >65 y, *consider* ASA (81 mg daily or 100 mg every other day) if BP is controlled and the benefit of ischemic stroke and MI prevention is likely to outweigh the risk of a GI bleed and hemorrhagic stroke.	Estrogen plus progestin hormone therapy should not be used or continued. Antioxidants (vitamins E, C, and β-carotene), folic acid, and B₁₂ supplementation are not recommended to prevent CHD. ASA is not indicated to prevent MI in low-risk women age <65 y.	*J Am Coll Cardiol.*2011;57(12): 1404–1423
	ESC	2007 2012	Adults at risk of CV disease	Smoking cessation. Weight reduction if BMI >25 kg/m² or waist circumference >88 cm in women and >102 cm in men. No further weight gain if waist circumference 80–88 cm in women and 94–102 cm in men. Thirty minutes of moderately vigorous exercise on most days of the week. Healthy diet. Antihypertensives when BP >140/90 mm Hg. Statins when total cholesterol >190 mg/dL or LDL >115 mg/dL. In patients with known CV disease: ASA and statins. In patients with DM: glucose-lowering drugs. Psychosocial risk factor Low socioeconomic status, lack of social support, stress at work and in family life, depression, anxiety, hostility, and the type D personality contribute both to the risk of developing CVD and the worsening of clinical course and prognosis of CVD. These factors act as barriers to treatment adherence and efforts to improve lifestyle, as well as to promoting health and well-being in patients and populations. In addition, distinct psychobiologic mechanisms have been identified, which are directly involved in the pathogenesis of CVD. Psychological interventions can counteract psychosocial stress and promote healthy behaviors and lifestyle. Cognitive-behavioral methods are effective in supporting persons in adopting a healthy lifestyle. More evidence on the impact of total diet/dietary patterns such as the Mediterranean type of diet has gained interest in recent years. Antihypertensive treatment is beneficial in patients age >80 y. Aspirin is no longer recommended for primary prevention in people with diabetes. Nurse-coordinated prevention programs are effective across a variety of practice settings.	European Society of Cardiology recommends using the SCORE Risk System to estimate risk of atherosclerotic CV disease.	*Eur Heart J.* 2007;28:2375 http://eurheartj.oxfordjournals.org. *Eur Heart J.* 2012;33:1635–1701

[a]High risk: CHD or risk equivalent or 10-y absolute CHD risk >20% based on Framingham risk score (see Appendix VI, pages 396–397).

NEURAL TUBE DEFECTS

Disease Prevention	Organization	Date	Population	Recommendations	Comments	Source
Neural Tube Defects	AAFP USPSTF ICSI	2010 2009 2010	Women planning or capable of pregnancy	Recommend that all women of childbearing age take a daily supplement containing 400–800 μg of folic acid.	1. Women planning a pregnancy should start folic acid supplementation at least 1 mo before conception and continue through the first 2–3 mo of pregnancy. 2. The ACOG and AAFP recommend 4 mg/d folic acid for women with a history of a child affected by a neural tube defect.	http://www.guideline.gov/content.aspx?id=38619 http://www.uspreventiveservicestaskforce.org/uspstf09/folicacid/folicacidrs.htm https://www.icsi.org/_asset/gjr9h/PrevServAdults.pdf

				OBESITY	
Disease Prevention	**Organization**	**Date**	**Population**	**Recommendations**	**Comments**	**Source**

Disease Prevention	Organization	Date	Population	Recommendations	Comments	Source
Obesity	ICSI	2009	Adolescents and adults	1. Recommends a team approach for weight management in all persons of normal weight (BMI 18.5–24.9) or overweight (BMI 25–29.9) including: a. Nutrition b. Physical activity c. Lifestyle changes d. Screen for depression e. Screen for eating disorders f. Review medication list and assess if any medications can interfere with weight loss 2. Recommend regular follow-up to reinforce principles of weight management.	1. Recommend 30–60 min of moderate physical activity on most days of the week. 2. Nutrition education focused on decreased caloric intake, encouraging healthy food choices, and managing restaurant and social eating situations. 3. Weekly weight checks. 4. Encourage nonfood rewards for positive reinforcement. 5. Stress management techniques.	http://www.guideline.gov/content.aspx?id=32825
	Endocrine Society	2008	Children	1. Recommends exclusive breast-feeding for at least 6 mo. 2. Educate children and parents about healthy diets and the importance of regular physical activity. 3. Encourage school systems to promote healthy eating habits and provide health education courses. 4. Clinicians should help educate communities about healthy dietary and activity habits.	1. Avoid the consumption of calorie-dense, nutrient-poor foods (eg, juices, soft drinks, "fast food" items, and calorie-dense snacks). 2. Control calorie intake by portion control. 3. Reduce saturated dietary fat intake for children age >2 y. 4. Increase dietary fiber, fruits, and vegetables. 5. Eat regular, scheduled meals and avoid snacking. 6. Limit television, video games, and computer time to 2 h daily.	http://www.guidelines.gov/content.aspx?id=13572

OSTEOPOROTIC HIP FRACTURES				

Disease Prevention	Organization	Date	Population	Recommendations	Comments	Source
Osteoporotic Hip Fractures	AAFP USPSTF	2010 2005	Postmenopausal women	Recommend against the routine use of combined estrogen and progestin for the prevention of osteoporotic fractures.	The results of studies including the WHI and the Heart and Estrogen/Progestin Replacement Study reveal that HRT probably reduces osteoporotic hip and vertebral fractures and may decrease the risk of colon CA; however, HRT may lead to an increased risk of breast CA, stroke, cholecystitis, dementia, and venous thromboembolism. HRT does not decrease the risk of coronary artery disease (CAD).	http://www.guideline.gov/content.aspx?id=38619 http://www.uspreventiveservicestaskforce.org/uspstf/uspspmho.htm
	AAFP USPSTF	2010 2005	Postmenopausal women who have had a hysterectomy	Recommend against the routine use of estrogen for the prevention of osteoporotic fractures in postmenopausal women who have had a hysterectomy.		http://www.guideline.gov/content.aspx?id=38619 http://www.uspreventiveservicestaskforce.org/uspstf/uspspmho.htm
Otitis Media, Recurrent	AAP	2013	Children 6 mo to 12 y	• Recommend against prophylactic antibiotics to reduce the frequency of episodes of AOM in children with recurrent AOM. • Recommend exclusive breast-feeding for at least the first 6 mo of life. • Vaccines recommended for all children to prevent bacterial AOM 　○ Pneumococcal vaccine 　○ Influenza vaccine	• Level of evidence B.	http://www.guidelines.gov/content.aspx?id=43892

| | POSTPARTUM HEMORRHAGE | | | | |

Disease Prevention	Organization	Date	Population	Recommendations	Comments	Source

Postpartum Hemorrhage	WHO	2012	Pregnant women	• Uterotonic medications should be given to all women during the third stage of labor.
				  ○ Oxytocin 10 IU IV or IM is first choice
				  ○ Methylergometrine or oral/rectal misoprostol is the alternative
				• Controlled cord traction is recommended for removal of the placenta.
						http://www.guidelines.gov/content.aspx?id=39383

Preterm Birth	ACOG	2012	Pregnant women	• Advise against the use of **maintenance** tocolytics to prevent preterm birth. • Avoid antibiotics for the purpose of prolonging gestation or improving neonatal outcome in preterm labor and **intact membranes.**	• No evidence to support the use of prolonged tocolytics for women with preterm labor. • No evidence to support strict bed rest for the prevention of preterm birth. • The positive predictive value of a positive fetal fibronectin test or a short cervix for preterm birth is poor in isolation.	http://www.guidelines.gov/content.aspx?id=38621

PREECLAMPSIA

Disease Prevention	Organization	Date	Population	Recommendations	Comments	Source
Preeclampsia	USPSTF	2014	Pregnant women at increased risk of preeclampsia	Recommends use of aspirin 81 mg/day after 12 wk of gestation in women who are at high risk of preeclampsia.		http://www.uspreventiveservicestaskforce.org/Page/Topic/recommendation-summary/low-dose-aspirin-use-for-the-prevention-of-morbidity-and-mortality-from-preeclampsia-preventive-medication

PRESSURE ULCERS

Disease Prevention	Organization	Date	Population	Recommendations	Comments	Source

Pressure Ulcers	ICSI
	WONCA
	NICE
		2010
		2010
		2014
			Adults or children with impaired mobility	1. Recommend a risk assessment of all persons in both outpatient and inpatient settings (eg, the Braden Scale in adults and Braden Q Scale in children).
				2. Recommend education of patient, family, and caregivers regarding the causes and risk factors of pressure ulcers.
				3. Recommend caution when using compression stockings with lower-extremity arterial disease.
				4. Avoid thigh-high stockings when compression stockings are used.
				  a. Avoid dragging patient when moving.
				  b. Pad skin-to-skin contact.
				  c. Lubricate or powder bed pans prior to placing under patient.
				  d. Keep skin moisturized
				5. Recommend minimizing pressure on skin, especially areas with bony prominences.
				  a. Turn patient side-to-side every 2 h.
				  b. Pad areas over bony prominences.
				  c. Use heel protectors or place pillows under calves.
				  d. Consider a bariatric bed for patients weighing over 300 lb.
				  e. Consider high-specification foam mattress for high risk patients admitted to secondary care or who are undergoing surgery
				6. Recommend managing moisture.
				  a. Moisture barrier protectant on skin
				  b. Frequent diaper changes
				  c. Scheduled toileting
				  d. Treat candidiasis if present
				  e. Consider a rectal tube for stool incontinence with diarrhea
				7. Recommend maintaining adequate nutrition and hydration.
				8. Recommend keeping the head of the bed at or <30° elevation.
					1. Outpatient risk assessment for pressure ulcers:
					  a. Is the patient bed or wheel chair bound?
					  b. Does the patient require assistance for transfers?
					  c. Is the patient incontinent of urine or stool?
					  d. Any history of pressure ulcers?
					  e. Does the patient have a clinical condition placing the patient at risk for pressure ulcers?
					    i. DM
					    ii. Peripheral vascular disease
					    iii. Stroke
					    iv. Polytrauma
					    v. Musculoskeletal disorders (fractures or contractures)
					    vi. Spinal cord injury
					    vii. Guillain-Barré syndrome
					    viii. Multiple sclerosis
					    ix. CA
					    x. Chronic obstructive pulmonary disease
					    xi. Coronary heart failure
					    xii. Dementia
					    xiii. Preterm neonate
					    xiv. Cerebral palsy
					  f. Does the patient appear malnourished?
					  g. Is equipment in use that could contribute to ulcer development (eg, oxygen tubing, prosthetic devices, urinary catheter)?
						http://www.guideline.gov/content.aspx?id=36059
						http://www.guidelines.gov/content.aspx?id=23868
						http://www.guideline.gov/content.aspx?id=48026

SEXUALLY TRANSMITTED INFECTIONS

Disease Prevention	Organization	Date	Population	Recommendations	Comments	Source
Sexually Transmitted Infections (STIs)	AAFP USPSTF	2010 2008	Sexually active adolescents and high-risk adults	Recommend high-intensity behavioral counseling to prevent STIs for all sexually active adolescents and for adults at increased risk for STIs.		http://www.guideline-gov/content.aspx?id=38619 http://www.uspreventiveservicestaskforce.org/uspstf/uspsstds.htm

STROKE

Disease Prevention[a]	Organization	Date	Population	Recommendations	Comments	Source
Stroke[a]	AHA/ASA	2011	Treat all known CV risk factors	Screen and treat BP to <140/90 mm Hg.	1. Strokes and nonfatal strokes are reduced in diabetic patients by lower BP targets (<130/80 mm Hg).In the absence of harm, this benefit appears to justify the lower BP goal. 2. Average stroke rate in patients with risk factors is approximately 5% per year. 3. Adjusted-dose warfarin and antiplatelet agents reduce absolute risk of stroke. 4. Women have a higher prevalence of stroke than men. 5. Women have unique risk factors for stroke, such as pregnancy, hormone therapy, higher prevalence of hypertension in older ages.	*Stroke.* 2011;42:517-584 *Chest.* 2004;126:429S-456S
	AHA/ASA	2011	HTN	If HTN with diabetes or renal disease, treat to <130/80 mm Hg.		
	FDA	2014	Atrial fibrillation Asymptomatic adults	Data do not support the use of Aspirin for primary prevention of a heart attack or stroke. Aspirin is associated with "serious risks," including increased risk of intracerebral and GI bleeding.		http://www.fda.gov/downloads/ForConsumers/Consumer Updates/UCM395477.pdf *J Am Coll Cardiol.* 2006;48:e149-246 *Circulation.* 2011;123(11):1243-1262 *Circulation.*2006;114:e257-e354 *N Engl J Med.*2009;360:2066-2078
	AHA/ACC	2014	Atrial fibrillation	1. Prioritize rate control; consider rhythm control if this is the first event, if it occurs in a young patient with minimal heart disease or if symptomatic. 2. Rate control goal is <110 beats/min in patients with stable ventricular function (ejection fraction [EF] >40%). 3. Antithrombotic therapy is required. Anticoagulation or antiplatelet therapy is determined by ACC/AHA or CHA_2DS_2 VASc (nonvalvular atrial fibrillation) guidelines. 4. For patients with AF who have mechanical valves, warfarin is recommended with an INR target of 2–3 or 2.5–3.5, depending on the type and location of prosthesis. 5. For patients with non-valvular AF with a history of stroke, TIA or CHA_2DS_2 VASc ≥2, oral anticoagulation is recommended: warfarin (INR: 2–3) or NOACs (novel oral anticoagulation agents)—see treatment. 6. In patients treated with warfarin, INR should be performed weekly until INR is stable and at least monthly when INR is in range and stable. 7. Renal function should be evaluated prior to initiation of direct thrombin or factor Xa inhibitors and should be reevaluated when clinically indicated and at least annually. 8. In non-valvular AF with CHA_2DS_2 VASc = 0 no antithrombotic therapy or treatment with ASA or an OAC may be considered. 9. Following coronary revascularization (PCI or surgical) in patients with CHA_2DS_2 VASc ≥2, may be reasonable to use Clopidogrel with OAC but without ASA.		AHA/ACC/HRS Guideline for the Management of Patients with Atrial Fibrillation. CT January. LS Wann, JS Alpert, et al. 2014 *Circulation.* 2014 http://circ.ahajournals.org/content/early/2014/04/10/CIR.0000000000000041

				STROKE		
Disease Prevention[a]	Organization	Date	Population	Recommendations	Comments	Source
Stroke[a] (continued)		2015		Initially clinicians should identify low-risk AF patients who do not require antithrombotic therapy (CHA$_2$DS$_2$ VASc score, 0 for men, 1 for women). Patients with at least 1 risk factor (except when the only risk is being a woman) should be offered OAC. The patient's individual risk of bleeding should be addressed (BP control, discontinuing unnecessary medications such as ASA or non-steroidal anti-inflammatory drugs).		*JAMA.* 2015:313(19):1950–1962. DOI:10.1001/jama.2015.4369
	ECS	2010 2012 2013	Atrial fibrillation	ESC recommends the CHA$_2$DS$_2$ VASc score as more predictive for stroke risk, especially with a low CHADS$_2$ score. NOACs offer better efficacy, safety, and convenience compared with OAC with VKAs. In high-risk patient unsuitable for anticoagulation, dual antiplatelet therapy (ASA plus clopidogrel) is reasonable.	Absolute cerebrovascular accident (CVA) risk reduction with dual antiplatelet Rx is 0.8% per year balanced by increased bleeding risk 0.7% ACTIVE Trial. In high-risk patients with history of TIA/minor ischemic stroke, dual antiplatelet therapy (ASA+Plavix), started in the first 24 h, is superior to ASA alone in preventing stroke in the first 90 d, without having increased risk of hemorrhage.	*Eur Heart J.* 2010;31:2369-2429 *Eur Heart J.* 2012;33:2719-2747 *N Engl J Med.* 2013;369:11-19
	FDA Warning	2011	Atrial fibrillation	Dronedarone should not be used in patients who have chronic AF wit associated severe HF or LV systolic dysfunction. See Management Algorithm, pages 159–169, Chapter 3, for pharmacologic and antithrombotic recommendations. Dronedarone is contraindicated in patients with NYHA Class IV heart failure or NYHA Class II –III heart failure with a recent decompensation requiring hospitalization or referral to a specialized heart failure clinic. Dronedarone reduces the incidence of AF recurrences, hospitalization, and death in patients with paroxysmal or persistent AF. However, dronedarone should not be used in high-risk patients with permanent AF or patients with unstable chronic heart failure (HF) due to safety concerns. *J Clin Pharm Ther.* 2014 Apr;39(2):112–117.	Dronedarone doubles rate of CV death, stroke, and heart failure in patients with chronic atrial fibrillation.	*Lancet.* 2006;367:1903-212 http://www.fda.gov/Drugs/ DrugSafety/ucm240011.htm
	HRS	2015		Given the impact of AF on stroke and the association of AF with cognitive dysfunction, brain imaging may improve the care of AF patients by helping to stratify stroke risk in AF patients. Presence of subclinical brain infarcts is robustly associated with the subsequent risk of stroke. Short-term risk of stroke after transient ischemic attack (TIA) was 3-fold higher in patients with a brain infarct on MRI compared to those without.		Van Wagoner DR, Piccini JP, Albert CM, et al. Progress toward the prevention and treatment of atrial fibrillation: A summary of the Heart Rhythm Society Research Forum on the Treatment and Prevention of Atrial Fibrillation, Washington, DC. December 9–10, 2013. *Heart Rhythm.* 2015 Jan;12(1): e5-e25.

				STROKE		
Disease Prevention[a]	**Organization**	**Date**	**Population**	**Recommendations**	**Comments**	**Source**
Stroke[a] (continued)		2014		Compared to warfarin, NOACs offer relative efficacy, safety, and convenience. Warfarin efficacy and safety depend on the quality of anticoagulation control, as reflected by the average time in therapeutic range (TTR). Due to the difficulty of achieving therapeutic international normalized ratios (INRs) quickly after starting warfarin, an increased risk of stroke has been observed in the 30 d after initiation of warfarin. SAMeTT2R2 seems predictive of labile INRs and consequently more thromboembolism, bleeding, and death.		*Am J Med.* 2014 Nov;127(11): 1383–1088. DOI: 10.1016/j.amjmed.2014. 05.023. Epub 2014 May 22.
				In patients with nonvalvular atrial fibrillation, a high SAMe-TT2R2 score (reflecting poor anticoagulation control) with poor time in therapeutic range) was associated with more bleeding, adverse cardiovascular events, and mortality during follow-up.		
	CCS	2012	Atrial fibrillation	All patients should be stratified using CHADS2 and HASBLED risk scores Patients with CHADS2 = 0 should have CHADS2-VaSc score calculated All patients with CHADS2 ≥ 2 and most of the ones with CHADS2 = 1 should have OAC therapy. When OAC therapy is recommended, dabigatran and rivaroxaban are preferred over warfarin. Rate control goal is <100 beats/min. In stable CAD, ASA (75–325 mg) for CHADS2 = 3, OAC for most CHADS2 = 1. In high-risk patients with ACS, ASA + clopidogrel + OAC might be required (with adequate assessment of risk of stroke, recurrent CAD events, and hemorrhage).		*Can J Cardiol.* 2012;28:125–136
	AHA/ASA	2011	DM	1. Six-fold increase of stroke. 2. Short-term glycemic control does not lower macro vascular events. 3. HgA1c goal is <6.5%. 4. BP goal is <130/80 mm Hg. 5. Statin therapy. 6. Consider ACE inhibitor or ARB therapy for further stroke risk reduction.		*Eur Heart J.* 2010;31:2369-2429 *Stroke.* 2011;42:517-584
		2015		Among NVAF patients, SAMe-TT2R2 could represent a useful clinical tool to identify patients who would have poor quality of anticoagulation control with VKAs. SAMe-TT2R2 successfully predicts the composite outcome of major bleeding, TE complications, and death. DOI: http://dx.doi.org/10.1093/europace/euu353 Abumuaileq RR, Abu-Assi E, Raposeiras-Roubin S et al.: Evaluation of SAMe-TT2R2 risk score for predicting the quality of anticoagulation control in a real-world cohort of patients with non-valvular atrial fibrillation on vitamin-K antagonists. Europace. 2015 May;17(5):711–717. doi: 10.1093/europace/euu353		

STROKE

Disease Prevention	Organization	Date	Population	Recommendations	Comments	Source
Stroke[a] (continued)		2014		SAMeTT2R2 scores ≥ 2 predict increased stroke risk in the 3 y following incident AF in patients commenced on VKA treatment. These findings suggest that patients with high SAMeTT2R2 scores may require intensified anticoagulation control or use of oral non-VKA anticoagulants. *Circulation.* 2014;130:A19565		
	USPSTF AHA/ASA	2007 2011	Asymptomatic CAS	1. No indication for general screening for CAS with ultrasonograph. 2. Screen for other stroke risk factors and treat aggressively. 3. ASA unless contraindicated. 4. Prophylactic carotid endarterectomy (CEA) for patients with high-grade (>70%) CAS by ultrasonography when performed by surgeons with low (<3%) morbidity/mortality rates may be useful in selected cases depending on life expectancy, age, sex, and comorbidities. 5. However, recent studies have demonstrated that "best" medical therapy results in a stroke rate <1%. 6. The number needed to treat (NNT) in published trials to prevent one stroke in 1 year in this asymptomatic group varies from 84 up to 2000. (*J Am Coll Cardiol.* 2011;57:e16-e94)	Medical treatment of asymptomatic CAS should be aggressive. Surgical intervention should be individualized guided by comparing comorbid medical conditions and life expectancy to the surgical morbidity and mortality. Atherosclerotic intracranial stenosis: ASA should be used in preference to warfarin. Warfarin—significantly higher rates of adverse events with no benefit over ASA. (*N Engl J Med.* 2005;352(13): 1305-1316) Qualitative findings (embolic signals and plaque ulceration) may identify patients who would benefit from asymptomatic CEA.	*J Am Coll Cardiol.* 2011;57(8): 1002-1038 *Ann Intern Med.* 2007;147: 860-870 *Neurology.* 2005;65(6):794-801 *Stroke.* 2077;42:517-584 *Neurology.* 2011;77:751-758 *Neurology.* 2011;77:744-750 *J Am Coll Cardiol.* 2011;57(8): 997-1001 *Stroke.* 2011;42:227-276
	ASA/ACCF/ AHA/AANN AANS/ACR CNS ASA/ACCF/ AHA/AANN AANS/ACR CNS		Symptomatic CAS	Optimal timing for CEA is within 2 wk posttransient ischemic attack. CEA plus medical therapy is effective within 6 mo of symptom onset with >70% CAS. Intense medical therapy alone is indicated if the occlusion is <50%. Intensive medical therapy plus CEA may be considered with obstruction 50%–69%. Surgery should be *limited* to male patients with a low perioperative stroke/ death rate (<6%) and should have a life expectancy of at least 5 y.		
			Cryptogenic CVA Hyperlipidemia	Carotid artery stenting is associated with increased nonfatal stroke frequency but this is offset by decreased risk of MI post-CEA. Cryptogenic CVA with patent foramen ovale should receive ASA 81 mg/day.	Consider referral to tertiary center for enrollment in randomized trial to determine optimal Rx. Closure I Trial demonstrated no benefit at 2 y of patent foramen ovale (PFO) closure device over medical therapy. In 2013, the PC Trial also failed to demonstrate significant benefit in reducing recurrent embolic events in patients undergoing PFO closure compared to medical therapy, at 4 y follow-up.	*Arch Intern Med.*2011;171(20): 1794-1795 *J Am Coll Cardiol.*2009;53(21): 2014-2018 *N Engl J Med.* 2012;366:991-999 *Stroke.* 2011;42:517-584 *N Engl J Med.* 2013;368: 1083-1091

STROKE

Disease Prevention[a]	Organization	Date	Population	Recommendations	Comments	Source
Stroke[a] (continued)			Sickle cell disease	See Cholesterol and Lipid Management (pages 192–196). Statin therapy post-CVA with intensive lipid-lowering goal after an ischemic stroke or transient ischemic attack with or without CHD reduced the risk of stroke and CV events (SPARCL Trial). Begin screening with transcranial Doppler (TCD) at age 2 y.	Transfusion therapy decreased stroke rates from 10% to <1% per year. (*N Engl J Med.* 1998;339:5) Transfusion therapy decreased stroke rates from 10% to <1% per year. (*N Engl J Med.* 1998;339:5)	*Stroke.* 2006;37:1583-1633 *Stroke.* 2008;39:1647-1652 *Stroke.* 2011;42:517-584
			Smoking	Transfusion therapy is recommended for patients at high-stroke risk per TCD (high cerebral blood flow velocity >200 cm/s). Frequency of screening not determined.		
	ACC/ASA	2014	Primary prevention in women	– Higher lifetime risk, third leading cause death for women, 53.5% of new recurrent strokes occur in women.		Guidelines for the Prevention of Stroke in Women A Statement for Healthcare Professionals From the American Heart Association/American Stroke Association. C Bushnell, LD McCullough, IA Awad et al. *Stroke.* 2014;45. DOI: 10.1161/01.str.0000442009. 06663.48
				– Sex-specific risk factors: pregnancy, preeclampsia, gestational diabetes, oral contraceptive use, postmenopausal hormone use, changes in hormonal status.		
				– Risk factors with a stronger prevalence in women: migraine with aura, atrial fibrillation, diabetes, hypertension, depression, psychosocial stress.		
			Cerebral venous thrombus (CVT)	– In patients with suspected CVT, routine blood studies consisting of a complete blood count, chemistry panel, prothrombin time, and activated partial thromboplastin time should be performed.		
				– Screening for potential prothrombotic conditions that may predispose a person to CVT (eg, use of contraceptives, underlying inflammatory disease, infectious process) is recommended in the initial clinical assessment.		
				– Women with CVT during pregnancy should continue taking full anticoagulant doses of low-molecular-weight heparin (LMWH) throughout pregnancy and should continue LMWH or vitamin K antagonists (INR target of 2.0 to 3.0) for at least 6 wk postpartum, for a total minimum treatment duration of 6 mo.		
			Oral contraceptives/ menopause, postmenopausal hormone therapy	– Stroke risk with low-dose OC users is about 1.4–2 times that of non-OC users.		
				– Measurement of BP is recommended prior to initiation of hormonal contraception therapy.		
				– Routine screening for prothrombotic mutations prior to initiation of hormonal contraception is not useful.		
				– Among OC users, aggressive therapy of stroke risk factors may be reasonable.		
				– Hormone therapy (conjugated equine estrogen) with or without medroxyprogesterone) should not be used for primary or secondary prevention of stroke in postmenopausal women.		
				– Selective estrogen receptor modulators, such as raloxifene, tamoxifen, or tibolone, should not be used for primary prevention of stroke.		

[a]Assess risk of stroke in all patients. See Appendix VII, pages 398–399 for risk assessment tool.

SAM$_e$TT$_2$R$_2$ SCORE	
Sex (female)	1
Age > 60	1
Medical history (> 2 comorbidities: HTN, DM, CAD/MI, PAD, CHF, history of stroke, pulmonary disease, hepatic or renal disease)	1
Treatment (rhythm control strategy) (interacting medications, eg, beta-blocker, verapamil, amiodarone)	1
Tobacco use (within 2 y)	2
Race (non-white)	2
Maximum points	8
Interpretation	Score > 2 = NOAC Score 0–2 = VKA with TTR > 65%–70%

Fauchier L, Angoulvant D, Lip GY. The SAMe-TT$_2$R$_2$ score and quality of anticoagulation in atrial fibrillation: a simple aid to decision-making on who is suitable (or not) for vitamin K antagonists. DOI: http://dx.doi.org/10.1093/europace/euv088

SUDDEN INFANT DEATH SYNDROME

Disease Prevention	Organization	Date	Population	Recommendations	Comments	Source
Sudden Infant Death Syndrome (SIDS)	ICSI	2010	Newborns and infants	Counsel all parents to place their infants on their backs to sleep.	Stomach and side sleeping have been identified as major risk factors for SIDS.	https://www.icsi.org/_asset/x1mmv1/PrevServKids.pdf

	TOBACCO USE				
Disease Prevention	Organization	Date	Population	Recommendations	Comments	Source
Tobacco Use	AAFP	2010	Children and adolescents	Recommends counseling that avoidance of tobacco products is desirable.	The efficacy of counseling to prevent tobacco use in children and adolescents is uncertain.	http://www.guideline.gov/content.aspx?id=38619
	USPSTF	2013	School-aged children and adolescents	Recommends that primary care clinicians provide interventions including education or brief counseling to prevent the initiation of tobacco use.		http://www.guideline.gov/content.aspx?id=47067

CLINICAL RECOMMENDATIONS FOR USE OF PROFESSIONALLY APPLIED OR PRESCRIPTION-STRENGTH, HOME-USE TOPICAL FLUORIDE AGENTS FOR CARIES PREVENTION IN PATIENTS AT ELEVATED RISK OF DEVELOPING CARIES

Age Group or Dentition Affected	Professionally Applied Topical Fluoride Agent	Prescription-Strength, Home-Use Topical Fluoride Agent
Younger than 6 y		
6–18 y	2.26% fluoride varnish at least every 3 to 6 mo (**In Favor**) or 1.23% fluoride (acidulated phosphate fluoride [APF]) gel for 4 min at least every 3 to 6 mo (**In Favor**)	0.09% fluoride mouthrinse at least weekly (**In Favor**) or 0.5% fluoride gel or paste twice daily (**Expert Opinion For**)
Older than 18 y	2.26% fluoride varnish at least every 3 to 6 mo (**Expert Opinion For**) or 1.23% fluoride (APF) gel for at least 4 min every 3 to 6 mo (**Expert Opinion For**)	0.09% fluoride mouthrinse at least weekly (**Expert Opinion For**) or 0.5% fluoride gel or paste twice daily (**Expert Opinion For**)
Adult Root Caries	2.26% fluoride varnish at least every 3 to 6 mo (**Expert Opinion For**) or 1.23% fluoride (APF) gel for 4 min at least every 3 to 6 mo (**Expert Opinion For**)	0.09% fluoride mouthrinse daily (**Expert Opinion For**) or 0.5% fluoride gel or paste twice daily (**Expert Opinion For**)

Additional Information:

- 0.1% fluoride varnish, 1.23% fluoride (APF) foam, or prophylaxis pastes are not recommended for preventing coronal caries in all age groups (**Expert Opinion Against or Against**). See American Dental Association (ADA) publication for recommendation strength by age group. The full report, which includes more details, is available at ebd.ada.org.
- No prescription-strength or professionally-applied topical fluoride agents except 2.26% fluoride varnish are recommended for children younger than 6 y (**Expert Opinion Against or Against**), but practitioners may consider the use of these other agents on the basis of their assessment of individual patient factors that alter the benefit to harm relationship.
- Prophylaxis before 1.23% fluoride (APF) gel application is not necessary for coronal caries prevention in all age groups (**Expert Opinion Against or Against**). See ADA publication for recommendation strength by age group. No recommendation can be made for prophylaxis prior to application of other topical fluoride agents. The full report, which includes more details, is available at the ebd.ada.org.

Patients at low risk of developing caries may not need additional topical fluorides other than over-the-counter fluoridated toothpaste and fluoridated water.

Source: Weyant RJ, et al. Topical fluoride for caries prevention. Chicago, IL.: American Dental Association; 2013. http://www.guideline.gov/content.aspx?id=47553.

	VENOUS THROMBOEMBOLISM				
Disease Prevention	Organization	Date	Population	Recommendations	Comments	Source
Venous Thromboembolism (VTE) Prophylaxis in Nonsurgical Patients	ACCP ACP	2012 2011	Medical patients with low risk (**Padua Prediction score—see Table I**) Medical patients with high risk (*JAMA.* 2012;307:306) (**Padua Prediction score—see Table I**)	Recommend against the use of pharmacologic prophylaxis or mechanical prophylaxis. Recommend for anticoagulant thromboprophylaxis with low-molecular-weight heparin (LMWH)—equivalent of enoxaparin 40 mg SQ daily; low-dose unfractionated heparin (UFH) 5000 units bid or tid; or fondaparinux 2.5 mg SQ daily. If patient bleeding or high risk of bleeding (see Table II), mechanical prophylaxis with graduated compression stockings (GCS) or intermittent pneumatic compression (IPC) recommended. When bleeding risk decreases, substitute pharmacologic thromboprophylaxis for mechanical prophylaxis—continue thromboprophylaxis for duration of hospital stay—extended prophylaxis after discharge not recommended for medical patients.	Routine ultrasound screening for DVT is not recommended in any group. 150–200,000 deaths from VTE in US per year. Hospitalized patients' VTE risk is 130-fold greater than that of community residents. (*Mayo Clin Proc.* 2001;76:1102) Neither heparin nor warfarin is recommended prophylactically for patients with central venous catheters. In higher risk long-distance travelers, frequent ambulation, calf muscle exercises, aisle seat, and below-the-knee graduated compression stockings (GCS) is recommended over aspirin or anticoagulants. Inpatients with solid tumors and additional risk factors for VTE (history of DVT, thrombophilic drugs, immobilization), prophylactic dose LMWH or UFH is recommended. Be cautious in patients with Ccr <30 mL/min—UFH or dalteparin (half dose) preferred. Consider adjusted LMWH dose in patients <50 kg or >110 kg in weight. Inferior vena cava (IVC) filter indicated in patients with diagnosed DVT or pulmonary embolism (PE) who cannot be anticoagulated because of bleeding—IVC filter should not be used prophylactically. Although several studies have shown survival benefit for VTE prophylaxis in surgical patients, this has not been proven in medical patients. (*N Engl J Med.* 2007;356:1438)	*Ann Intern Med.* 2011; 155:625-632 http://ChestJournal. chestpubs.org/ content/suppl/2012

TABLE I   RISK FACTORS FOR VTE IN HOSPITALIZED MEDICAL PATIENTS—PADUA PREDICTIVE SCALE

Risk Factor	Points
Active cancer[a]	3
Previous VTE	3
Reduced mobility[b]	3
Underlying thrombophilic disorder[c]	3
Recent (<1 mo) trauma or surgery	2
Age (>70 y)	1
Congestive heart failure (CHF) or respiratory failure	1
Acute MI or stroke	1
Acute infection or inflammatory disorder	1
Obesity (BMI > 30)	1
Thrombophilic drugs (hormones, tamoxifen, erythroid stimulating agents, lenalidomide, bevacizumab)	1
High risk: >4 points–11% risk of VTE without prophylaxis	
Low risk: <3 points–0.3% risk of VTE without prophylaxis	

[a]Local or distant metastasis, chemotherapy or radiation within last 6 mo
[b]Bed rest for >3 d
[c]Hereditary thrombophilia (see **Table III**) and antiphospholipid antibody syndrome, nephrotic syndrome, hemolytic anemia

TABLE II   RISK FACTORS FOR BLEEDING (*CHEST*. 2011;134:69-79)

Risk Factor[c,d]	N = 10,866 % of Patients	Overall Risk
Active gastroduodenal ulcer	2.2	4.15
GI bleed <3 mo previous	2.2	3.64
Platelet count <50 K	1.7	3.37
Age ≥85 y (vs 40 y)	10	2.96
Hepatic failure (INR[a] >1 5)	2	2.18
Renal failure (GFR[b] <30 mL/min)	11	2.14
ICU admission	8.5	2.10
Current cancer	10.7	1.78
Male sex	49.4	1.48

[a]International normalized ratio
[b]Glomerular filtration rate
[c]Although not studied in medical patients, antiplatelet therapy would be expected to increase risk of bleeding.
[d]Go to www.outcomes-umassmed.org/IMPROVE/risk_score/vte/index.html to calculate the risk of bleeding for individual patients.

TABLE III   HEREDITARY THROMBOPHILIC DISORDERS

Disorder	% of US Population	Increase in Lifetime of Risk of Clot
Resistance to activated protein C (factor V Leiden mutation)	5–6	3×
Prothrombin gene mutation	2–3	2.5×
Elevated Factor 8 (>175% activity)	6–8	2–3×
Elevated Homocysteine	10–15	1.5–2×
Protein C deficiency	0.37	10×
Protein S deficiency	0.5	10×
Antithrombin deficiency	0.1	25×
Homozygous factor V Leiden	0.3	60×

VENOUS THROMBOEMBOLISM (VTE)

Disease Prevention	Organization	Date	Population	Recommendations	Comments	Source
Venous Thromboembolism (VTE) in Surgical Patients	ACCP	2012	SURGICAL—Low risk (<40 y, minor surgery,[a] no risk factor,[b] Caprini score <2) (see Table IV) —Intermediate risk (minor surgery plus risk factors, age 40–60 y, major surgery with no risk factors; Caprini score 3–4) —High risk (Major surgery plus risk factors, high-risk medical patient, major trauma, spinal cord injury, craniotomy, total hip or knee arthroplasty (THA, TKA) thoracic, abdominal, pelvic cancer surgery)	Early ambulation—consider mechanical prophylaxis (intermittent pneumatic compression—IPC or GCS). UFH 5000 U SQ q8h starting 2 h preoperative. or LMWH equivalent to enoxaparin 40 mg SQ 2 h before surgery then daily or 30 mg q12h SQ starting 8–12 h postop. —Fondaparinux 2.5 mg SQ daily starting 8–12 h postop. UFH 5000 U SQ q8h starting 2 h preoperative or LMWH—equivalent to enoxaparin 40 mg SQ 2 h preoperative then daily or 30 mg SQ q12h starting 8–12 h postop and also use mechanical prophylaxis with IPC or GCS. —Extend prophylaxis for as long as 28–35 d in high-risk patients. In THA, TKA ortho patients, acceptable VTE prophylaxis also includes rivaroxaban 10 mg/d, dabigatran 225 mg/d, adjusted dose warfarin and aspirin, although LMWH is preferred. If high risk of bleeding, use IPC alone. (*Ann Intern Med.* 2012;156:710. *Ann Intern Med.* 2012;156:720. *JAMA.* 2012;307:294)	1. 75%–90% of surgical bleeding is structural. VTE prophylaxis adds minimally to risk of bleeding. 2. With creatinine clearance <30 cc/min UFH with partial thromboplastin time (PTT) monitoring is preferred (decrease dose if PTT prolonged). 3. Patients with liver disease and prolonged INR are still at risk for clot. Risk-to-benefit ratio of VTE prophylaxis should be individualized. 4. Epidural anesthesia—wait 10–12 h after bid prophylactic dose of LMWH, 18 h after daily prophylactic dose of LMWH, and 24 h after prophylactic dose of fondaparinux. 5. Prophylactic IVC filter for high-risk surgery is *not* recommended. 6. For cranial and spinal surgery patients at low risk for VTE use mechanical prophylaxis—high-risk patients should have pharmacologic prophylaxis added to mechanical prophylaxis once hemostasis is established and bleeding risk decreased. 7. Patients at high risk of bleeding[c] with major surgery should have mechanical prophylaxis (IPC, GCS)— initiate anticoagulant prophylaxis if risk lowered. 8. Surgical patients receive indicated prophylaxis 60% of the time compared to 40% in medical patients.	*Chest.* 2012;141:7s–47s

[a]Eye, ear, laparoscopy, cystoscopy, arthroscopic operations.

[b]Prior VTE, cancer, stroke, obesity, congestive heart failure pregnancy, thrombophilic medications (tamoxifen, raloxifene, lenalidomide, thalidomide, erythroid-stimulating agents).

[c]SELECTED RISK FACTORS RAISING RISK OF MAJOR BLEEDING COMPLICATIONS.

General Risk Factors

Active bleeding, previous major bleed, known untreated bleeding disorder, renal or liver failure, thrombocytopenia, acute stroke, uncontrolled high BP, concomitan use of anticoagulants, or antiplatelet therapy

Procedure-Specific Risk Factors

Major abdominal surgery—extensive cancer surgery, pancreaticoduodenectomy, hepatic resection, cardiac surgery (pneumonectomy or extended resection). Procedures where bleeding complications have especially severe consequences: craniotomy, spinal surgery, spinal trauma.

TABLE IV CAPRINI RISK ASSESSMENT MODEL			
1 Point	**2 Points**	**3 Points**	**5 Points**
• Age 41–60 y • Minor surgery • BMI >251 g/m^2 • Swollen legs • Varicose veins • Pregnancy or postpartum • History of recurrent spontaneous abortion • Sepsis (<1 mo) • Lung disease • History of acute MI • Congestive heart failure (CHF) (<1 mo) • History of inflammatory bowel disease • Medical patient at bed rest	• Age 61–74 y • Arthroscopic surgery • Major open surgery >45 min • Laparoscopic surgery • Malignancy • Confined to bed • Immobilizing cast • Central venous catheter	• Age >75 y • History VTE • Family history of VTE • Factor V Leiden • Prothrombin gene mutation • Lupus anticoagulant • Elevated homocysteine • Other congenital or acquired thrombophilia	• Stroke (<1 mo) • Elective arthroplasty; hip, pelvis, or leg fracture • Acute spinal cord injury (<1 mo)
		Caprini Score <3: low risk Caprini Score 3–4: intermediate risk Caprini Score >5: high risk	

ABDOMINAL AORTIC ANEURYSM (AAA)

Risk factors of developing AAA:
- Age >60 y. About 1 person in 1000 develops an abdominal aortic aneurysm between the ages of 60 and 65. Screening studies have shown that abdominal aortic aneurysms occur in 2% to 13% of men and 6% of women >65 y.
- Smoking markedly increases risk for AAA. The risk is directly related to number of years smoking and decreases in the years following smoking cessation.
- Men develop AAA 4 to 5 times more often than women.
- AAA is more common in white population compared to other ethnicities.
- History of CHD, PAD, HTN, hypercholesterolemia.
- Family history of AAA increases the risk of developing the condition and accentuates the risks associated with age and gender. The risk of developing an aneurysm among brothers of a person with a known aneurysm who are >60 y of age is as high as 18%.

Risk of expansion:
- Age >70 y, cardiac or renal transplant, previous stroke, severe cardiac disease, tobacco use.

Risk of AAA rupture:
The evidence suggests that aneurysms expand at an average rate of 0.3 to 0.4 cm y.
The annual risk of rupture based upon aneurysm size is estimated as follows:
- <4.0 cm in diameter = <0.5%
- Between 4.0 and 4.9 cm in diameter = 0.5%–5%
- Between 5.0 and 5.9 cm in diameter = 3%–15%
- Between 6.0 and 6.9 cm in diameter = 10%–20%
- Between 7.0 and 7.9 cm in diameter = 20%–40%
- ≥8.0 cm in diameter = 30%–50%

Aneurysms that expand rapidly (>0.5 cm over 6 mo) are at high risk of rupture.
Growth tends to be more rapid in smokers and less rapid in patients with peripheral artery disease or diabetes mellitus.
The risk of rupture of large aneurysms (≥5.0 cm) is significantly greater in women (18%) than in men (12%).
Other risk factors for rupture: cardiac or renal transplant, decreased forced expiratory volume in 1 second, higher mean BP, larger initial AAA diameter, current tobacco use—length of time smoking is more significant than amount smoked.

ACCF/AHA 2005/2011 recommendations:
Pharmacologic therapy:
- All patients with AAA should have BP and fasting serum lipids monitored and controlled as recommended for patients with atherosclerotic disease (Class I, LOE C).
- Smoking cessation: counseling and medications should be provided to all patients with AAA or family history of AAA.
- Patients with infrarenal or juxtarenal AAA 4.0 to 5.4 cm in diameter should be monitored by ultrasounds or CT scans every 6 to 12 mo to detect expansion (Class I, LOE A).
- In patients with AAA <4.0 cm in diameter, monitoring by ultrasound every 2 to 3 y is reasonable (Class IIa, LOE B).
- Perioperative administration of β-adrenergic blocking agents, in the absence of contraindications, is indicated to reduce the risk of adverse cardiac events and mortality in patients with coronary artery disease undergoing surgical repair of atherosclerotic aortic aneurysms (Class I, LOE A).
- β-adrenergic blocking agents may be considered to reduce the rate of aneurysm expansion in patients with aortic aneurysms (Class IIb, LOE B).

Surgical therapy:
- Patients with infrarenal or juxtarenal AAAs ≥5.5 cm in diameter should undergo repair to eliminate risk of rupture (Class I, LOE B).
- Repair can be beneficial in patients with infrarenal or juxtarenal AAA 4.0 to 5.4 cm in diameter (Class IIa, LOE B).
- Repair is probably indicated in patients with suprarenal or type IV thoracoabdominal aortic aneurysm >5.5–6.0 cm in diameter (Class IIa, LOE B).
- Intervention is not indicated for asymptomatic infrarenal or juxtarenal AAA if <5.0 cm in diameter in men or <4.5 cm in diameter in women (Class III, LOE A).
- In patients with clinical triad of abdominal and/or back pain, a pulsatile abdominal mass, and hypotension, immediate surgical evaluation is indicated (Class I, LOE B).
- In patients with symptomatic AAA, repair is indicated regardless of diameter (Class I, LOE C).
- Open or endovascular repair of infrarenal AAAs and/or common iliac aneurysms is indicated in patients who are good surgical candidates (Class I, LOE A).
- Periodic long-term surveillance imaging should be performed to monitor for vascular leak, document shrinkage/stability of the excluded aneurysm sac, confirm graft position, and determine the need for further intervention in patients who have undergone endovascular repair of infrarenal aortic and/or iliac aneurysms (Class I, LOA A).
- Open aneurysm repair is reasonable to perform in patients who are good surgical candidates but who cannot comply with the periodic long-term surveillance required after endovascular repair (Class IIa, LOE C).
- Endovascular repair of infrarenal aortic aneurysm in patients who are at high surgical or anesthetic risk (presence of coexisting severe cardiac, pulmonary, and/or renal disease) is of uncertain effectiveness (Class IIb, LOE B).

ABDOMINAL AORTIC ANEURYSM (AAA) (CONTINUED)

ESC 2014 recommendations:

Pharmacologic therapy:

- Smoking cessation is recommended to slow the growth of the AAA.
- Patients with HTN and AAA should be treated with β-blockers as a first-line treatment.
- ACEI and statins should be considered in patients with AAA to reduce risk of cardiovascular risk.
- Enlargement of AAA is usually associated with the development of an intraluminal mural thrombus. Overall data on the benefits of ASA in reducing AAA growth are contradictory; however, given the strong association between AAA and other atherosclerotic diseases, the use of ASA may be considered according to the presence of other cardiovascular comorbidities.
- Surveillance is indicated and safe in patients with AAA with a maximum diameter <5.5 cm and slow growth <1 cm/y
- In patients with small AAA, imaging should be considered:
  - Every 4 y for AAA 2.5–2.9 cm diameter
  - Every 3 y for AAA 3.0–3.9 cm diameter
  - Every 2 y for AAA 4.0–4.4 cm diameter
  - Every year for AAA >4.5 cm diameter

Surgical therapy:

- AAA repair is indicated if:
  - AAA >5.5 cm in diameter
  - Aneurysm growth >1 cm/y
- If a large aneurysm is anatomically suitable for EVAR[a], either open or endovascular repair is recommended in patients with acceptable surgical risk.
- If a large aneurysm is anatomically unsuitable for EVAR, open aortic repair is recommended.
- In patients with asymptomatic AAA, who are unfit for open repair, EVAR, along with best medical treatment may be considered.
- In patients with suspected rupture of AAA, immediate abdominal ultrasound or CT is recommended.
- In case of ruptured AAA, emergency repair is indicated.
- In case of symptoms but non-ruptured AAA, urgent repair is indicated.
- In case of symptomatic AAA anatomically suitable for EVAR, either open or endovascular aortic repair is recommended.

[a]EVAR = endovascular aortic repair.

Sources: Adapted from http://www.uptodate.com/contents/abdominal-aortic-aneurysm-beyond-the-basics.

Hirsch AT, Haskal ZJ, Hertzer NR, et al. ACC/AHA guidelines for the management of patients with peripheral arterial disease (lower extremity, renal, mesenteric, and abdominal aortic). *J Vasc Inter Radiol* 2006;17:1383-1398.

Rooke TW, Hirsch AT, Misra S, et al. 2011 ACCF/AHA focused update of the guideline for the management of patients with peripheral artery disease (updating the 2005 guideline). *JACC.* 2011 Nov 1;58(19):2020-2045.

Erbel R, Aboyans V, Boileau C, et al. 2014 ESC guidelines on the diagnosis and treatment of aortic diseases. Document covering acute and chronic aortic diseases of the thoracic and abdominal aorta of the adult. The Task Force for the diagnosis and treatment of aortic disease of the European Society of Cardiology (ESC). *Eur Heart J.* 2014;35:2873-2926. doi:10.1093/eurheartj/ehu281.

ADRENAL INCIDENTALOMAS

Disease Management	Organization	Date	Population	Recommendations	Comments	Source
Adrenal Incidentalomas	AACE	2009	Adults	1. Recommends clinical, biochemical, and radiographic evaluation for evidence of hypercortisolism, aldosteronism, the presence of pheochromocytoma, or a malignant tumor. 2. Patients who will be managed expectantly should have reevaluation at 3–6 mo and then annually for 1–2 y.	1. A 1-mg overnight dexamethasone suppression test can be used to screen for hypercortisolism. 2. Measure plasma-fractionated metanephrines and normetanephrines to screen for pheochromocytoma. 3. Measure plasma renin activity and aldosterone concentration to assess for primary or secondary aldosteronism.	https://www.aace.com/files/adrenal-guidelines.pdf

ALCOHOL USE DISORDERS					

Disease Management	Organization	Date	Population	Recommendations	Comments	Source
Alcohol Use Disorders	ICSI NICE VA/DoD	2010 2010 2009	Adults	1. For patients identified with alcohol dependence, schedule a referral to a substance use disorders specialist before the patient has left the office. 2. Refer all patients with alcohol abstinence syndrome to a hospital for admission. 3. Recommend prophylactic thiamine for all harmful alcohol use or alcohol dependence. 4. Refer suitable patients with decompensated cirrhosis for consideration of liver transplantation or ce they have been sober from alcohol for ≥3 mo. 5. Recommend pancreatic enzyme supplerentation for chronic alcoholic pancreatitis with steatorrhea and malnutrition.	1. Assess all patients for a coexisting psychiatric disorder (dual diagnosis). 2. Addiction-focused psychosocial intervention is helpful for patients with alcohol dependence. 3. Consider adjunctive pharmacotherapy under close supervision for alcohol dependence: 　a. Naltrexone 　b. Acamprosate	https://www.icsi.org/_asset/gtjr9h/PrevServAdults.pdf http://www.guidelines.gov/content.aspx?id=23784 http://www.guidelines.gov/content.aspx?id=15676

ANAPHYLAXIS

Disease Management	Organization	Date	Population	Recommendations	Comments	Source
Anaphylaxis	NICE EACCI	2011 2014	Children and adults	• Blood samples for mast cell tryptase testing should be obtained at onset and after 1–2 h. • All people ≥16 y suspected of having an anaphylactic reaction should be observed for at least 6–12 h before discharge. • All children younger than age 16 y suspected of having an anaphylactic reaction should be admitted for observation. • Patients treated for an anaphylactic reaction should be referred to an allergy specialist. • Treat anaphylaxis with epinephrine (1:1000) 0.01 mg/kg (maximum 0.5 mg) SC; may repeat as necessary IM every 15 minutes. • Patients should be prescribed an epinephrine injector (eg, EpiPen). • Patients with circulatory instability should be placed supine with lower extremities raised and given intravenous saline 20 mL/kg bolus. • Recommend inhaled β-2 agonists and glucocorticoids for wheezing or signs of bronchoconstriction. • H_1- and H_2-blockers can be added for cutaneous signs of anaphylaxis.	Anaphylaxis is defined as a severe, life-threatening, generalized hypersensitivity reaction. It is characterized by the rapid development of: • Airway edema • Bronchospasm • Circulatory dysfunction	http://www.nice.org.uk/nicemedia/live/13626/57474/57474.pdf http://www.guideline.gov/content.aspx?id=48690

ANDROGEN DEFICIENCY SYNDROME

Disease Management	Organization	Date	Population	Recommendations	Comments	Source
Androgen Deficiency Syndrome	Endocrine Society	2010	Adult men	1. Recommends an AM total testosterone level for men with symptoms and signs of androgen deficiency.[a] 2. Measure a serum luteinizing hormone (LH) and follicular stimulating hormone (FSH) in all men with testosterone deficiency. 3. Recommends a dual-energy x-ray absorptiometry scan for all men with testosterone deficiency. 4. Testosterone therapy indicated for androgen deficiency syndrome unless contraindications exist.[b]	1. Testosterone therapy options: a. Testosterone enanthate or cypionate 150–200 mg IM every 2 weeks b. Testosterone patch 5–10 mg qhs c. 1% testosterone gel 5–10 g daily d. Testosterone 30 mg to buccal mucosa q12h	http://www.guidelines.gov/content.aspx?id=16326

[a]Lethargy, easy fatigue, lack of stamina or endurance, reduced libido, mood changes, irritability, and loss of libido and motivation.

[b]Breast cancer (CA), prostate CA, hematocrit >50%, untreated severe obstructive sleep apnea, severe obstructive urinary symptoms, or uncontrolled heart failure.

ANXIETY

Disease Management	Organization	Date	Population	Recommendations	Comments	Source
Anxiety	NICE	2011	Adults	1. Recommends cognitive behavioral therapy for generalized anxiety disorder (GAD). 2. Recommends sertraline if drug treatment is needed. 3. If sertraline is ineffective, recommend a different selective serotonin reuptake inhibitor (SSRI) or selective noradrenergic reuptake inhibitor (SNRI). 4. Avoid long-term benzodiazepine use or antipsychotic therapy for GAD.		http://www.nice.org.uk/nicemedia/live/13314/52599/52599.pdf

APNEA						

Disease Management	Organization	Date	Population	Recommendations	Comments	Source

Apnea, Central Sleep (CSAS)	American Academy of Sleep Medicine	2012	Adults	• Primary CSAS
				  ○ Positive airway pressure therapy may be used to treat primary CSAS
				  ○ Limited evidence to support the use of acetazolamide for CSAS
				  ○ Zolpidem or triazolam may be used to treat CSAS if patients are not at high risk for respiratory depression
				• CSAS related to CHF
				  ○ Nocturnal oxygen therapy
				  ○ CPAP therapy targeted to normalize the apnea-hypopnea index
				• CSAS related to ESRD
				  ○ Options for therapy include CPAP, nocturnal oxygen, and bicarbonate buffer use during dialysis
						http://www.guideline.gov/content.aspx?id=35175

Apnea, Obstructive Sleep (OSA)	ACP	2013	Adults	• All overweight adults diagnosed with OSA should lose weight. • Recommends nocturnal CPAP (continuous positive airway pressure) therapy as first-line therapy for OSA. • Option to use mandibular advancement devices for those patients intolerant of CPAP.		http://www.guideline.gov/content.aspx?id=47136

ASCITES, DUE TO CIRRHOSIS

Disease Management	Organization	Date	Population	Recommendations	Comments	Source

Ascites, Due to Cirrhosis	AASLD	2013	Adults with cirrhosis	• Diagnostic paracentesis is recommended for all patients with new-onset ascites.
				• The routine use of platelets or fresh frozen plasma prior to a paracentesis is not recommended.
				  ○ Ascitic fluid analysis
				    ○ Cell count with differential
				    ○ Albumin
				    ○ Protein
				    ○ Bedside inoculation of aerobic and anaerobic culture bottles
				• Management of cirrhotic ascites
				  ○ Alcohol cessation
				  ○ <2 g sodium/day
				  ○ Oral furosemide and spironolactone in a 2:5 ratio
				  ○ Fluid restriction not necessary unless serum sodium <125 mmol/L
				  ○ All patients with cirrhosis and ascites should be considered for liver transplantation
				  ○ Avoid NSAIDs
				  ○ Cautious use of ACEI or ARB
				• Management of refractory cirrhotic ascites
				  ○ Avoid propranolol
				  ○ Avoid ACEI or ARB
				  ○ Consider use of oral midodrine
				  ○ Serial therapeutic paracenteses is a treatment option
				  ○ Transjugular intrahepatic portosystemic shunt (TIPSS) is a therapeutic option in carefully selected patients
				  ○ Albumin 6–8 g/L ascitic fluid removed indicated for large volume paracentesis >5 L.
				• Management of spontaneous bacterial peritonitis (SBP)
				  ○ Recommend cefotaxime 2 g IV q8h
				  ○ Alternative is ofloxacin 400 mg PO bid
				  ○ Add albumin 1.5 g/kg/day on day 1 and 1 g/kg/day on day 3 if creatinine >1 mg/dL, BUN >30 mg/dL, or bilirubin >4 mg/dL
				• SBP prophylaxis
				  ○ Cefotaxime or oral norfloxacin for 7 days in patients admitted for upper gastrointestinal bleed
				  ○ Long-term oral trimethoprim-sulfamethoxazole or norfloxacin for any patient with a history of SBP
				  ○ Consider SBP prophylaxis if ascitic fluid protein <1.5 g/dL in association with creatinine >1.2 mg/dL or sodium <130 mmol/L or bilirubin >3 mg/dL
				• Hepatorenal syndrome options for treatment:
				  ○ Midodrine + SQ Octreotide + albumin
				  ○ Norepinephrine infusion + albumin
				  ○ Referral for liver transplantation
				• Hepatic hydrothorax
				  ○ Chest tube is contraindicated
				  ○ Dietary sodium restriction and diuretics is first-line therapy
				  ○ TIPSS is an option for refractory cases
				• Avoid percutaneous gastrotomy tube placement in patients with ascites.
						http://www.guideline.gov/content.aspx?id=45103

Disease Management	Organization	Date	Population	Recommendations	Comments	Source
					ASTHMA	

Asthma	GINA ICSI	2012	Children age >5 y; adolescents, and adults	1. Recommend classification of asthma by level of control.
				2. Recommend a chest radiograph at the initial visit to exclude alternative diagnoses.
				3. Recommend assessing for tobacco use and strongly advise smokers to quit.
				4. Recommend spirometry with bronchodilators to determine the severity of airflow limitation and its reversibility.
				  a. Repeat spirometry at least every 1–2 y for asthma monitoring.
				5. Consider allergy testing for history of atopy, rhinitis, rhinorrhea, and seasonal variation or specific extrinsic triggers.
				6. Recommend an asthma action plan based on peak expiratory flow (PEF) monitoring for all patients.
				7. Recommend allergen and environmental trigger avoidance.
				8. Physicians should help educate patients, assist them in self-management, develop goals of treatment, create an asthma action plan, and regularly monitor asthma control.
				9. Asthma exacerbations should be treated with:
				  a. Corticosteroids
				    – Prednisolone 0.5–1 mg/kg PO daily or equivalent × 7 days for mild-moderate exacerbations
				    – Methylprednisolone 1 mg/kg IV q6h initially for severe exacerbations
				  b. Oxygen to keep SpO_2 >90%
				  c. Rapid-acting β-agonists
				  d. Ipratropium bromide
				  e. Consider bilevel positive airway pressure (Bi-PAP) for acute asthma exacerbations
				10. Develop a chronic medication regimen for patients adjusted based on their asthma action plan.
					1. Controlled asthma defined by:
					  a. Daytime symptoms ≤2×/week
					  b. No limitations of daily activities
					  c. No nocturnal symptoms
					  d. Need for reliever medicines ≤2×/week
					  e. Normal or near-normal lung function
					  f. No exacerbations
					2. Partially controlled asthma if:
					  a. Daytime symptoms >2×/week
					  b. Any limitations of daily activities or any nocturnal symptoms
					  c. Need for reliever medicines ≤2×/week
					  d. <80% predicted PEF or forced expiratory volume at 1 second (FEV_1)
					  e. Any exacerbations
					3. Uncontrolled asthma if there are ≥3 features of partially controlled asthma in any week.
					4. Risk factors for adverse asthma events:
					  a. Poor clinical control
					  b. Frequent asthma exacerbations
					  c. History of ICU admission for asthma exacerbation
					  d. FEV_1 <60% predicted
					  e. Exposure to cigarette smoke
					  f. Need for high-dose medications
					5. Recommend an inhaled corticosteroid for partially controlled or uncontrolled asthma.
					6. Add a long-acting β-agonist or leukotriene inhibitor for incomplete control with inhaled corticosteroid alone.
					7. Short-acting $β_2$-agonists should be used as needed for relief of acute asthma symptoms or 20 minutes prior to planned exertion in exercise-induced. Alternatives for exercise-induced asthma include a leukotriene inhibitor or cromolyn.
					8. For difficult-to-control asthma:
					  a. Treat potentially aggravating conditions: rhinitis, gastroesophageal reflux disease (GERD), nasal polyps
					  b. Consider alternative diagnoses: chronic obstructive pulmonary disease (COPD) or vocal cord dysfunction
						http://www.guidelines.gov/content.aspx?id=39409 http://www.guidelines.gov/content.aspx?id=38255

ATOPIC DERMATITIS

Disease Management	Organization	Date	Population	Recommendations	Comments	Source
Atopic Dermatitis (AD)	AAD	2014	Adults and children	1. Generous application of skin moisturizers after bathing. 2. Recommend limited use of hypoallergenic non-soap cleansers. 3. Consider wet-wrap therapy with topic corticosteroids for moderate-severe AD during flares. 4. Twice daily topical corticosteroids are the first-line therapy for AD. 5. Topical calcineurin inhibitors (tacrolimus or pimecrolimus) can be used for maintenance AD therapy. 6. Recommend against topical antihistamine therapy for AD. 7. Phototherapy is second-line treatment for refractory cases. 8. Consider systemic immunomodulating agents for severe cases refractory to topical agents and phototherapy.	Systemic immunomodulating agents that have been studied in AD are: azathioprine, cyclosporine, or methotrexate.	http://www.guideline.gov/content.aspx?id=48409 http://www.guideline.gov/content.aspx?id=48410

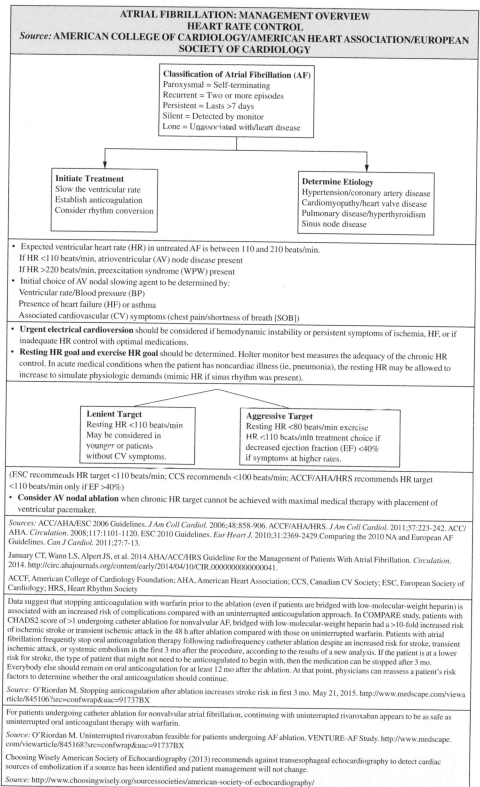

ATRIAL FIBRILLATION: MANAGEMENT OVERVIEW
HEART RATE CONTROL
Source: **AMERICAN COLLEGE OF CARDIOLOGY/AMERICAN HEART ASSOCIATION/EUROPEAN SOCIETY OF CARDIOLOGY**

Classification of Atrial Fibrillation (AF)
Paroxysmal = Self-terminating
Recurrent = Two or more episodes
Persistent = Lasts >7 days
Silent = Detected by monitor
Lone = Unassociated with heart disease

Initiate Treatment
Slow the ventricular rate
Establish anticoagulation
Consider rhythm conversion

Determine Etiology
Hypertension/coronary artery disease
Cardiomyopathy/heart valve disease
Pulmonary disease/hyperthyroidism
Sinus node disease

- Expected ventricular heart rate (HR) in untreated AF is between 110 and 210 beats/min.
  If HR <110 beats/min, atrioventricular (AV) node disease present
  If HR >220 beats/min, preexcitation syndrome (WPW) present
- Initial choice of AV nodal slowing agent to be determined by:
  Ventricular rate/Blood pressure (BP)
  Presence of heart failure (HF) or asthma
  Associated cardiovascular (CV) symptoms (chest pain/shortness of breath [SOB])

- **Urgent electrical cardioversion** should be considered if hemodynamic instability or persistent symptoms of ischemia, HF, or if inadequate HR control with optimal medications.
- **Resting HR goal and exercise HR goal** should be determined. Holter monitor best measures the adequacy of the chronic HR control. In acute medical conditions when the patient has noncardiac illness (ie, pneumonia), the resting HR may be allowed to increase to simulate physiologic demands (mimic HR if sinus rhythm was present).

Lenient Target
Resting HR <110 beats/min
May be considered in
younger or patients
without CV symptoms.

Aggressive Target
Resting HR <80 beats/min exercise
HR <110 beats/min treatment choice if
decreased ejection fraction (EF) <40%
if symptoms at higher rates.

(ESC recommends HR target <110 beats/min; CCS recommends <100 beats/min; ACCF/AHA/HRS recommends HR target <110 beats/min only if EF >40%)
- **Consider AV nodal ablation** when chronic HR target cannot be achieved with maximal medical therapy with placement of ventricular pacemaker.

Sources: ACC/AHA/ESC 2006 Guidelines. *J Am Coll Cardiol.* 2006;48:858-906. ACCF/AHA/HRS. *J Am Coll Cardiol.* 2011;57:223-242. ACC/AHA. *Circulation.* 2008;117:1101-1120. ESC 2010 Guidelines. *Eur Heart J.* 2010;31:2369-2429.Comparing the 2010 NA and European AF Guidelines. *Can J Cardiol.* 2011;27:7-13.

January CT, Wann LS, Alpert JS, et al. 2014 AHA/ACC/HRS Guideline for the Management of Patients With Atrial Fibrillation. *Circulation.* 2014. http://circ.ahajournals.org/content/early/2014/04/10/CIR.0000000000000041.

ACCF, American College of Cardiology Foundation; AHA, American Heart Association; CCS, Canadian CV Society; ESC, European Society of Cardiology; HRS, Heart Rhythm Society

Data suggest that stopping anticoagulation with warfarin prior to the ablation (even if patients are bridged with low-molecular-weight heparin) is associated with an increased risk of complications compared with an uninterrupted anticoagulation approach. In COMPARE study, patients with CHADS2 score of >1 undergoing catheter ablation for nonvalvular AF, bridged with low-molecular-weight heparin had a >10-fold increased risk of ischemic stroke or transient ischemic attack in the 48 h after ablation compared with those on uninterrupted warfarin. Patients with atrial fibrillation frequently stop oral anticoagulation therapy following radiofrequency catheter ablation despite an increased risk for stroke, transient ischemic attack, or systemic embolism in the first 3 mo after the procedure, according to the results of a new analysis. If the patient is at a lower risk for stroke, the type of patient that might not need to be anticoagulated to begin with, then the medication can be stopped after 3 mo. Everybody else should remain on oral anticoagulation for at least 12 mo after the ablation. At that point, physicians can reassess a patient's risk factors to determine whether the oral anticoagulation should continue.

Source: O'Riordan M. Stopping anticoagulation after ablation increases stroke risk in first 3 mo. May 21, 2015. http://www.medscape.com/viewarticle/845106?src=confwrap&uac=91737BX

For patients undergoing catheter ablation for nonvalvular atrial fibrillation, continuing with uninterrupted rivaroxaban appears to be as safe as uninterrupted oral anticoagulant therapy with warfarin.

Source: O'Riordan M. Uninterrupted rivaroxaban feasible for patients undergoing AF ablation. VENTURE-AF Study. http://www.medscape.com/viewarticle/845168?src=confwrap&uac=91737BX

Choosing Wisely American Society of Echocardiography (2013) recommends against transesophageal echocardiography to detect cardiac sources of embolization if a source has been identified and patient management will not change.

Source: http://www.choosingwisely.org/sourcessocieties/american-society-of-echocardiography/

2014 AHA/ACC/HRS GUIDELINES FOR PREVENTION OF THROMBOEMBOLISM IN PATIENTS WITH AF

- Antithrombotic therapy based on shared decision making, discussion of risks of stroke and bleeding, and patient's preferences
- Antithrombotic therapy selection based on risk of thromboembolism
- CHA_2DS_2-VASc score recommended to assess stroke risk
- Warfarin recommended with mechanical heart valves. Target INR intensity should be based on the type and location of prosthesis
- With prior stroke, TIA, or CHA_2DS_2-VASc score ≥2, oral anticoagulants are recommended. Options include warfarin or NOACs: dabigatran, rivaroxaban, or apixaban
- With warfarin, determine INR at least weekly during initiation and monthly when stable
- Direct thrombin or factor Xa inhibitor recommended, if unable to maintain therapeutic INR
- Reevaluate the need for anticoagulation at periodic intervals
- Bridging therapy with LMWH or UFH recommended with a mechanical heart valve if warfarin is interrupted. Bridging therapy should balance risks of stroke and bleeding
- Without a mechanical heart valve, bridging therapy decisions should balance stroke and bleeding risks against the duration of time patient will not be anticoagulated
- Evaluate renal function prior to initiation of direct thrombin or factor Xa inhibitors, and reevaluate when clinically indicated and at least annually
- For atrial flutter, antithrombotic therapy is recommended as for AF

Adapted from January CT, Wann LS, Alpert JS, et al. 2014 AHA/ACC/HRS guideline for the management of patients with atrial fibrillation. *Circulation*. 2014. http://circ.ahajournals.org/content/early/2014/04/10/CIR.0000000000000041.

ATRIAL FIBRILLATION: NONVALVULAR NEW ORAL ANTICOAGULATION AGENTS EUROPEAN HEART RHYTHM EXECUTIVE SUMMARY 2013 EUROPEAN SOCIETY OF CARDIOLOGY 2012 AMERICAN HEART ASSOCIATION AND AMERICAN STROKE ASSOCIATION 2012

- New oral anticoagulation agents (NOAC) are alternative agents to the use of warfarin.
- *Quantitative* indicators of the function **are not clinically available** for direct thrombin inhibitors (DTI) or factor X inhibitors (FXa).
- *Qualitative* indicators of the *presence* for DTI agent (dabigatran) and FXa inhibitors (rivaroxaban and apixaban) are available.
    - Activated partial thromboplastin time (aPTT) is a measure of DTI presence.
    - Prothrombin time (PT) is a measure of FXa inhibitor presence.
- Drug interactions with NOAC agents are generally less than with warfarin but still need to be considered.
- Rivaroxaban should be taken with food to optimize absorption and bioavailability. No other NOAC agents are influenced to food ingestion.
- No interaction is noted between NOAC agents and proton pump inhibitor (PPI) agents and H_2 blockers exist.
- All NOAC agents require dose reduction with renal dysfunction.
- NOAC agents have a short action of duration of 12 to 24 hours and therefore should be avoided in patients with poor medicine adherence.
- No specific antidotes for NOAC agents exist.
    - If no bleeding, hold subsequent doses and observe.
    - If clinical bleeding noted expert opinion suggests the use of prothrombin complex concentrates (PCC) 25 U/kg is recommended.
- Preoperatively with normal renal function should hold NOAC agent ≥24 h before surgery with minor bleeding risk expected; hold ≥48 h with major bleeding risk.
- NOAC agents have demonstrated noninferiority to warfarin with less ICH. However, no head-to-head trials are available. May consider newer agents if: difficult-to-control international normalized ratio (INR) resistance in obtaining frequent INR levels, no renal disease present and good adherence as newer agents have a short half-life. The European and Canadian Guidelines favor use of the newer agents, whereas the ACCF/AHA/HRS reports no preference.

Sources: Heidbuchel H, Verhamme P, Alings M, et al. EHRA Practice Guide on the use of new oral anticoagulants in patients with nonvalvular atrial fibrillation: executive summary. *Eur Heart J.* 2013;34:2094-2106. Furie KL, Goldstein LB, Albers GW, et al; American Heart Association Stroke Council; Council on Quality of Care and Outcomes Research; Council on Cardiovascular Nursing; Council on Clinical Cardiology; Council on Peripheral Vascular Disease. Oral antithrombotic agents for the prevention of stroke in nonvalvular atrial fibrillation: a science advisory for healthcare professionals from the American Heart Association/American Stroke Association. *Stroke.* 2012;43:3442-3453. Gonsalves WI, Pruthi RK, Patnaik MM. The new oral anticoagulants in clinical practice. *Mayo Clin Proc.* 2013;88:495-511. Camm AJ, Lip GY, De Caterina R, et al; ESC Committee for Practice Guidelines, et al. 2012 focused update of the ESC Guidelines for the management of atrial fibrillation: an update of the 2010 ESC Guidelines for the management of atrial fibrillation. Developed with the special contribution of the European Heart Rhythm Association. *Eur Heart J.* 2012;33:2719-2747.

DABIGATRAN ETEXILATE (PRADAXA®)

- Direct thrombin inhibitor
- Dosage:
  - 150 mg 1 tab bid (ClCr >50 mL/min)
  - 75 mg 1 tab bid (ClCr 15–30 mL/min)
  - Not recommended in end-stage CKD on or not on dialysis
- Pharmacokinetics/pharmacodynamics: Cytochrome P450 metabolism: none; half-life: 12 to 14 h; renal elimination: 80%
- ACC/AHA recommends it as a useful alternative to warfarin in patients who have nonvalvular AF and do not have severe renal and liver disease.
- ESC recommends it in patients with nonvalvular AF with at least one moderate risk factor.
- RE-LY Trial (150 mg bid)—similar reduction in stroke and systemic embolism vs warfarin (2.07% vs 2.78% per year). Increased GI bleeds compared to warfarin, especially in patients ≥75 y old.
- By FDA 12/2012, risk of bleeding did not appear to be higher in patients with new use of dabigatran compared to new use of warfarin.
- **Switching patients from warfarin to dabigatran**, discontinue warfarin and start dabigatran when the INR is <2.0.
- **Switching patients from dabigatran to warfarin**, adjust the starting time of warfarin based on creatinine clearance as follows:
  - For CrCl ≥50 mL/min, start warfarin 3 days before discontinuing dabigatran.
  - For CrCl 30–50 mL/min, start warfarin 2 days before discontinuing dabigatran.
  - For CrCl 15–30 mL/min, start warfarin 1 day before discontinuing dabigatran.
- **Converting from/to parenteral anticoagulants**:
  - For patients currently receiving a parenteral anticoagulant, start dabigatran 0 to 2 h before the time that the next dose of parenteral drug was to have been administered or at the time of discontinuation of a continuously administered parenteral drug (eg, intravenous unfractionated heparin).
  - For patients currently taking dabigatran, wait 12 h (CrCl ≥30 mL/min) or 24 h (CrCl <30 mL/min) after the last dose of dabigatran, before initiating treatment with a parenteral anticoagulant.
- If possible, **discontinue dabigatran 1 to 2 days (CrCl ≥50 mL/min) or 3 to 5 days (CrCl <50 mL/min) before invasive or surgical procedures.** Consider longer times for patients undergoing major surgery, spinal puncture, or placement of a spinal or epidural catheter or port, in whom complete hemostasis may be required. Restart as soon as possible.
- Discontinuation on Pradaxa without adequate continuous anticoagulation increases the risk of stroke.
- To measure adherence for dabigatran, measure thrombin level. If low, the patient is not taking the medicine.
- Idarucizumab, an investigational fully humanized antibody fragment (FAB) intended to be used as an antidote for dabigatran etexilate mesylate, currently undergoing a phase 3 study RE-VERSE AD.

Source: http://www.medscape.com/viewarticle/827433

+ (XARELTO®)

- Direct factor X_a inhibitor
- FDA indication: Nonvalvular AF, DVT, PE.
- Dosage in nonvalvular AF:
  - 20 mg 1 tab qhs with meal (CrCl >50 mL/min)
  - 15 mg 1 tab qhs with meal (CrCl 15–50 mL/min)
  - Not recommended in end-stage CKD on or not on dialysis
- Pharmacokinetics/pharmacodynamics: Cytochrome P450 metabolism: 32%; half-life: 9 to 13 h; renal elimination: 33%
- ROCKET AF trial: Noninferior to warfarin regarding prevention of stroke and systemic embolism. No reduction in rates of mortality or ischemic stroke, but a significant reduction in hemorrhagic stroke and intracranial hemorrhage. Compared to warfarin it was nonsignificantly different in nonmajor bleeding; had significant reduction in fatal bleeding but increased GI bleeding and bleeds requiring transfusion.
- 5 phase III trials dabigatran vs warfarin: Patients with major bleeding on dabigatran required more red cell transfusions but received less plasma, required a shorter stay in ICU, and had a trend to lower mortality compared with those who had major bleeding on warfarin.
- Switching from warfarin to rivaroxaban: Discontinue warfarin and start XARELTO as soon as INR <3.
- **Switching from rivaroxaban to warfarin:** No clinical trial data are available to guide converting patients. Company recommends to d/c rivaroxaban and begin both a parenteral anticoagulant and warfarin at the time the next dose of rivaroxaban would be taken.
- **Rivaroxaban should be stopped at least 24 h before surgeries** or other invasive procedures and should be resumed as soon as possible. If oral medication cannot be taken, consider administering a parenteral anticoagulant.
- Premature discontinuation of rivaroxaban increases the risk of stroke.
- To measure adherence for rivaroxaban, measure factor Xa activity. If low, the patient is not taking the medicine.

Andexanet alfa = an antidote to the factor Xa inhibitor, ANNEXA-R trial, awaiting results of phase 3 summer 2015.
Source: http://www.annalsoflongtermcare.com/content/rivaroxaban-reversal-agent-safe-and-effective-trial-finds-potential-universal-antidote

APIXABAN (ELIQUIS®)

- Direct factor X_a inhibitor
- Indication: Nonvalvular AF, DVT prophylaxis after hip or knee replacement surgery.
- Dosage:
  - 5 mg 1 tab bid
  - 2.5 mg 1 tab bid on patients ≥80 y old, weight ≤60 kg, Cr ≥1.5 mg/dL or patients taking P450 and P-glycoprotein inhibitors
  - Not recommended in severe CKD or end-stage CKD on or not-on dialysis
  - Avoid concomitant use of rivaroxaban with strong CYP3A4 inhibitors and combined P-gp.
- Pharmacokinetics/pharmacodynamics: Cytochrome P450 metabolism: 15%; half-life: 8 to 15 h; renal elimination: 40%.
- AVERROES trial: Apixaban was superior in preventing stroke vs ASA in patients who could not tolerate/were intolerant to warfarin.
- ARISTOTLE trial: Apixaban was superior to warfarin in reducing stroke or systemic embolism by 21%. Also 31% reduction in major bleeding and 11% reduction in all-cause mortality (not CV). Rates of hemorrhagic stroke and ISH (but not ischemic stroke) were lower in apixaban group. GI bleeding was similar in both groups. Apixaban was better tolerated than warfarin with slightly fewer discontinuations.
- **Switching from warfarin to apixaban**: Warfarin should be discontinued and apixaban started when INR <2.
- **Switching from apixaban to warfarin**: Discontinue apixaban and begin both a parenteral anticoagulant and warfarin at the time the next dose of apixaban would have been taken, discontinuing the parenteral anticoagulant when INR reaches an acceptable range.
- **Discontinue apixaban at least 48 h prior to elective surgeries** or invasive procedures with high risk of bleeding and 24 h prior to invasive procedures with low risk of bleeding. Bridging is not generally required. Resume after surgery as soon as possible.
- Premature discontinuation of apixaban has increased risk of thrombotic events.
- To measure adherence for apixaban, measure factor Xa activity. If low, the patient is not taking the medicine.

Andexanet alfa = an antidote to the factor Xa inhibitor, ANNEXA-A Study, currently seeking approval to FDA.
http://www.medscape.com/viewarticle/832648
Sources: January CT, Wann LS, Alpert JS, et al. 2014 AHA/ACC/HRS Guideline for the Management of Patients With Atrial Fibrillation. *Circulation.* 2014. http://circ.ahajournals.org/content/early/2014/04/10/CIR.0000000000000041.
Ruff CR, Giugliano RP. *Hot topics in cardiology.* 2010;4:7-14.
Ericksson BI, et al. *Clin Pharmacokinet.* 2009;48:1-22.
Ruff CR, et al. *Am Heart J.* 2010;160:635-641
www.pradaxa.com
www.xarelto-us.com
www.eliquis.com

EDOXABAN (SAVAYSA®)

- Factor X_a inhibitor
- FDA indication: nonvalvular AF, DVT, PE
- Dosage in non-valvular AF:
  - 60 mg once daily in patients with CrCl >50 to ≤95 mL/min (CrCl with Cockcroft–Gault equation)
  - 30 mg daily in patients with CrCl 15 to 50 mL/min
  - Do not use in patients with CrCl >95 mL/min because of increased risk of ischemic stroke compared to warfarin
  - Not recommended in patients with moderate or severe hepatic impairment (Child–Pugh B and C)
- Contraindications: active pathological bleeding.
- There is no established way to reverse the anticoagulant effects of edoxaban, which can be expected to persist for approximately 24 h after the last dose. The anticoagulant effect of edoxaban cannot be reliably monitored with standard laboratory testing. Hemodialysis does not significantly contribute to edoxaban clearance.
- Epidural or spinal hematomas may occur in patients treated with edoxaban who are receiving neuroaxial anesthesia or undergoing spinal puncture.
- Concomitant use of drugs affecting hemostasis may increase the risk of bleeding. These include aspirin and other antiplatelet agents, other anti-thrombotic agents, fibrinolytic therapy, and chronic use of nonsteroidal anti-inflammatory drugs.
- Pharmacokinetics/pharmacodynamics: peak plasma concentration: 1 to 2 h, half-life: 10–14 h; Renal elimination: 50%. Steady-state concentrations are achieved in 3 days.
- **The ENGAGE AF-TIMI 48 Study:** The median study drug exposure for the edoxaban and warfarin treatment groups was 2.5 y. Bleeding led to treatment discontinuation in 3.9% and 4.1% of patients in the edoxaban 60 mg and warfarin treatment groups, respectively. Treatment arms of edoxaban were noninferior to warfarin for the primary efficacy endpoint of stroke or systemic embolism. However, the 30 mg (15 mg dose-reduced) treatment arm was numerically less effective than warfarin for the primary endpoint, and was also markedly inferior in reducing the rate of ischemic stroke. Approximately half of the edoxaban dose is eliminated by the kidney, and edoxaban blood levels are lower in patients with better renal function, averaging about 30% less in patients with CrCl of >80 mL/min, and 40% less in patients with CrCl >95 mL/min when compared to patients with a CrCl of >50 to ≤80 mL/min. Given the clear relationship of dose and blood levels to effectiveness in the ENGAGE AF-TIMI 48 study, it could be anticipated that patients with better renal function would show a smaller effect of edoxaban compared to warfarin than would patients with mildly impaired renal function, and this was in fact observed.
- **Switching to Edoxaban**
  - **Switching patients from warfarin to edoxaban:** Discontinue warfarin and start edoxaban when INR ≤2.5.
  - **Switching patients from OAC other than warfarin or other VKA:** Discontinue the current oral anticoagulant and start edoxaban at the time of the next scheduled dose of the other oral anticoagulant.
  - **Switching patients from LMWH to edoxaban:** Discontinue LMWH and start edoxaban at the time of the next scheduled administration of LMWH.
  - **Switching patients from unfractionated heparin to edoxaban:** Discontinue the infusion and start edoxaban 4 h later.
- **Switching from Edoxaban:**
  - **Switching patients from edoxaban to warfarin:**
    ORAL For patients taking 60 mg of edoxaban reduce the dose to 30 mg and begin warfarin concomitantly. For patients receiving 30 mg of edoxaban, reduce the dose to 15 mg and begin warfarin concomitantly. INR must be measured at least weekly and just prior to the daily dose of edoxaban to minimize the influence of edoxaban on INR measurements. Once a stable INR ≥2.0 is achieved, edoxaban should be discontinued and the warfarin continued.
    PARENTERAL Discontinue edoxaban and administer a parenteral anticoagulant and warfarin at the time of the next scheduled edoxaban dose. Once a stable INR ≥2.0 is achieved the parenteral anticoagulant should be discontinued and the warfarin continued.
  - **Switching patients from edoxaban to non-VKA anticoagulants:** Discontinue edoxaban and start the other oral anticoagulant at the time of the next dose of edoxaban.
  - **Switching patients from edoxaban to parenteral anticoagulants:** Discontinue edoxaban and start the parenteral anticoagulant at the time of the next dose of edoxaban.
- If possible, discontinue edoxaban at least 24 h before invasive or surgical procedures because of the risk of bleeding. It can be restarted after the surgical or other procedure as soon as adequate hemostasis has been established noting that the time to onset of pharmacodynamic effect is 1 to 2 h. Administer a parenteral anticoagulant and then switch to oral edoxaban, if oral medication cannot be taken during or after surgical intervention.
- Discontinuation of edoxaban without adequate continuous anticoagulation increases the risk of stroke.

Source: http://www.savaysa.com/.

NOAC COMPARISON CHART					
	Warfarin	**Dabigatran**	**Rivaroxaban**	**Apixaban**	**Edoxaban**
Molecular target	Vitamin-dependent clotting factor	Thrombin	Factor X_a	Factor X_a	Factor X_a
Dosing in AF	Once daily	Twice daily	Once daily	Twice daily	Once daily
Time to peak plasma concentration (min)	240	85–150	30–180	30–120	30–60
Time to peak effect (h)	96–120	2	2–3	1–2	1–2
Half-life (h)	40	14–17	5–9 (increased to 11–13 in elderly)	8–15	9–11
Renal clearance	<1%	80%	33%	25%	35%
Hepatic excretion		20%	66%	75% (Hepatic-biliary-intestinal)	65%
Food and drug interactions	Foods rich in vitamin K, substrates of CYP2C9, CYP3A4, and CYP1A2	Strong P-gp inhibitors and inducers	Strong CYP3A4 inducers, strong inhibitors of both CYP3A4 and P-gp	Strong inhibitors and inducers of CYP3A4 and P-gp	Strong P-gp inhibitors
Creatinine clearance below which drug is contraindicated	n/a	<30 mL/min	<15 mL/min	<15 mL/min	<30 mL/min (Japan)

Sources: Lip et al. *J Intern Med.* 2015.
Lau YC, Lip GY. Which drug should we use for stroke prevention in atrial fibrillation? *Curr Opin Cardiol.* 2014 Jul;29(4):293–300.

ANTITHROMBOTIC STRATEGIES FOLLOWING CORONARY ARTERY STENTING IN PATIENTS WITH AF AT MODERATE TO HIGH THROMBOEMBOLIC RISK (IN WHOM ORAL ANTICOAGULATION THERAPY IS REQUIRED)

Hemorrhagic Risk	Clinical Setting	Stent Implanted	Anticoagulation Regimen
Low or intermediate (eg, HAS-BLED score 0–2)	Elective	Bare metal	1 mo: triple therapy of VKA (INR 2.0–2.5) + aspirin ≤100 mg/d + clopidogrel 75 mg/d (or aspirin 100 mg/d). Up to 12th mo: combination of VKA (INR 2.0–2.5) + clopidogrel 75 mg/d[b] Lifelong: VKA (INR 2.0–3.0) alone
	Elective	Drug eluting	3 (–olimus[a] group) to 6 (paclitaxel) mo: triple therapy of VKA (INR 2.0–2.5) + aspirin ≤100 mg/d + clopidogrel 75 mg/d. Up to 12th mo: combination of VKA (INR 2.0–2.5) + clopidogrel 75 mg/day[b] (or aspirin 100 mg/d). Lifelong: VKA (INR 2.0–3.0) alone
	ACS	Bare metal/drug eluting	6 mo: triple therapy of VKA (INR 2.0–2.5) + aspirin ≤100 mg/d + clopidogrel 75 mg/d. Up to 12th mo: combination of VKA (INR 2.0–2.5) + clopidogrel 75 mg/d[b] (or aspirin 100 mg/d). Lifelong: VKA (INR 2.0–3.0) alone
High (eg, HAS-BLED score ≥3)	Elective	Bare metal[c]	2–4 wk: triple therapy of VKA (INR 2.0–2.5) + aspirin ≤100 mg/d + clopidogrel 75 mg/d. Lifelong: VKA (INR 2.0–3.0) alone
	ACS	Bare metal[c]	4 wk: triple therapy of VKA (INR 2.0–2.5) + aspirin ≤100 mg/day + clopidogrel 75 mg/d. Up to 12th mo: combination of VKA (INR 2.0–2.5) + clopidogrel 75 mg/d[b] (or aspirin 100 mg/d). Lifelong: VKA (INR 2.0–3.0) alone

ACS, acute coronary syndrome; AF, atrial fibrillation; INR, international normalized ratio; VKA, vitamin K antagonist. Gastric protection with a proton pump inhibitor (PPI) should be considered where necessary.
[a]Sirolimus, everolimus, and tacrolimus.
[b]Combination of VKA (INR 2.0–3.0) + aspirin ≤100 mg/d (with PPI, if indicated) may be considered as an alternative.
[c]Drug-eluting stents should be avoided as far as possible, but, if used, consideration of more prolonged (3–6 mo) triple antithrombotic therapy is necessary.
Adapted from Lip GY, Huber K, Andreotti F, et al; European Society of Cardiology Working Group on Thrombosis. Management of antithrombotic therapy in atrial fibrillation patients presenting with acute coronary syndrome and/or undergoing percutaneous coronary intervention/stent. *Thromb Haemost.* 2010;103:13-28.

ATRIAL FIBRILLATION: MANAGEMENT, RHYTHM CONTROL DRUG NONPHARMACOLOGIC THERAPY
Source: AMERICAN COLLEGE OF CARDIOLOGY/AMERICAN HEART ASSOCIATION/EUROPEAN SOCIETY OF CARDIOLOGY

- **AFFIRM, RACE, PIAF,** and **STAF** Trials found no difference in quality of life between rate and rhythm control in atrial fibrillation (AF). The AFFIRM and RACE Trials demonstrated no difference in stroke rate or mortality between rate and rhythm control in AF.

Favors Rate Control	vs	**Favors Rhythm Control**
Asymptomatic in AF		Continued symptoms in AF
Older patients		Younger patients
Advanced heart disease		LONE or minimal heart disease
Comorbid conditions		Few comorbid conditions
Persistent AF		Recent onset/paroxysmal AF

- **Rhythm control**
  Fifty percent of patients with new-onset AF spontaneously convert to sinus in 48 h.
- **2, 3, 4 Cardioversion rule**
  - New-onset AF <**2 days** in duration—may be considered for acute electrical or drug conversion to sinus rhythm while on heparin.
  - Onset of AF >**2 days** or of unknown duration—requires either **3 weeks** of therapeutic oral anticoagulation (INR 2–3) or a negative transesophageal echocardiogram (TEE) to exclude clot before conversion while on heparin should be considered.
  - In either approach to conversion, oral anticoagulation (OAC) must be continued at least **4 weeks** postconversion because of the possibility of delayed return of atrial contraction and clot release. In high-risk patients, lifelong OAC should be considered.
- (LONE, no associated disease; HTN, hypertension; CAD, coronary artery disease; HF, heart failure; LVH, left ventricular hypertrophy.)
- FDA Warning 2011: Dronedarone should not be used in chronic atrial fibrillation; it doubles rate of cardiovascular (CV) death, stroke, and HF.
- **Nonpharmacologic approach:**
- AF catheter ablation/MAZE procedure (open surgical approach)
  Consider if antiarrhythmic drug therapy fails or if AF coexists with preexcitation pathway. AF ablation is more effective in younger patients with paroxysmal AF; catheter ablation maintains sinus rhythm approximately 80% as opposed to approximately 40% with drugs at 5 y. May require repeat procedures (average: 1.8 procedures).
  Long-term anticoagulation should be continued even after successful ablation in patients at high risk for thromboembolism. In low-embolic-risk patients, warfarin may be converted to aspirin (ASA) therapy after 3 mo. (*J Am Coll Cardiol.* 2010;55:735-743)
- Consider MAZE procedure if performing open heart surgery for other reasons or if vascular or cardiac anatomy prevents the less-invasive catheter approach.
- Consider implantable atrial defibrillators: least commonly used treatment.
- **Prevention of atrial remodeling**
  - Calcium channel blockers
  - Angiotensin-converting enzyme (ACE) inhibitors
  - Angiotensin receptor blocker (ARB) agents
  - Statins

Sources: ACC/AHA/ESC 2006 Guidelines. *J Am Coll Cardiol.* 2006;48:858-906. ACCF/AHA/HRS. *J Am Coll Cardiol.* 2011;57:223-242. ACC/AHA. *Circulation.* 2008;117:1101-1120. ESC 2010 Guidelines. *Eur Heart J.* 2010;31:2369-2429. *Circulation.* 2009;119:606-618. January CT, Wann LS, Alpert JS, et al. 2014 AHA/ACC/HRS Guideline for the Management of Patients With Atrial Fibrillation. *Circulation.* 2014. http://circ.ahajournals.org/content/early/2014/04/10/CIR.0000000000000041.

STRATEGIES FOR RHYTHM CONTROL IN PATIENTS WITH PAROXYSMAL[a] AND PERSISTENT AF[b] FROM 2014 AHA/ACC/HRS GUIDELINE FOR THE MANAGEMENT OF PATIENTS WITH ATRIAL FIBRILLATION

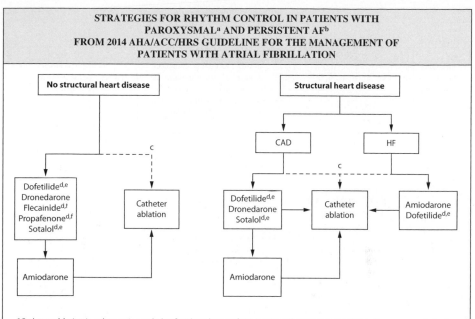

[a]Catheter ablation is only recommended as first-line therapy for patients with paroxysmal AF (Class IIa recommendation).
[b]Drugs are listed alphabetically.
[c]Depending on patient preference when performed in experienced centers.
[d]Not recommended with severe LVH (wall thickness >1.5 cm).
[e]Should be used with caution in patients at risk for torsades de pointes ventricular tachycardia.
[f]Should be combined with AV nodal blocking agents. AF indicates atrial fibrillation; CAD, coronary artery disease; HF, heart failure; and LVH, left ventricular hypertrophy.
Source: January CT, Wann LS, Alpert JS et al. *Circulation*. 2014 http://circ.ahajournals.org/content/early/2014/04/10/cir.0000000000000041

HEART RHYTHM SOCIETY

Disease Management	Organization	Date	Population	Recommendations	Comments	Source
Atrial Fibrillation	Heart Rhythmn Society	2014		Recommends against use of Class Ic antiarrhythmic drugs (Vaughan–Williams) as a first-line agent for the maintenance of sinus rhythm in patients with ischemic heart disease who have experienced prior MI.		http://www. choosingwisely.org/ societies/heart-rhythm-society/

HAS-BLED BLEEDING RISK SCORE FOR WARFARIN THERAPY

Letter	Clinical Characteristics	Points Awarded
H	**Hypertension** (systolic blood pressure [SBP] >160 mm Hg)	1
A	**Abnormal renal function** (presence of chronic dialysis or renal transplantation or serum creatinine ≥2.6 mg/mL μmol/L) and abnormal liver function (chronic hepatic disease or biochemical evidence of significant hepatic derangement (bilirubin >2× upper limit of normal, in association with glutamic-oxaloacetic transaminase [GOT]/glutamic-pyruvic transaminase [GPT] >3× upper limit normal) *1 point each*	1 or 2
S	**Stroke**	1
B	**Bleeding** (previous bleeding history and/or predisposition to bleeding, eg, bleeding diathesis, anemia)	1
L	**Labile INRs** (unstable/high INRs or poor time in therapeutic range, eg, <60%)	1
E	**Elderly** (age >65 y)	1
D	**Drugs or alcohol** (concomitant use of drugs such as antiplatelet agents, nonsteroidal antiinflammatory drugs, or alcohol abuse) *1 point each*	1 or 2
		Maximum 9 points

Interpretation

The risk of (spontaneous) major bleeding (intracranial, hospitalization, hemoglobin decrease 2 g/L, and/or transfusion) within 1 y in patients with atrial fibrillation enrolled in the Euro Heart Survey, expressed as bleeds per 100 patient-years:
- score 0:1.13
- score 1:1.02
- score 2:1.88
- score 3:3.74
- score 4:8.70
- score 5:12.50
- score 6–9: insufficient data to quantify risk

Information adapted from:
– 2010 Guidelines for the management of atrial fibrillation. *Eur Heart J.* 2010;31:2369-2429; Table 10.
– Pisters R, Lane DA, Nieuwlaat R, de Vos CB, Crijns HJ, Lip GY. A novel user-friendly score (HAS-BLED) to assess 1-y risk of major bleeding in atrial fibrillation patients: the Euro Heart Survey. *Chest.* 2010;138:1093-1100; Table 5.

THROMBOEMBOLIC RISK SCORES IN NONVALVULAR ATRIAL FIBRILLATION

	CHADS$_2$	Points	CHA$_2$DS$_2$-VASc	Points
C	Congestive heart failure	1	Congestive heart failure (**or *left ventricular systolic dysfunction [LVEF] ≤40%***)	1
H	Hypertension (blood pressure [BP] consistently >140/90 mm Hg or treated hypertension [HTN] on medication)	1	Hypertension (BP consistently >140/90 mm Hg or treated HTN on medication)	1
A	Age ≥75 y	1	Age ≥75 y	2
D	Diabetes mellitus	1	Diabetes mellitus	1
S$_2$	Prior stroke or transient ischemic attack (TIA)	2	Prior stroke or TIA or ***thromboembolism***	2
V			*Vascular disease (eg, coronary artery disease, peripheral artery disease, myocardial infarction [MI], aortic plaque)*	1
A			*Age 65–74 years*	1
Sc			*Sex category (ie, female gender)*	1
Max.		6		9

STROKE RISK STRATIFICATION WITH THE CHADS$_2$ AND CHA$_2$DS$_2$-VASC SCORES

	Adjusted stroke rate (% per year)
CHADS$_2$ acronym[a]	
0	1.9%
1	2.8%
2	4.0%
3	5.9%
4	8.5%
5	12.5%
6	18.2%
CHA$_2$DS$_2$-VAS$_c$ acronym[b]	
0	0%
1	1.3%
2	2.2%
3	3.2%
4	4.0%
5	6.7%
6	9.8%
7	9.6%
8	6.7%
9	15.20%

RISK FACTORS FOR STROKE AND THROMBOEMBOLISM IN NONVALVULAR AF

"Major" Risk Factors	"Clinically Relevant Nonmajor" Risk Factors
Previous • Stroke • TIA • Systemic embolism • Age ≥75 y	• Heart failure or moderate-to-severe left ventricular (LV) systolic dysfunction (LVEF ≤40%) • Hypertension • Diabetes mellitus • Female sex • Age 65–74 y • Vascular disease

Information adapted from:
– 2010 Guidelines for the management of atrial fibrillation. *Eur Heart J.* 2010;31:2369-2429; Tables 8(a) and (b).
– Gage BF, Waterman AD, Shannon W, Boechler M, Rich MW, Radford MJ. Validation of clinical classification schemes for predicting stroke. Results from the National Registry of Atrial Fibrillation. *JAMA.* 2001;285:2864-2870.

ATTENTION-DEFICIT HYPERACTIVITY DISORDER (ADHD)

Disease Management	Organization	Date	Population	Recommendations	Comments	Source
Attention-Deficit Hyperactivity Disorder (ADHD)	AAP	2011	Children 4–18 y old	• Initiate an evaluation for ADHD in any child who presents with academic or behavioral problems and symptoms of inattention, hyperactivity, or impulsivity. • Consider children with ADHD as children with special health care needs. • For children age 4–5 y, parent- or teacher-administered behavior therapy is the treatment of choice. • Methylphenidate is reserved for severe refractory cases. • For children ages 6–18 y, first-line treatment is with FDA-approved medications for ADHD ± behavior therapy.	• Essential to assess any child with ADHD for concomitant emotional, behavioral, developmental, or physical conditions (eg, mood disorders, tic disorders, seizures, sleep disorders, learning disabilities, or disruptive behavioral disorders). • For children 6–18 y, evidence is best to support stimulant medications and less strong to support atomoxetine, ER guanfacine, and ER clonidine for ADHD.	http://pediatrics.aappublications.org/content/early/2011/10/14/peds.2011-2654.full.pdf

	NICE	2013	Children, young adults, and adults	• Health care and education professionals require training to better address the needs of people with ADHD.
				• Recommend against universal screening for ADHD in nursery, primary, and secondary schools.
				• A diagnosis of ADHD should only be made by a specialist psychiatrist, pediatrician, or other appropriately qualified health care professional with training and expertise in the diagnosis of ADHD.
				• Health care professionals should stress the value of a balanced diet, good nutrition, and regular exercise for children, young people, and adults with ADHD.
				• Drug treatment is not recommended for preschool children with ADHD.
				• Drug treatment is not indicated as the first-line treatment for all school-age children and young people with ADHD. It should be reserved for those with severe symptoms and impairment or for those with moderate levels of impairment who have refused nondrug interventions.
				• Where drug treatment is considered appropriate, methylphenidate, atomoxetine, and dexamfetamine are recommended, within their licensed indications, as options for the management of ADHD in children and adolescents.
				• For adults with ADHD, drug treatment should be the first-line treatment.
				  ○ Following a decision to start drug treatment in adults with ADHD, methylphenidate should normally be tried first.
				  ○ Atomoxetine or dexamfetamine should be considered in adults unresponsive or intolerant to an adequate trial of methylphenidate.
						http://www.guideline.gov/content.aspx?id=14325

AUTISM

Disease Management	Organization	Date	Population	Recommendations	Comments	Source

Autism	NICE	2011	Children and young adults	• Consider autism for regression in language or social skills in children <3 y.
				• Clinical signs of possible autism have to be seen in the context of a child's overall development, and cultural variation may pertain.
				• An autism evaluation by a specialist is indicated for any of the following signs of possible autism:
				  ○ Language delay
				  ○ Regression in speech
				  ○ Echolalia
				  ○ Unusual vocalizations or intonations
				  ○ Reduced social smiling
				  ○ Rejection of cuddles by family
				  ○ Reduced response to name being called
				  ○ Intolerance of others entering into their personal space
				  ○ Reduced social interest in people or social play
				  ○ Reduced eye contact
				  ○ Reduced imagination
				  ○ Repetitive movements like body rocking
				  ○ Desire for unchanged routines
				  ○ Immature social and emotional development
					• Differential diagnosis of autism includes:
					  ○ Neurodevelopmental disorders
					  ○ Mood disorders
					  ○ ADHD
					  ○ Oppositional defiant disorder
					  ○ Conduct disorder
					  ○ Obsessive-compulsive disorder (OCD)
					  ○ Rett syndrome
					  ○ Hearing or vision impairment
					  ○ Selective mutism
						http://www.nice.org.uk/nicemedia/live/13572/56428/56428.pdf

	Cochrane database of systematic reviews	2014		• Recommend against chelation therapy for autism spectrum disorders.		http://www.cochrane.org/CD010766/BEHAV_chelation-for-autism-spectrum-disorder-asd

AUTISM SPECTRUM DISORDERS (ASD)

Disease Management	Organization	Date	Population	Recommendations	Comments	Source

Autism Spectrum Disorders (ASD)	American College of Medical Genetics and Genomics	2013	Children with autism spectrum disorders	• Every child with an ASD should have a medical home.
				• A genetic consultation should be offered to all patients with an ASD and their families.
				• Three-generation family history with pedigree analysis.
				• Initial evaluation to identify known syndromes or associated conditions
				  ○ Examination with special attention to dysmorphic features
				  ○ If specific syndromic diagnosis is suspected, proceed with targeted testing
				  ○ If appropriate clinical indicators present, perform metabolic and/or mitochondrial testing (alternatively, consider a referral to a metabolic specialist)
				  ○ Chromosomal microarray: oligonucleotide array-comparative genomic hybridization or single-nucleotide polymorphism array
				  ○ Deoxyribonucleic acid (DNA) testing for fragile X (to be performed routinely for male patients only)
				• *Methyl-CPG-binding protein 2 (MECP2)* sequencing to be performed for all females with autism spectrum disorders (ASDs).
				• *MECP2* duplication testing in males, if phenotype is suggestive.
				• *Phosphatase and tensin homolog (PTEN)* testing only if the head circumference is >2.5 standard deviation (SD) above the mean.
						http://www.guideline.gov/content.aspx?id=47137

BACK PAIN, LOW

Disease Management	Organization	Date	Population	Recommendations	Comments	Source

Back Pain, Low	NICE	2009	Adults	1. Educate patients and promote self-management of low back pain.
				 2. Recommends offering one of the following treatment options:
				   a. Structure exercise program
				   b. Manual therapy[a]
				   c. Acupuncture
				 3. Consider a psychology referral for patients with a high disability and/or who experience significant psychological distress from their low back pain.
				 4. Recommends against routine lumbar spine x-rays.
				 5. Recommends an MRI scan of lumbar spine only if spinal fusion is under consideration.
				 6. Consider a referral for surgery in patients with refractory, severe nonspecific low back pain who have completed the programs above and would consider spinal fusion.
					1. Analgesic ladder for low back pain
					   a. Recommend scheduled acetaminophen
					   b. Add NSAIDs and/or weak opioids
					   c. Consider adding a tricyclic antidepressant
					   d. Consider a strong opioid for short-term use for people in severe pain
					   e. Refer for specialist assessment for people who may require prolonged use of strong opioids
						http://www.nice.org.uk/nicemedia/live/11887/44343/44343.pdf

	ICSI	2010	Adults	See table.		https://www.icsi.org/health_initiatives/other_initiatives/low_back_pain/

[a]Manual therapy includes spinal manipulation, spinal mobilization, and massage.

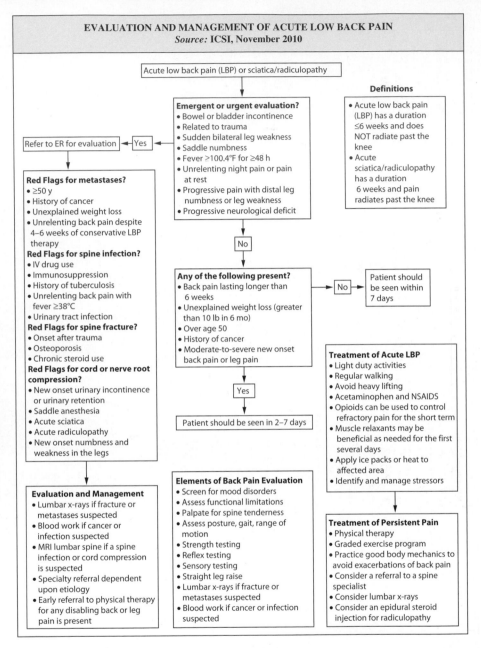

EVALUATION AND MANAGEMENT OF ACUTE LOW BACK PAIN
Source: ICSI, November 2010

Acute low back pain (LBP) or sciatica/radiculopathy

Emergent or urgent evaluation?
- Bowel or bladder incontinence
- Related to trauma
- Sudden bilateral leg weakness
- Saddle numbness
- Fever ≥100.4°F for ≥48 h
- Unrelenting night pain or pain at rest
- Progressive pain with distal leg numbness or leg weakness
- Progressive neurological deficit

Refer to ER for evaluation ◄— Yes

No

Definitions
- Acute low back pain (LBP) has a duration ≤6 weeks and does NOT radiate past the knee
- Acute sciatica/radiculopathy has a duration 6 weeks and pain radiates past the knee

Red Flags for metastases?
- ≥50 y
- History of cancer
- Unexplained weight loss
- Unrelenting back pain despite 4–6 weeks of conservative LBP therapy

Red Flags for spine infection?
- IV drug use
- Immunosuppression
- History of tuberculosis
- Unrelenting back pain with fever ≥38°C
- Urinary tract infection

Red Flags for spine fracture?
- Onset after trauma
- Osteoporosis
- Chronic steroid use

Red Flags for cord or nerve root compression?
- New onset urinary incontinence or urinary retention
- Saddle anesthesia
- Acute sciatica
- Acute radiculopathy
- New onset numbness and weakness in the legs

Any of the following present?
- Back pain lasting longer than 6 weeks
- Unexplained weight loss (greater than 10 lb in 6 mo)
- Over age 50
- History of cancer
- Moderate-to-severe new onset back pain or leg pain

No ► Patient should be seen within 7 days

Yes

Patient should be seen in 2–7 days

Treatment of Acute LBP
- Light duty activities
- Regular walking
- Avoid heavy lifting
- Acetaminophen and NSAIDS
- Opioids can be used to control refractory pain for the short term
- Muscle relaxants may be beneficial as needed for the first several days
- Apply ice packs or heat to affected area
- Identify and manage stressors

Evaluation and Management
- Lumbar x-rays if fracture or metastases suspected
- Blood work if cancer or infection suspected
- MRI lumbar spine if a spine infection or cord compression is suspected
- Specialty referral dependent upon etiology
- Early referral to physical therapy for any disabling back or leg pain is present

Elements of Back Pain Evaluation
- Screen for mood disorders
- Assess functional limitations
- Palpate for spine tenderness
- Assess posture, gait, range of motion
- Strength testing
- Reflex testing
- Sensory testing
- Straight leg raise
- Lumbar x-rays if fracture or metastases suspected
- Blood work if cancer or infection suspected

Treatment of Persistent Pain
- Physical therapy
- Graded exercise program
- Practice good body mechanics to avoid exacerbations of back pain
- Consider a referral to a spine specialist
- Consider lumbar x-rays
- Consider an epidural steroid injection for radiculopathy

BARRETT ESOPHAGUS

Disease Management	Organization	Date	Population	Recommendations	Comments	Source
Barrett Esophagus	AGA	2011	Patients with biopsy diagnosis of Barrett esophagus (metaplastic columnar epithelium in distal esophagus)	• **No dysplasia** ○ Endoscopic surveillance (ES) every 3–5 y • **Low-grade dysplasia** ○ ES every 6–12 mo—consider radiofrequency ablation (RFA)—90% complete eradication of dysplasia • **High-grade dysplasia** ○ ES every 3 mo if no eradication therapy • **Eradication therapy** ○ RFA, photodynamic therapy (PDT), or endoscopic mucosal resection (EMR) is preferred over ES in high-grade dysplasia (strong recommendation)	• In patients with Barrett esophagus without dysplasia, 0.12% develop esophageal cancer per year compared to 0.5% with low-grade dysplasia • Progression from high-grade dysplasia to cancer is 6% per year (*N Engl J Med.* 2011;365:1375) • Esophagectomy for high-grade dysplasia is an option, but less morbidity with ablation therapy (*N Engl J Med.* 2009;360:2277) • 40% of patients with Barrett esophagus and esophageal cancer have no history of chronic GERD symptoms • Long-term high-dose PPIs or antireflux therapy has been shown to decrease risk of neoplastic progression in patients with Barrett esophagus. (*Clin Gastroenteral Hepatol.* 2013;11:382)	*Gastrointestinal Endoscopy.* 2012;76:1087. *Gastroenterology.* 2011;140:1084. *N Engl J Med.* 2014;371:836. *N Engl J Med.* 2014;371:2499.

BELL PALSY

Disease Management	Organization	Date	Population	Recommendations	Comments	Source

Bell Palsy	AAN	2012	Adults with Bells Palsy	• For patients with recent-onset Bells Palsy (<72 h of symptoms)
				  ○ Steroids are recommended to increase the probability of facial nerve recovery
				    – Prednisone 1 mg/kg PO daily × 7 d
				  ○ Antivirals (eg, acyclovir or valacyclovir) × 7 d given with steroids might improve outcomes and can be offered.
					• Antivirals are thought to have a marginal effect at best of facial nerve recovery when added to steroids. The benefit is <7%.	www.guideline.gov/content.aspx?id=38700

	AAO	2013	Adult and children with Bells Palsy	• No routine lab studies needed for unequivocal Bells Palsy. • Recommend against routine diagnostic imaging for straightforward Bells Palsy. • Recommend oral steroids for Bells Palsy with or without antiviral medications if initiated within 72 h of symptom onset in patients 16 y and older. • Recommend against antiviral monotherapy for Bells Palsy. • Recommend eye protection for patients with incomplete eye closure. • Inadequate evidence to support surgical decompression with Bells Palsy. • Recommend against electrodiagnostic testing for Bells Palsy with incomplete facial paralysis. • Recommend against physical therapy or acupuncture for Bells Palsy.	• Cochrane analysis found no benefit of adding antivirals to corticosteroids vs corticosteroid monotherapy.	http://www.guideline.gov/content.aspx?id=47483
	Cochrane database of systematic reviews	2015				http://www.cochrane.org/CD001869/NEUROMUSC_antiviral-treatment-for-bells-palsy

BENIGN PROSTATIC HYPERPLASIA (BPH)

Disease Management	Organization	Date	Population	Recommendations	Comments	Source

Benign Prostatic Hyperplasia (BPH)	AUA	2010	Adult men	1. Routine measurement of serum creatinine is not indicated in men with BPH.
				2. Do not recommend dietary supplements or phytotherapeutic agents for lower urinary tract symptoms (LUTS) management.
				3. Patients with LUTS with no signs of bladder outlet obstruction by flow study should be treated for detrusor overactivity.
				  a. Alter fluid intake
				  b. Behavioral modification
				  c. Anticholinergic medications
				4. Options for moderate-severe LUTS from BPH (AUA symptom index score ≥8)
				  a. Watchful waiting
				  b. Medical therapies
				    i. α-blockers[a]
				    ii. 5-Alfa-reductase inhibitors[b]
				    iii. Anticholinergic agents
				    iv. Combination therapy
				  c. Transurethral needle ablation
				  d. Transurethral microwave thermotherapy
				  e. Transurethral laser ablation or enucleation of the prostate
				  f. Transurethral incision of the prostate
				  g. Transurethral vaporization of the prostate
				  h. Transurethral resection of the prostate
				  i. Laser resection of the prostate
				  j. Photoselective vaporization of the prostate
				  k. Prostatectomy
				5. Surgery is recommended for BPH causing renal insufficiency, recurrent urinary tract infections (UTIs), bladder stones, gross hematuria, or refractory LUTS.
					1. Combination therapy with alfa-blocker and 5-alfa-reductase inhibitor is effective for moderate-severe LUTS with significant prostate enlargement.
					2. Men with planned cataract surgery should have cataract surgery before initiating alfa-blockers.
					3. 5-Alfa-reductase inhibitors should not be used for men with LUTS from BPH without prostate enlargement.
					4. Anticholinergic agents are appropriate for LUTS that are primarily irritative symptoms and patient does not have an elevated postvoid residual (>250 mL).
					5. The choice of surgical method should be based on the patient's presentation, anatomy, surgeon's experience, and patient's preference.
						http://www.guidelines.gov/content.aspx?id=25635&search=aua+2010+bph

[a]Alfa-blockers: alfuzosin, doxazosin, tamsulosin, and terazosin. All have equal clinical effectiveness.
[b]5-Alfa-reductase inhibitors: dutasteride and finasteride.

BREAST CANCER FOLLOW-UP

Disease Management	Organization/ Population	Recommendations	Comments	Source
Breast Cancer Follow-up and Management After Primary Treatment	American Society of Clinical Oncology (ASCO) clinical practice guidelines update *J Clin Oncol.* 2013;31:961-965 Early-stage women with curable breast cancer	**Mode of Surveillance** 1. Careful history and physical examination every 3–6 mo for first 3 y after primary therapy (with or without adjuvant treatment), then every 6–12 mo for next 2 y and then annually. 2. Counsel patients about symptoms of recurrence including new lumps, bone pain, chest pain, dyspnea, abdominal pain, or persistent headaches. 3. High-risk women for familial breast CA syndromes should be referred for genetic counseling–high-risk criteria include Ashkenazi Jewish heritage, history of ovarian CA at any age in patient or any first-degree relatives; any first-degree relatives with breast CA before age 50; two or more first- or second-degree relatives diagnosed with breast CA at any age; patient or relative with bilateral breast CA; history of breast CA in male relative. 4. All women should be counseled to perform monthly self-breast examinations. 5. Mammography—women treated with breast conserving therapy should have first posttreatment mammogram no earlier than 6 mo after radiation. Subsequent mammograms every 6–12 mo for surveillance (yearly preferred if stability of mammogram achieved). 6. Regular gynecology follow-up with pelvic examination. Tamoxifen increases risk of uterine cancer and patients should be advised to report any vaginal bleeding. 7. Coordination of care: risk of recurrence continues through more than 15 y. Continuity of care by physician experienced in surveillance of patients and in breast examination is recommended. Follow-up by a primary care physician (PCP) leads to the same outcome as specialist follow-up. If the patient desires transfer of care to PCP, 1 y after definitive therapy is appropriate.	1. The following routine studies are NOT recommended for routine breast cancer surveillance: a. CBC and automated chemistry studies b. Routine chest x-ray c. Bone scans d. Liver ultrasound e. Routine CT scanning f. Routine FDG-PET scanning g. Breast MRI (unless patient has $BRCA_1$ or $BRCA_2$ mutation or previous mediastinal radiation at young age). h. Tumor markers including CA27.29, CA 15-3, or CEA are not recommended for routine surveillance. *JAMA.* 1994; 27:1587-1592. 2. Although studies have shown no survival benefit for routine surveillance testing, many oncologists will do routine blood studies including tumor markers especially in higher risk women. The most important follow-up strategy is to make certain patients know and report early signs or symptoms that may reflect recurrent disease. 3. There is a significant difference in the behavior of hormone receptor (HR) positive vs hormone receptor negative disease. HR negative disease tends to recur earlier (2–3 y) than HR positive breast cancer (>50% of relapses occur after 5 y). There is also a 3- to 4-fold increase risk of brain metastasis in HR negative women. Overexpression of Her2 is found in 20% of breast cancer patients and targeted therapy in this group has significantly improved prognosis. Her2 overexpressed patients, however, are also at increased risk for brain metastasis. HR positive patients have a 4-fold increased risk of bone metastasis compared to HR negative patients in whom metastasis to liver, lung, and brain are more common (*N Engl J Med.* 2007;357:39).	*NCCN Guidelines.* 2015;BINV-16:27

BRONCHITIS, ACUTE

Disease Management	Organization	Date	Population	Recommendations	Comments	Source

Bronchitis, Acute	Michigan Quality Improvement Consortium	2010	Adults age ≥18 y	1. Recommends against a chest x-ray if all the following are present:
				  a. Heart rate <100 beats/min
				  b. Respiratory rate <24 breaths/min
				  c. Temperature <100.4°F (38°C)
				2. Recommends against antibiotics.
					1. Consider antitussive agents for short-term relief of coughing.
					2. β_2 agonists or mucolytic agents should not be used routinely to alleviate cough.
						http://www.guideline.gov/content.aspx?id=38688

CANCER

Disease Management	Organization	Date	Population	Recommendations	Comments	Source
Non-Small Cell Lung Cancer (NSCLC) Follow-up Care	ACCP (American College of Chest Physicians)	2013	Non-small cell lung cancer patients treated with curative intent	1. Chest CT scan should be performed every 6 months for first 2 years after resection then once a year thereafter. 2. Routine imaging with PET scanning is not recommended. 3. Patients should be seen every 3–4 months for 2 years then less frequently. Health-related quality of life should be assessed with each visit. 4. Surveillance biomarker testing should not be done outside of clinical trials. 5. Smoking cessation interventions recommended. Annual influenza vaccine and every 5 year pneumococcal vaccinations encouraged.	1. Only 30%–35% of patients diagnosed with NSCLC are candidates for surgery with curative intent. Lung CA is responsible for 165,000 deaths/year. 2. Cure rates are reflective of stage: Stage I—70% Stage II— 40% Stage IIA—24% Stage IIIA—24% 3. Platinum-based chemotherapy is standard of care for NSCLC resected for cure. This adjuvant therapy reduces recurrence risk by 5%–10%. 4. Symptoms of local recurrence include increase or change in cough, dyspnea, or chest pain. 5. Lung cancer is the most common malignancy to metastasize to brain—headache or neurologic symptoms should be an indication for brain MRI with gadolinium. 6. In older, compromised patients with a Stage I lung cancer, less than 3 cm in size, treated with radiosteriotactic body radiation have a 70%–75% chance of prolonged disease-free survival.	*JAMA* 2010;303:1070

CANCER

Disease Management	Organization	Date	Population	Recommendations	Comments	Source
Use of Epoetin and Darbepoetin in Adult Patients with Cancer	American Society of Hematology/American Society of Clinical Oncology (ASH/ASCO)	2010	Adult patients with cancer and anemia	1. History, physical exam, and diagnostic studies to exclude other causes of anemia aside from chemotherapy or malignant marrow infiltration. 2. The FDA label now limits the use of Erythrocyte Stimulating Agents (ESA) ONLY to anemic cancer patients receiving chemotherapy with palliative intent. (*N Engl J Med.* 2007;356:2448) ESA is NOT to be used in patients with curable malignancies or in patients with cancer not on chemotherapy. Side effects of thrombosis and potentially increased cancer growth should be discussed with the patient. (*J Natl Cancer Inst.* 2013;105:1018) 3. Epoetin and darbepoetin are equal in efficacy. 4. ESA should not be used if hemoglobin >10 g/dL. The main benefit of ESA is to reduce transfusion need. (*Br J Cancer.* 2010;102:301) 5. FDA-approved starting dose of epoetin is 150 U/kg 3 times/week or 40,000 U weekly. For darbepoetin the dose is 2.25 µg/kg weekly or 500 µg every 3 weeks subcutaneously. 6. Stop ESAs at 6–8 weeks if no evidence of a response. Check for underlying tumor progression, iron deficiency, or other causes of anemia. 7. Dose of ESAs should be lowest concentration needed to avoid transfusion. Keep hemoglobin <12. 8. Periodic monitoring of ferritin and iron studies is recommended since ESAs will not work in iron deficiency. 9. Use of ESAs in lower-risk myelodysplastic syndrome to decrease transfusions is approved if erythropoietin level is <500 mµ/mL.	1. Early studies raising hemoglobin level to >12 g/dL resulted in significant increased risk of venous thromboembolus. 2. Beware of clot risk when using ESAs with other thrombophilic drugs (tamoxifen, BCP, lenalidomide). 3. The molecular structure of darbepoetin increases its half-life, allowing for less frequent injections. 4. 50% of cancers will have erythropoietin receptors on the cell surface. It has NOT been proven that ESAs interaction with cell surface receptors leads to cellular proliferation. 5. When patients stop chemotherapy for whatever reason, ESAs must be stopped and transfusion therapy substituted. 6. The addition of intravenous iron to ESAs will increase hemoglobin more rapidly since iron is sequestered in the reticuloendothelial system in the cancer-associated anemia of chronic disease. (*N Engl J Med.* 2005; 352:1011) 7. ESAs widely used in chronic renal insufficiency, reducing need for transfusion significantly. Iron often given to these patients to keep ferritin level between 100 and 500 ng/mL and transferrin saturation 20% to 50%. (*N Engl J Med.* 2010;362:3)	*Blood.* 2010;116:4045–4059. ASH/ASCO guidelines update on use of epoetin and darbepoetin.

CANCER

Disease Management	Organization	Date	Population	Recommendations	Comments	Source
Ovarian Cancer Follow-up	NCCN	2015	Women treated for ovarian cancer with complete response (Stage I–IV)	1. Office visits every 2–4 months for 2 years, then 3–6 months for 3 years, then annually after 5 years. 2. Physical exam including pelvic exam and measurement of CA-125 with each visit. 3. Refer for genetic risk evaluation if not previously done. 4. Chest/abdominal/pelvic CT, MRI, PET-CT, or PET as clinically indicated due to symptoms or rising CA-125.	1. All patients with ovarian cancer should be screened for BRCA 1 and 2 mutations. 10% of patients with Lynch syndrome will develop ovarian cancer. 2. 23,000 new cases of ovarian cancer in the United States with 14,000 deaths. Survival is related to stage: Stage I— 86% Stage II— 68% Stage III—38% Stage IV—19% 3. Relapsed ovarian cancer rarely curable but sequential treatments and intraperitoneal chemotherapy has extended survival to 50–60 months.	NCCN Guidelines version 1.2015; OV-5. http://www.NCCN.org/professionals/physician-gls/pdf/ovarian.gdf

Disease Management	Organization	Date	Population	Recommendations	Comments	Source
				CANCER		
Colorectal Cancer Follow-up Care	American Society of Clinical Oncology Cancer Care Ontario (CCO)	2013	Adults with non-metastatic colorectal cancer (Stage II and III)	1. Surveillance guided by risk of recurrence and functional status of the patient. Early detection of relapse would lead to treatment including surgery for possible cure. 2. Highest risk of recurrence during first 4 years after diagnosis. 95% of relapses occur in first 5 years. 3. Medical history, physical exam, and CEA testing every 3–6 months for 5 years. The higher the risk, the more frequent the follow-up. 4. Abdominal and chest CT scan is recommended annually for 3 years. Highest risk patients (Stage III, >4 nodes+) should consider imaging every 4–6 months. 5. Routine PET scan not recommended for surveillance. 6. Patients with rectal cancer should also have pelvic CT annually for 3–5 years. 7. A surveillance colonoscopy should be performed 1 year after initial surgery. If normal repeat colonoscopy every 5 years. If complete colonoscopy not performed before diagnosis do as soon as the patient recovers from adjuvant therapy. 8. Any new or persistent worsening of symptoms warrant consideration of recurrence	1. Stage I colon cancer with very low risk of recurrence. Colonoscopy follow-up every 5 years but CEA and imaging not needed. 2. Colon Cancer with >90% to liver as the first site of metastasis. In rectal cancer 50% of first metastasis is to lung. (*CA Cancer J Clin.* 2015;65:5) 3. Patients found to have resectable metastatic disease (liver, lungs) or local recurrence who are rendered disease free by surgical or radio-frequency ablation (RFA) should be followed with frequent surveillance. 10-year survival in 30%–40% range. (*J Clin Onc.* 2010;28: 2300) 4. BRAF mutation prognostic for early relapse and chemotherapy resistance with shortened survival. (*PloS One.* 2013;8:eb5995) 5. Patients with CRC younger than 50 y/o or with significant family history should be evaluated for Lynch syndrome with microsatellite instability and immune histochemistry testing. (*N Engl J Med.* 2009;361:2449) 6. Patients with Stage II CRC with microsatellite instability will have a shorter survival if given 5-fluorouracil compared to placebo. (*Clin Genet.* 2009;76:1) 7. Uncertainty remains regarding use of aspirin or cyclooxygenase inhibitor to reduce risk of recurrence. 8. Exercise (>150 minutes/week) weight loss for high BMI, smoking cessation, and healthy diet advised.	*J Clin Oncol.* 2013;31: 4465–4470

CANCER

Disease Management	Organization	Date	Population	Recommendations	Comments	Source
Malignant Spinal Cord Compression (MSCC)	Scottish Palliative Care Guidelines National Collaborating Centre for Cancer —Metastatic spinal cord compression	2014 2012	Adults with MSCC	1. Patients presenting with >48 hours for paraplegia—radiation for pain control, surgery only if spine unstable – Chance for neuro recovery is zero. (*Lancet Oncology*. 2005;6:15) 2. Patients presenting with significant or progressing weakness of lower extremities—if no previous history of cancer biopsy non-neural cancer if accessible. If biopsy not possible and lymphoma or myeloma unlikely give decadron 40–100 mg daily and take to surgery to make tissue diagnosis and relieve compression. (*Neurology*. 1989;39:1255. *Lancet Neurol*. 2008; 7:459) If unstable, the spine should be stabilized. Taper steroids (decrease by ½ every 3 days) and begin radiation in 2–3 weeks. If tumor is lymphoma or myeloma consider initiating chemotherapy and high-dose decadron. Recovery of lower extremity strength dependent on degree of paraparesis initially. 3. Patients presenting with back pain but mild neurologic symptoms—if no previous cancer find site to biopsy, check PSA, serum protein electrophoresis, beta-2 microglobulin, alfa beta protein. Begin moderate dose decadron (16 mg/day) with radiation therapy initially. Surgery reserved for progression of symptoms after starting radiation especially in radioinsensitive cancers (renal cell, sarcoma, melanoma). Recovery of neurologic function in 80%–90% range. 4. Patients presenting with back pain but no neurologic symptoms—if no previous diagnosis of cancer search for site to biopsy (physical exam, PET,CT) and consult Radiation Therapy. If myeloma or lymphoma treat with systemic chemotherapy. Radiation is primary treatment with surgery only on progression. Low dose or no steroids is acceptable. Chance of continued lower extremity strength approaches 100%.	1. MRI with and without gadolinium of the entire spine is mandatory. 30% of patients will have cord compression in more than 1 area. 2. 20% of patients presenting with MSCC have not had a previous diagnosis of cancer. 3. 5%–8% of patients with known cancer will develop MSCC during their course of disease. 4. Most common tumors associated with MSCC are lung, breast, prostate, myeloma, and lymphoma. 5. Most common site of MSCC is the thoracic spine (70%) and least common cervical spine (10%). 6. Back pain present in 95% of patients with average time to MSCC being 6–7 weeks. Once motor, sensory, or autonomic dysfunction occur—time to total paraplegia is rapid (hours to days). 7. Indications for surgery in MSCC include lack of diagnosis, progression on radiation, unstable fracture or bone in spinal canal, and previous radiation to site of MSCC. (*Int J Oncol*. 2011;38:5. *J Clin Onc*. 2011;29:3072) 8. Posterior decompression using a laminectomy was standard surgery for MSCC but now resection of tumor with bone reconstruction and stabilization is done most commonly. 9. Stereotactic body radiation therapy is being used more commonly with improved results especially in radiation resistant cancers. (*Cancer*. 2010;116:2258)	*Int J Radiat Oncol Biol Phys*. 2012;84:312 *Quarterly J of Med*. 2014;107:277–282

CANCER SURVIVORSHIP: LATE EFFECTS OF CANCER TREATMENTS

CA Treatment History	Late Effects	Periodic Evaluation
Any CA experience	Psychosocial disorders[b]	
Any chemotherapy	Oral and dental abnormalities	Dental examination and cleaning (every 6 mo)
Chemotherapy (alkylating agents)[a]	Gonadal dysfunction Hematologic disorders[c] Ocular toxicity[d] Pulmonary toxicity[f] Renal toxicity[f] Urinary tract toxicity[g]	Pubertal assessment (yearly) in adults if symptoms of hypogonadism present History, examination for bleeding disorder; CBC/differential (yearly) Visual acuity, funduscopic examination, evaluation by ophthalmologist (yearly if ocular tumors, TBI, or $\geq$30 Gy; otherwise, every 3 y) CXR, PFTs (at entry into long-term follow-up, then as clinically indicated) Blood pressure (yearly); electrolytes, BUN, creatinine, Ca^{++}, Mg^{++}, PO_4, urinalysis (at entry into long-term follow-up, then clinically as indicated)
Chemotherapy (anthracycline antibiotics)[a]	Cardiac toxicity[h]	ECHO or MUGA; ECG at entry into long-term follow-up, periodic thereafter ($\uparrow$ frequency if chest radiation); fasting glucose, lipid panel (every 3–5 y)[i]
	Hematologic disorders[c]	See "Chemotherapy (alkylating agents)"[i]
Chemotherapy antitumor antibiotics mitomycin C[i], bleomycin[i]	Pulmonary toxicity[e] Renal injury[f]	CXR and PFTs end of exposure then reevaluation as clinically indicated Monitor urinalysis and creatinine
Chemotherapy–antimetabolites (cytarabine, high-dose IV; MTX, high-dose IV, intrathecal)	Clinical leukoencephalopathy[j] Neurocognitive deficits	Full neurologic examination (yearly) Neuropsychological evaluation (at entry into long-term follow-up, then as clinically indicated)
Chemotherapy (epipodophyllotoxins)[a]	Hematologic disorders (causes AML with specific 11q 23 translocation[c])	See "Chemotherapy (alkylating agents)"[i]
Chemotherapy (heavy metals Cis-platinum, Carboplatin)	Dyslipidemia/hypertension and increased risk of cardiovascular disease Gonadal dysfunction Hematologic disorders[c] Ototoxicity[j] Peripheral sensory neuropathy Renal toxicity[f]	See "Chemotherapy (alkylating agents)"[i] Fasting lipid panel at entry. Complete pure tone audiogram or brainstem auditory-evoked response (yearly × 5 y, then every 5 y); Examination yearly for 2–3 y
Chemotherapy—microtubular inhibitors (taxanes, ixabepilone, eribulin)	Peripheral neuropathy	Examination yearly for 2–3 y
Chemotherapy (nonclassical alkylators)	Gonadal dysfunction Reduced CD4 count Hematologic disorders[c]	See "Chemotherapy (alkylating agents)"[i]
Chemotherapy (plant alkaloids) dacarbazine	Peripheral sensory neuropathy Raynaud phenomenon	See "Chemotherapy (heavy metals)"[i] Yearly history/examination
Chemotherapy (purine agonists)	Hematologic disorders[c] Reduction in CD4 count	See "Chemotherapy (alkylating agents)"[i] Monitor for infection
Corticosteroids (dexamethasone, prednisone)	Ocular toxicity[d] Avascular osteonecrosis Osteopenia/osteoporosis	Musculoskeletal examination (yearly)

CANCER SURVIVORSHIP: LATE EFFECTS OF CANCER TREATMENTS (CONTINUED)

CA Treatment History	Late Effects	Periodic Evaluation
Targeted biologic therapy – Monoclonal antibodies 　– Trastuzumab (anti–HER-2) 　– Rituximab (anti-CD20 antibody on B lymphocytes) 　– Panitumumab, cetuximab (anti-EGFR)	Cardiac dysfunction is usually reversible Reduction in immunoglobulins and increased risk of infection	Monitor 2D echo for ejection fraction every 3 mo during therapy and as needed for symptoms Monitor quantitative immunoglobulins if increased frequency of infection
Multi-targeted Tyrosine kinase inhibitors (TKI's) – erlotinib – sunitinib – sorafenib – axitinib – pazopanib – imatinib	Fatigue, diarrhea, hypertension, liver injury while on drug but little long-term toxicity	Routine monitoring for end-organ damage after completion of therapy not indicated
Immune-mediated therapy – ipilimumab – Nivolumab – Pembrolizumab	Autoimmunity—colitis, hepatitis, dermatitis, thyroiditis, hypophysitic pneumonitis—often reversible but not always Gonadal dysfunction Growth hormone deficiency (children and adolescents) Hyperthyroidism Hyperprolactinemia Hypothyroidism Neurocognitive deficits Ocular toxicity[d] Oncologic disorders[k] Oral and dental abnormalities Ototoxicity[j] Overweight/obesity/metabolic syndrome Pulmonary toxicity[e] Renal toxicity[f] Urinary tract toxicity[g]	Check hormone levels every 6 months See "Chemotherapy (alkylating agents)" Height, weight, BMI (every 6 mo until growth completed, then yearly); Tanner staging (every 6 mo until sexually mature) TSH, free thyroxine (T_4) (yearly) Prolactin level (as clinically indicated) TSH, free T_4 See "Chemotherapy (cytarabine)" See "Chemotherapy (alkylating agents)" See "Hematopoietic cell (bone marrow) transplant" See "Any chemotherapy" See "Chemotherapy (heavy metals)" Fasting glucose, fasting serum insulin, fasting lipid profile (every 2 y if overweight or obese; every 5 y if normal weight) See "Chemotherapy (alkylating agents)" See "Chemotherapy (alkylating agents)" See "Chemotherapy (alkylating agents)"
Hematopoietic cell (bone marrow) transplant	Hematologic disorders[c] Oncologic disorders Avascular osteonecrosis Osteopenia/osteoporosis	See "Chemotherapy (alkylating agents)" Inspection/examination targeted to irradiation fields (yearly) See "Corticosteroids (dexamethasone, prednisone)" See "Chemotherapy (antimetabolites)"

CANCER SURVIVORSHIP: LATE EFFECTS OF CANCER TREATMENTS (CONTINUED)

CA Treatment History	Late Effects	Periodic Evaluation
Chemotherapy drugs with minimal long-term toxicity effects – Topoisomerase I inhibitors (Camptosar, topotecan) – Antibiotics (actinomycin) – Antimetabolites (L-asparaginase, 5-fluorouracil (5-FU), capecitabine, gemcitabine, 6-mercaptopurine)	Mild reduction in bone marrow reserve	Routine monitoring for end-organ dysfunction is not indicated
Radiation therapy (field- and dose-dependent)	Cardiac toxicity[h] Central adrenal insufficiency (pediatric brain tumors) Cerebrovascular complications[j] Chronic sinusitis Functional asplenia	See "Chemotherapy (alkylating agents)" 8 AM serum cortisol (yearly × 15 y, and as clinically indicated) Neurologic examination (yearly) Head/neck examination (yearly) Blood culture when temperature ≥101 °F (38.3 °C), rapid institution of empiric antibiotics

AML, acute myelocytic leukemia; BMI, body mass index; BUN, blood urea nitrogen; CBC, complete blood count; CXR, chest x-ray; ECG, electrocardiogram; ECHO, echocardiogram; IV, intravenous; MTX, methotrexate; MUGA, multiple-gated acquisition scan; PFTs, pulmonary function tests; TBI, total-body irradiation; TSH, thyroid-stimulating hormone.

[a]Chemotherapeutic agents, by mechanism of action:
- Alkylating agents: busulfan, carmustine (BCNU), chlorambucil, cyclophosphamide, ifosfamide, lomustine (CCNU), mechlorethamine, melphalan, procarbazine, thiotepa
- Antimetabolites: MTX, cytosine arabinoside, gemcitabine
- Heavy metals: carboplatin, cisplatin, oxaliplatin
- Nonclassical alkylators: dacarbazine (DTIC), temozolomide
- Anthracycline antibiotics: daunorubicin, doxorubicin, epirubicin, idarubicin, mitoxantrone
- Antitumor antibiotics: bleomycin, mitomycin C
- Plant alkaloids: vinblastine, vincristine, vinorelbine
- Purine agonists: fludarabine, pentostatin, cladribine
- Microtubular inhibitors: docetaxel, paclitaxel, cabazitaxel, ixabepilone
- Epipodophyllotoxins: etoposide (VP16), teniposide (VM26)

[b]Psychosocial disorders: mental health disorders, risky behaviors, psychosocial disability because of pain, fatigue, limitations in health care/insurance access, "chemo brain" syndrome

[c]Hematologic disorders: acute myeloid leukemia, myelodysplasia

[d]Ocular toxicity: cataracts, orbital hypoplasia, lacrimal duct atrophy, xerophthalmia, keratitis, telangiectasias, retinopathy, optic chiasm neuropathy, endophthalmos, chronic painful eye, maculopathy, glaucoma

[e]Pulmonary toxicity: pulmonary fibrosis, interstitial pneumonitis, restrictive lung disease, obstructive lung disease. Increased sensitivity to oxygen toxicity—keep FiO₂ ≤28% in patients with bleomycin exposure

[f]Renal toxicity: glomerular and tubular renal insufficiency, hypertension, hemolytic uremic syndrome

[g]Urinary tract toxicity: hemorrhagic cystitis, bladder fibrosis, dysfunctional voiding, vesicoureteral reflux, hydronephrosis, bladder malignancy

[h]Cardiac toxicity: cardiomyopathy, arrhythmias, left ventricular dysfunction, congestive heart failure, pericarditis, pericardial fibrosis, valvular disease, myocardial infarction, atherosclerotic heart disease

[i]Clinical leukoencephalopathy: spasticity, ataxia, dysarthria, dysphagia, hemiparesis, seizures

[j]Ototoxicity: sensorineural hearing loss, tinnitus, vertigo, tympanosclerosis, otosclerosis, eustachian tube dysfunction, conductive hearing loss

[k]Oncologic disorders: secondary benign or malignant neoplasm, especially breast CA after mantle radiation, gastrointestinal malignancy after paraaortic radiation for seminoma of the testis

[l]Cerebrovascular complications: stroke, and occlusive cerebral vasculopathy

Note: Guidelines for surveillance and monitoring for late effects after treatment for adult CAs available via the National Comprehensive Cancer Network, Inc. (NCCN). (http://www.nccn.org/professionals/physician_gls)

Source: Long-Term Follow-Up Guidelines for Survivors of Childhood, Adolescent, and Young Adult Cancers. Children's Oncology Group. Version 3.0 October 2008. (For full guidelines and references, see http://www.survivorshipguidelines.org)
See also: *N Engl J Med.* 2006;355:1722-1782; *J Clin Oncol.* 2007;25:3991-4008. *JAMA.* 2011;305:2311.

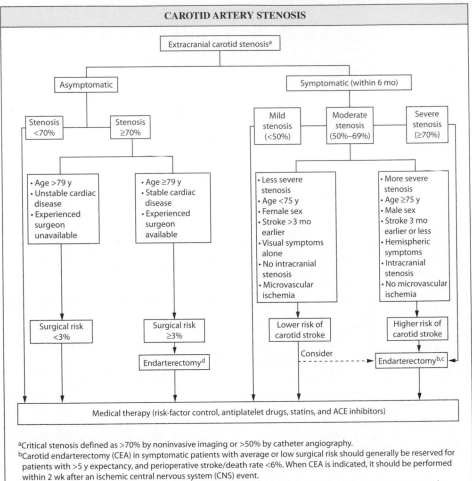

CAROTID ARTERY STENOSIS

[Flowchart content:]

Extracranial carotid stenosis[a]

Asymptomatic | Symptomatic (within 6 mo)

Asymptomatic branch:
- Stenosis <70%
- Stenosis ≥70%

Stenosis ≥70% branches:
- Age >79 y; Unstable cardiac disease; Experienced surgeon unavailable → Surgical risk <3%
- Age ≥79 y; Stable cardiac disease; Experienced surgeon available → Surgical risk ≥3% → Endarterectomy[d]

Symptomatic branch:
- Mild stenosis (<50%)
- Moderate stenosis (50%–69%)
- Severe stenosis (≥70%)

Moderate/Severe:
- Less severe stenosis; Age <75 y; Female sex; Stroke >3 mo earlier; Visual symptoms alone; No intracranial stenosis; Microvascular ischemia → Lower risk of carotid stroke → Consider ⇢ Endarterectomy[b,c]
- More severe stenosis; Age ≥75 y; Male sex; Stroke 3 mo earlier or less; Hemispheric symptoms; Intracranial stenosis; No microvascular ischemia → Higher risk of carotid stroke → Endarterectomy[b,c]

Medical therapy (risk-factor control, antiplatelet drugs, statins, and ACE inhibitors)

[a]Critical stenosis defined as >70% by noninvasive imaging or >50% by catheter angiography.
[b]Carotid endarterectomy (CEA) in symptomatic patients with average or low surgical risk should generally be reserved for patients with >5 y expectancy, and perioperative stroke/death rate <6%. When CEA is indicated, it should be performed within 2 wk after an ischemic central nervous system (CNS) event.
[c]Carotid artery stenting (CAS) with an embolic protection device is an alternative to CEA in symptomatic patients with average or low surgical risk when >70% obstruction is present, and the periprocedural stroke and mortality rate is <6%. CAS may be chosen over CEA if the neck anatomy is surgically unfavorable or if comorbid conditions make CEA a very high risk.
[d]The annual rate of stroke in asymptomatic patients treated with optimal medical therapy for carotid artery stenosis has decreased to <1%. Therefore the benefit of CEA or CAS remains controversial in asymptomatic patients. (*Stroke.* 2010;41:975-979)

Source: AHA/ASA 2005 Guidelines. *Circulation.* 2006;113:e872. *Stroke.* 2006;37:577. ASA/ACCF/AHA/AANN/AANS/ACR/ASNR/CNS/SAIP/SCAI/SIR/SNIS/SVM/SVS 2011 Guidelines. *J Am Coll Cardiol.* 2011;57:e16-e94. ACCF/SCAI/SVMB/SIR/ASITN 2007 Consensus. *J Am Coll Cardiol.* 2007;49(1):126-168.

CAROTID ARTERY STENOSIS
SURGICAL MANAGEMENT POST-CVA OR STROKE—2014

- CAS (carotid artery stenting) is indicated as an alternative to CEA (carotid endarterectomy) for symptomatic patients at average or low risk of complications associated with endovascular intervention when the diameter of the lumen of the internal carotid artery is reduced by >70% by noninvasive imaging or >50% by catheter-based imaging or noninvasive imaging with corroboration, and the anticipated rate of periprocedural stroke or death is <6% (Class IIa; Level of Evidence B).
- It is reasonable to consider patient's age in choosing between CAS and CEA. For older patients (≥70 y), CEA may be associated with improved outcome compared with CAS, particularly when arterial anatomy is unfavorable for endovascular intervention. For younger patients, CAS is equivalent to CEA in terms of risk for periprocedural complication (ie, stroke, MI, or death) and long-term risk for ipsilateral stroke (Class IIa; Level of Evidence B).
- CAS and CEA in the above settings should be performed by operators with established periprocedural stroke and mortality rates of <6% for symptomatic patients, similar to that observed in trials comparing CEA to medical therapy and more recent observational studies (Class I; Level of Evidence B).
- Routine, long-term follow-up imaging of the extracranial carotid circulation with carotid duplex ultrasonography is not recommended (Class III; Level of Evidence B).
- For patients with recurrent or progressive ischemic symptoms ipsilateral to a stenosis or occlusion of a distal (surgically inaccessible) carotid artery, or occlusion of a midcervical carotid artery after institution of optimal medical therapy, the usefulness of EC/IC bypass is considered investigational (Class IIB; Level of Evidence C).

Women only:

- For women with recent TIA or IS and ipsilateral moderate (50%–69%) carotid stenosis, CEA is recommended depending on patient-specific factors, such as age and comorbidities, if the perioperative morbidity and mortality risk is estimated to be <6%.
- In women who are to undergo CEA, aspirin is recommended unless contraindicated, because aspirin was used in every major trial that demonstrated efficacy of CEA.
- For women with recent TIA or IS within the past 6 mo and ipsilateral severe (70%–99%) carotid artery stenosis, CEA is recommended if the perioperative morbidity and mortality risk is estimated to be <6%.
- If a high-risk female patient (ie, 10-y predicted CVD risk ≥10%) has an indication for aspirin but is intolerant to it, the patient should be placed on clopidogrel.
- Aspirin therapy (75–325 mg/d is reasonable in women with diabetes mellitus unless contraindicated.
- When CEA is indicated for women with TIA or stroke, surgery within 2 w is reasonable rather than delaying surgery if there are no contraindications to early revascularization.
- Aspirin therapy can be useful in women >65 y of age (81 mg daily or 100 mg every other day) if blood pressure is controlled and benefit for ischemic and myocardial infarction prevention is likely to outweigh risk of gastrointestinal bleeding and hemorrhagic stroke (Class IIa; Level of Evidence B) and may be reasonable for women <65 y of age for ischemic stroke prevention.

Sources:
1. Guidelines for the Prevention of Stroke in Patients With Stroke and Transient Ischemic Attack. A Guideline for Healthcare Professionals From the American Heart Association/American Stroke Association. *Stroke.* 2014;45.
2. Bushnell C, McCullough LD, Awad IA, et al. Guidelines for the Prevention of Stroke in Women A Statement for Healthcare Professionals From the American Heart Association/American Stroke Association. *Stroke.* 2014;45.DOI; 10 1161/01.str.0000442009.06663.48.

CATARACT IN ADULTS: EVALUATION AND MANAGEMENT ALGORITHM
Source: AAO AND AOA

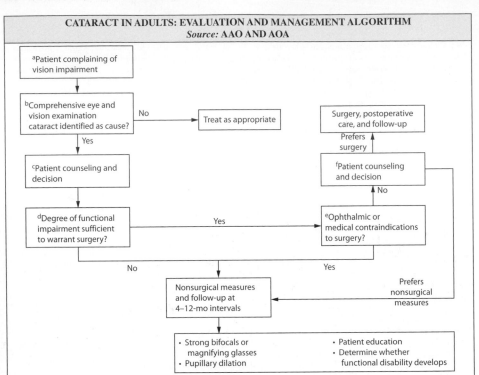

Notes:

[a]Begin evaluation only when patients complain of a vision problem or impairment.

Identifying impairment in visual function during routine history and physical examination constitutes sound medical practice.

[b]Essential elements of the comprehensive eye and vision exam:

- *Patient history:* Consider cataract if: acute or gradual onset of vision loss; vision problems under special conditions (eg, low contrast, glare); difficulties performing various visual tasks. Ask about: refractive history, previous ocular disease, amblyopia, eye surgery, trauma, general health history, medications, and allergies. It is critical to describe the actual impact of the cataract on the person's function and quality of life. There are several instruments available for assessing functional impairment related to cataract, including VF-14, Activities of Daily Vision Scale, and Visual Activities Questionnaire.
- *Ocular examination* Including: Snellen acuity and refraction; measurement of intraocular pressure; assessment of pupillary function; external exam; slit-lamp exam; and dilated exam of fundus.
- *Supplemental testing:* May be necessary to assess and document the extent of the functional disability and to determine whether other diseases may limit preoperative or postoperative vision. Most elderly patients presenting with visual problems do not have a cataract that causes functional impairment. Refractive error, macular degeneration, and glaucoma are common alternative etiologies for visual impairment.

[c]Once cataract has been identified as the cause of visual disability, patients should be counseled concerning the nature of the problem, its natural history, and the existence of both surgical and nonsurgical approaches to management. The principal factor that should guide decision making with regard to surgery is *the extent to which the cataract impairs the ability to function in daily life.*

The findings of the physical examination should corroborate that the cataract is the major contributing cause of the functional impairment, and that there is a reasonable expectation that managing the cataract will positively impact the patient's functional activity. Preoperative visual acuity is a poor predictor of postoperative functional improvement:

The decision to recommend cataract surgery should not be made solely on the basis of visual acuity.

[d]Patients who complain of mild-to-moderate limitation in activities due to a visual problem, those whose corrected acuities are near 20/40, and those who do not yet wish to undergo surgery may be offered nonsurgical measures for improving visual function. Treatment with nutritional supplements is not recommended. Smoking cessation retards cataract progression. Indications for surgery: cataract-impaired vision no longer meets the patient's needs; evidence of lens-induced disease (eg, phacomorphic glaucoma, phacolytic glaucoma); necessary to visualize the fundus in an eye that has the potential for sight (eg, diabetic patient at risk of diabetic retinopathy).

[e]*Contraindications to surgery*: the patient does not desire surgery; glasses or vision aids provide satisfactory functional vision; surgery will not improve visual function; the patient's quality of life is not compromised; the patient is unable to undergo surgery because of coexisting medical or ocular conditions; a legal consent cannot be obtained; or the patient is unable to obtain adequate postoperative care. Routine preoperative medical testing (12-lead EKG, CBC, measurement of serum electrolytes, BUN, creatinine, and glucose), while commonly performed in patients scheduled to undergo cataract surgery, does not appear to measurably increase the safety of the surgery.

[f]Patients with significant functional and visual impairment due to cataract who have no contraindications to surgery should be counseled regarding the expected risks and benefits of and alternatives to surgery.

Sources: American Academy of Ophthalmology Preferred Practice Pattern: Cataract in the Adult Eye. (2006) (http://www.aao.org)
American Optometric Association Consensus Panel on Care of the Adult Patient with Cataract. Optometric Clinical practice guideline: Care of the Adult Patient with Cataract. (2004) (http://www.aoa.org)

CERUMEN IMPACTION

Disease Management	Organization	Date	Population	Recommendations	Comments	Source

Cerumen Impaction	AAO-HNS	2008	Children and adults	1. Strongly recommended treating cerumen impaction when it is symptomatic or prevents a needed clinical examination.
				2. Clinicians should treat the patient with cerumen impaction with an appropriate intervention:
				  a. Ceruminolytic agents
				  b. Irrigation
				  c. Manual removal
					Ceruminolytic agents include Cerumenex, addax, Debrox, or dilute solutions of acetic acid, hydrogen peroxide, or sodium bicarbonate.	http://www.entnet.org/practice/cerumenimpaction.cfm

2013 ACC/AHA Guidelines on the Treatment of Cholesterol to Reduce Atherosclerotic CV Risk in Adults
MAJOR STATIN BENEFIT GROUPS
ALL SHOULD RECEIVE Rx UNLESS CONTRAINDICATED

1) *Clinical ASCVD*
   Rx: High-intensity statin unless contraindicated or if age >70 y (moderate Rx)
2) *Primary elevation of LDL-C ≥190 mg/dL*
   Rx: High-intensity statin unless contraindicated then moderate Rx
3) *Diabetes (type 1 or 2) aged 40–75 y with LDL-C 70–189 mg/dL and without clinical ASCVD*
   Rx: Moderate-intensity statin; high-intensity statin Rx if 10-y ASCVD risk ≥7.5%
4) *Without clinical ASCVD or diabetes with LDL-C 70–189 mg/dL and estimated 10-y ASCVD ≥7.5%*[a]
   Rx: Moderate to high intensity statin

[a]The Pooled Cohort Equation
http://tools.cardiosource.org/ASCVD-Risk-Estimator/
Also available as "ASCVD Risk" app from iTunes and GooglePlay.
https://itunes.apple.com/us/app/ascvd-risk-estimator/id808875968?mt=8
https://play.google.com/store/apps/details?id=org.acc.cvrisk&hl=en

INTENSITY STATIN DRUG LEVELS	
High-Intensity Rx (lowers LDL-C >50%)	Atorvastatin 80 mg
	Rosuvastatin 40 mg
Moderate-Intensity Rx (lowers LDL-C 30%–50%)	Atorvastatin 10–20 mg
	Rosuvastatin 5–10 mg
	Simvastatin[a] 20–40 mg
	Pravastatin 40–80 mg
	Lovastatin 40 mg
	Fluvastatin *XL* 80 mg
	Fluvastatin 40 mg bid
	Pitavastatin 2–4 mg
	[a]*Simvastatin 80 mg should be avoided due to high risk of drug interactions*
Low-Intensity Rx	Simvastatin 10 mg
	Pravastatin 10–20 mg
	Lovastatin 20 mg
	Fluvastatin 20–40 mg
	Pitavastatin 1 mg

- If unable to tolerate moderate to high intensity statin therapy, consider the use of low-intensity dosages to reduce ASCVD risk.
- No RCTs have been identified that demonstrate that **titration of the drug dose** to specific LDL-C level improved ASCVD outcomes in primary or secondary prevention.

PRIMARY PREVENTION—GLOBAL RISK ASSESSMENT

1) Identify higher risk patients with a 10-y ASCVD risk as these are the patients mostly likely to benefit from Rx. The absolute benefit in ASCVD risk reduction is proportional to the baseline risk of the individual.
2) However, not all high-risk patients benefit, therefore a **"patient-centered"** approach is required. The potential of ASCVD risk reduction, adverse effects, drug-drug interaction, and patient's preference all must be considered. Age ≥70 y should not restrict the use of moderated-intensity statin therapy if otherwise indicated.
3) Adults ≥21 y with primary LDL-C >190 mg/dL should receive high-intensity statin Rx (10-y risk estimate not required).
4) Diabetes (type 1 or 2) aged 40–75 y with LDL-C 70–189 mg/dL and without clinical ASCVD. Rx: moderate intensity statin; high-intensity statin Rx if 10-year ASCVD risk ≥7.5%
5) Without clinical ASCVD or diabetes with LDL-C 70–189 mg/dL and estimated 10-year ASCVD ≥7.5%. Rx: moderate to high intensity statin
6) Nontraditional risk factors to consider: LDL-C ≥160 mg/dL, genetic hyperlipidemia, premature family history of ASCVD with onset <55 y in first-degree male relative or <65 y in first-degree female relative; high-sensitivity CRP ≥2 mg/L, coronary artery calcium score score >300 Agatston units or >75% for age, sex and ethnicity, ankle brachial index <0.9, or elevated lifetime risk of ASCVD. These should be considered when:
   a) Patients who are not in the 1 of the 4 statin benefit groups.
   b) Patients in whom the decision to start statin Rx remains unclear.
7) The panel emphasizes that the benefit of statin therapy outweighs the risk of newly diagnosed diabetes.
8) No RCTs have been identified that demonstrate that **titration of the drug dose** to specific LDL-C level improved ASCVD outcomes in primary or secondary prevention

Stone NJ, Robinson J, Lichtenstein AH, et al. 2013 ACC/AHA Guideline on the Treatment of Blood Cholesterol to Reduce Atherosclerotic Cardiovascular Disease Risk in Adults: A Report of the American College of Cardiology/American Heart Association Task Force on Practice Guidelines.
Circulation published online November 12, 2013. http://circ.ahajournals.org/content/early/2013/11/11/01.cir.0000437738.63853.7a.full.pdf
http://circ.ahajournals.org/content/early/2013/11/11/01.cir.0000437738.63853.7a.full.pdf+html.

LIPID AND STATIN MONITORING

Initial

- Prior to initiating statin, consider fasting lipid panel, ALT, HbA1C (to R/O DM).
- Baseline CK levels if the patient is at increased risk of adverse muscle events based on personal or family history of statin intolerance, muscle disease, or concomitant drugs which may have interactions with statins.

Chronic

- Routine CK is not indicated unless symptoms.
- Follow-up hepatic function if symptoms suggesting hepatic toxicity arise.
- If confusion or memory impairment occurs while on statin, evaluate for nonstatin causes or drug interactions with statin.
- Repeat second lipid panel 4–12 weeks after initiating therapy to determine patient's adherence. Then repeat lipid panel every 3–12 mo as clinically indicated.
- 2015 Statin use was associated with an increased likelihood of new diagnoses of DM, diabetic complications, and overweight/ obesity in healthy people taking statin for primary prevention. *Source:* Mansi I, Frei CR, Wang CP, et al. Statins and new-onset diabetes mellitus and diabetic complications: a retrospective cohort study of US healthy adults. *J Gen Intern Med.* 2015. DOI:10.007/s11606-015-3335-1
- In METSMIN (Metabolic Syndrome in Men) cohort, statin therapy (simvastatin, atorvastatin) was associated with a 46% increased risk of type 2 diabetes (after adjustment for confounding factors, worsening of hyperglycemia, a 24% reduction in insulin sensitivity, and a 12% reduction in insulin secretion). The risk of diabetes was increased in a dose-dependent and time-dependent manner by both simvastatin and atorvastatin. *Source: Diabetologia.* 2015;58:1109-1117. DOI 10.1007/s00125-015-3528-5

NON-STATIN CHOLESTEROL LOWERING AGENTS

- No data have demonstrated that adding a **nonstatin lipid drug** to statin therapy further reduces ASCVD events.
- In high-risk patients (clinical ASCVD, age <75 y; LDL-C ≥190 mg/dL; 40–75 y old with DM) who are intolerant to statins, may consider the use of nonstatin cholesterol lowering drugs.
- *Niacin*: indicated for LDL-C elevation or fasting triglyceride ≥500 mg/dL; should be avoided with liver disease, persistent hyperglycemia, acute gout, or new onset AF.
- *BAS*: indicated for LDL-C elevation; should be avoided with triglycerides ≥300 mg/dL.
- *Ezetimibe*: indicated for LDL-C elevation when combine with statin monitor transaminase levels.
- *Fibrates*: indicated for fasting triglycerides ≥500 mg/dL; should avoid the addition of Gemfibrozil to statin agent due to increased risk of muscle symptoms. Fenofibrate should be avoided if moderate/severe renal impairment. If needed, fenofibrate should only be added to a low- or moderate-intensity statin.
- *Omega-3 fatty acids*: indicated in severe fasting triglycerides ≥500 mg/dL.
- *New class of LDL lowering agent*: PCSK9 (proprotein convertase subtilisin kexin 9)
- FDA Advisory Panel (June 2015) recommended approval of:
  1. Alirocumab (Praluent®) for lowering LDL cholesterol in patients with hypercholestcrolemia, citing likely benefit especially for patients with heterozygous familial hypercholesterolemia (HeFH). Other groups predicted to get special benefit include those at high CV risk or who don't tolerate statin.
  2. Evolocumab (Repatha®) for lowering LDL-cholesterol. Studies have shown decrease in LDL-cholesterol most notably in patients with heterozygous familial hypercholesterolemia.
- FOURIER trial is an ongoing study which is testing the use of evolocumab in combination with statin therapy against placebo plus statin therapy in patients with elevated cholesterol levels and existing cardiovascular disease.

Source: http://www.medscape.com/viewarticle/846143

http://www.medscape.com/viewarticle/846236

2014 NLA (NATIONAL LIPID ASSOCIATION) GUIDELINES

- Population: adults >20 y old
- **Targets of therapy: non-HDL-C is more predictive than LDL-C, both are primary targets. Apolipoprotein B (apo B) is considered a secondary, optional target for therapy.**
- If low/moderate ASCVD risk: Trial of lifestyle management prior to initiate drug therapy. Reduction of saturated fat and cholesterol intake, moderate physical activity, weight loss, consider adding plant stanols/sterols, increase viscous fiber intake. Evaluate every 6 wk for atherogenic cholesterol response. If after 12 wk, goal is not achieved, consider adding drug therapy/referral to dietician. Once goal achieved, follow every 4–6 mo to monitor adherence to lifestyle therapies.
- High/very high ASCVD risk: Lifestyle management concomitant with drug therapy. A moderate or high intensity statin should be first-line drug therapy for treatment, unless contraindicated. In patients with very high TG, may consider TG-lowering drug (fibrates, high-dose omega 3 fatty acids, nicotinic acid) for first-line use to prevent pancreatitis. Follow every 6 wk, increasing the dosage/ intensity if not at goal. If not at goal after 12 wk, refer to lipid specialist. Once at goal, follow every 4–6 mo for treatment adherence. Involve patient when making the decision to start statin.
- If TG ≥500, may consider TG-lowering drug as first-line therapy.
- If TG 500–1000 mg/dL, may start with statin if no history of pancreatitis.
- Nonstatin therapies (BAS, CAI, fibrate, nicotinic acid) may be considered (alone or in combination) in those with contraindications to statin therapy.
- For patients with statin intolerance, reducing the dose of statin, switching to a different statin or every other day statin may be considered.
- Goals: attain levels below the goal cut points, non-HDL-C.
- For patients with ASCVD or DM, consideration should be given to use of moderate- or high-intensity statin therapy irrespective of baseline atherogenic cholesterol levels.
- Women with FH of childbearing age should receive prepregnancy counseling and instructions to stop statins, ezetimibe, and niacin at least 4 wk before discontinuing contraception and should not use these medications during pregnancy and lactation.
- During pregnancy in women with FH: consider LDL-apheresis if there is significant atherosclerotic disease or if the patient has homozygous FH.

Risk Category	Treatment Goal Non-HDL-C (LDL-C)	Consider Drug Therapy Non-HDL-C (LDL-C)
Low	<130 (<100)	≥190 (≥160)
Moderate	<130 (<100)	≥160 (≥130)
High	<130 (<100)	≥130 (≥100)
Very High	<100 (<70)	≥100 (≥70)

Source: NLA recommendations for patient-centered management of dyslipidemia. https://www.lipid.org/
*J Clin Lipidol.*2011;5: S1-S8. doi:10.1016/j.jacl.2011.04.003.

2014 AMERICAN DIABETES ASSOCIATION HYPERLIPIDEMIA GUIDELINES

- In all patients with hyperlipidemia and DM recommend lifestyle modifications including:
  - Diet: focusing on the reduction of saturated fat, trans fat, and cholesterol intake; increase of n-3 fatty acids, viscous fiber, and plant stanols/sterols
  - Weight loss: if indicated
  - Physical activity
  - Smoke cessation
- Regardless of baseline lipid levels, statin therapy should be added to lifestyle therapy in all patients with hyperlipidemia and DM who have overt CVD or who are without CVD, but are age >40, ≥1 CVD risk factors (family history of CVD, hypertension, smoking, dyslipidemia, or albuminuria).
- For low-risk patients: without overt CVD, age <40; consider statin in addition to lifestyle therapy if LDL-C remains >100 mg/dL or if >1 CVD risk factors.
- LDL-C targeted statin therapy remains the preferred strategy.
- LDL-C therapy goals:
  - Individuals without overt CVD: <100 mg/dL (2.6 mmol/L).
  - Individuals with overt CVD: <70 mg/dL (1.8 mmol/L) with high dose of statin is an option.
  - If drug-treated patients do not reach the above targets on maximum tolerated statin therapy, a reduction in LDL-C of 30%–40% from baseline is an alternative therapeutic goal.
- First priority treatment if severe hypertriglyceridemia at risk for pancreatitis, then focus on reducing the LDL-C.
- Triglyceride levels <150 mg/dL (1.7 mmol/L) and HDL-C >40 mg/dL (1 mmol/L) in men and >50 mg/dL (1.3 mmol/L) in women are desirable.
- Combination therapy has been shown not to provide additional CV benefit above statin therapy alone and is not generally recommended.
- Statin therapy is contraindicated in pregnancy.
- Although there is an increased risk of incident diabetes with statin use, the CV rate reduction with statins outweighed the risk of incident diabetes even for patient a highest risk for diabetes.

Standards of Medical Care in Diabetes 2014. *Diabetes Care.* 2014;37(1):S14-S80.

CHOLESTEROL GUIDELINES DIFFERENCES 2014

Guidelines	ACC/AHA 2013	ESC/EAS 2011
Risk stratification tools	ASCVD	SCORE
Scope of evidence	Randomized control trials	All data covering dyslipidemia
Therapy	Statin Rx only	Statin + additional cholesterol agents
F/U LDL-C levels	Only for evaluation of adherence	To evaluate adherence, allow risk stratification and consider additional cholesterol-lowering therapies
Quality risk scores	Not evaluated in Asia-Pacific population	European country specific
Present usage	USA	Europe

Adapted from: Ray KK, Kastelein JJP, Boekholdt SM, et al. The ACC/AHA 2013 guideline on the treatment of blood cholesterol to reduce atherosclerotic cardiovascular disease risk in adults: the good the bad and the uncertain: a comparison with ESC/EAS guidelines for the management of dyslipidemias 2011. 2014.

2011 EUROPEAN SOCIETY OF CARDIOLOGY/EUROPEAN ATHEROSCLEROSIS SOCIETY GUIDELINES FOR THE MANAGEMENT OF DYSLIPIDEMIA

ESC/EAS GUIDELINES

1. Screen with lipid profile:

   Men ≥40 y

   Women ≥50 y or postmenopausal with additional risk factors

   Evidence of atherosclerosis in any vascular bed

   Diabetes type 2

   Family history of premature cardiovascular disease (CVD)

2. Estimate total CV 10-year risk by *SCORE* (Systemic Coronary Risk Estimation), which has a large European cohort database, or the *Framingham Risk Score*.

   If the 10-y risk is ≥5% at increased risk, recommend heart score modified to include HDL-C.

VERY HIGH RISK—LDL-C goal <70 mg/dL

   Documented CVD by invasive or noninvasive testing, previous MI, percutaneous coronary intervention (PCI), coronary artery bypass graft (CABG), other arterial revascularization procedures, ischemic cardiovascular accident (CVA), or peripheral arterial disease (PAD)

   Type 2 diabetes; type 1 with end-organ disease (microalbinuria)

   Moderate-to-severe chronic kidney disease (CKD) GRF <60 mL/min/1.73 m^2

   Calculated 10-year risk SCORE ≥10%; FRS ≥20%

HIGH RISK—LDL-C goal <100 mg/dL

   Markedly elevated lipids or BP

   SCORE ≥5% and <10% for the 10-y risk of fatal cardiovascular disease (CVD); Framingham Risk Score (FRS) ≥20%

MODERATE RISK—LDL-C goal <115 mg/dL

   SCORE ≥1% and <5% at 10 y; FRS 10%–20%.

   Family history (FH) of premature CAD

   Obesity

   Physical inactivity

   Low HDL-C, high TGs

LOW RISK

SCORE <1 %; FRS ≤5%

3. Lipid analysis

   LDL-C is the primary marker

   TGs, HDL-C, non-HDL-C, apolipoprotein B (apoB) (with diabetes and MetS), lipoprotein a (LpA) in selected high-risk patients with FH of premature disease. Total cholesterol (TC) adds little to assessment

4. Lifestyle management—same as ATP recommendations with additional use of phytosterols, soy protein, red yeast rice, polycosanol supplements

5. Secondary causes for hypercholesterolemia

   Hypothyroidism, nephrotic syndrome, pregnancy, Cushing syndrome, anorexia nervosa, immunosuppressant agents, corticosteroids

6. Drug therapy

   LDL-C

   Statins—initial agent in moderate-, high-, or very-high-risk patients

   Statin therapy in primary prevention should be limited to patients with moderate or high risk.

   Combined therapy: bile acid sequestrant (BAS) + nicotinic acid, cholesterol absorption inhibitor + BAS + nicotinic acid

   TG >880 mg/dL—pancreatitis

   Fibrates, nicotinic acid, n-3 fatty acids

   HDL-C

   Nicotinic acid, statin, nicotinic acid + statin

   CKD stages 1–2

   Statin well tolerated; stage >3; more adverse events—use atorvastatin, fluvastatin, gemfibrozil

Source: European Association for Cardiovascular Prevention & Rehabilitation, Reiner Z, Catapano AL, De Backer G, et al; ESC Committee for Practice Guidelines (CPG) 2008–2010 and 2010–2012 Committees. ESC/EAS Guidelines. *Eur Heart J.* 2011;32:1769-1818.

2014 MANAGEMENT OF DYSLIPIDEMIA FOR CARDIOVASCULAR DISEASE RISK REDUCTION VETERAN AFFAIRS AND US DEPARTMENT OF DEFENSE CLINICAL PRACTICE GUIDELINE

- Screen all men >35, women >45, and all patients with atherosclerotic CVD (ASCVD) or equivalents
- Equivalents of ASCVD: ACS or MI, CABG or PCI, sable obstructive CAD, CVA/TIA, atherosclerotic PVD (claudication or AAA)
- If the patient has a history of CVD or ACS, calculate 10-y CVD risk, measure lipid levels and BP

10-year risk	Statin dose
ASCVD (second prevention)	Moderate to high
>12 %	Moderate
6%–12% (with shared decision making)	Moderate
<6%	None

- Statin dose

Statin	Moderate (mg)	High (mg)
Atorvastatin	10–20	40–80
Rosuvastatin	5–10	20–40
Simvastatin	20–40	
Pravastatin	40	
Lovastatin	40–80	
Fluvastatin	80 (80 daily or 40 bid)	

- If risk between 6% and 12%, the 10-y CVD risk should be repeated every 2 years. If risk <6%, the 10-y CVD risk should be repeated every 5 y.
- All patients should be encouraged to make positive lifestyle changes, to follow Mediterranean diet and to optimize comorbid conditions.

EXPERT PANEL ON INTEGRATED GUIDELINES FOR CARDIOVASCULAR HEALTH AND RISK REDUCTION IN CHILDREN AND ADOLESCENTS: SUMMARY REPORT 2013

SUMMARY:
- All children should have cholesterol screening once between ages 9 and 11 y and once between ages 17 and 21 y.
- Nonfasting total cholesterol and HDL cholesterol should be used as the screening tests.
- Clinicians may recommend low-fat or nonfat dairy at age 1 y for high-risk patients.
- If lifestyle changes are not effective, a lipid-lowering agent should be considered at age 10 y.

EVIDENCE-BASED RECOMMENDATIONS FOR DIETARY MANAGEMENT OF ELEVATED LDL-C, NON-HDL-C AND TGs

Grades reflect the findings of the evidence review.

Recommendation levels reflect the consensus opinion of the Expert Panel.

Supportive actions represent expert consensus suggestions from the Expert Panel provided to support implementation of the recommendations; they are not graded.

NOTE: Values given are in mg/dL. To convert to SI units, divide the results for TC, LDL-C, HDL-C, and non–HDL-C by 38.6; for TGs, divide by 88.6.

ELEVATED LDL-C: CHILD 2—LDL		
2–21 y	Refer to a registered dietitian for family medical nutrition therapy:	Grade B Strongly Recommend
	• 25%–30% of calories from fat, ≤7% from saturated fat, approximately 10% from monounsaturated fat; <200 mg/d of cholesterol; avoid trans fats as much as possible *Supportive actions:* • Plant sterol esters and/or plant stanol esters[a] up to 2 g/d as replacement for usual fat sources can be used after age 2 y in children with familial hypercholesterolemia. • Plant stanol esters as part of a regular diet are marketed directly to the public. Short-term studies show no harmful effects in healthy children. • The water-soluble fiber psyllium can be added to a low-fat, low-saturated-fat diet as cereal enriched with psyllium at a dose of 6 g/d for children 2–12 y, and 12 g/d for those ≥12 y. • As in all children, 1 h/d of moderate-to-vigorous physical activity and <2 h/d of sedentary screen time are recommended.	Grade A Recommend
[a]Can be found added to some foods, such as some margarines.		

ELEVATED TGs OR NON–HDL-C: CHILD 2—TGs		
2–21 years	Refer to a registered dietitian for family medical nutrition therapy:[a]	Grade B Strongly Recommend
	• 25%–30% of calories from fat, ≤7% from saturated fat, ~10% from monounsaturated fat; <200 mg/day of cholesterol; avoid trans fats as much as possible	Grade A Recommend

	• Decrease sugar intake:
	  ◦ Replace simple with complex carbohydrates
	  ◦ No sugar sweetened beverages
		Grade B
		Recommend

	• Increase dietary fish to increase omega-3 fatty acids[b]	Grade D Recommend

[a]If child is obese, nutrition therapy should include calorie restriction, and increased activity (beyond that recommended for all children).

[b]The Food and Drug Administration (FDA) and the Environmental Protection Agency are advising women of childbearing age who may become pregnant, pregnant women, nursing mothers, and young children to avoid some types of fish and shellfish and eat fish and shellfish that are low in mercury. For more information, call the FDA's food information line toll free at 1-888-SAFEFOOD or visit http://www.fda.gov/downloads/Food/FoodborneIllnessContaminants/UCM312787.pdf - page=21.

Source: Expert Panel on Integrated Guidelines for Cardiovascular Health and Risk Reduction in Children and Adolescents: Summary Report *Pediatrics* 2011;128(5):S213–S258.

EVIDENCE-BASED RECOMMENDATIONS FOR PHARMACOLOGIC TREATMENT OF DYSLIPIDEMIA		
Grades reflect the findings of the evidence review.		
Recommendation levels reflect the consensus opinion of the Expert Panel.		
When medication is recommended, this should always be in the context of the complete cardiovascular risk profile of the patient and in consultation with the patient and the family.		
NOTE: Values given are in mg/dL. To convert to SI units, divide the results for TC, LDL-C, HDL-C, and non–HDL-C by 38.6; for TGs, divide by 88.6.		

Birth—10 y	Pharmacologic treatment is limited to children with severe primary hyperlipidemia (homozygous familial hypercholesterolemia, primary hypertriglyceridemia with TG ≥500 mg/dL) or a high-risk condition or evident cardiovascular disease; all under the care of a lipid specialist.	Grade C Recommend
≥10–21 y	Detailed FH and risk factor (RF) assessment required before initiation of drug therapy.[a] High- to moderate-level RFs and risk conditions (RCs).	Grade C Strongly recommend
	LDL-C:	
	If average LDL-C ≥250 mg/dL[a], consult lipid specialist.	Grade B Strongly recommend
	If average LDL-C ≥130–250 mg/dL, or non–HDL ≥145 mg/dL: • Refer to dietitian for medical nutrition therapy with Cardiovascular Health Integrated Lifestyle Diet (CHILD 1) → CHILD 2-LDL × 6 mo → repeat fasting lipid panel (FLP)	Grade A Strongly recommend
	Repeat FLP:	
	• → LDL-C <130 mg/dL, continue CHILD 2-LDL, reevaluate in 12 mo	Grade A Strongly recommend
	• → LDL-C ≥190[b] mg/dL, consider initiation of statin therapy	Grade A Strongly recommend
	• → LDL-C ≥130–189 mg/dL, FH (–), no other RF or RC, continue CHILD 2-LDL, reevaluate q 6 mo	Grade B Recommend
	• → LDL-C = 160–189 mg/dL + FH positive *or* ≥1 high-level RF/RC *or* ≥2 moderate-level RFs/RCs, consider statin therapy	Grade B Recommend
	• → LDL-C ≥130–159 mg/dL + ≥2 high-level RFs/RCs *or* 1 high-level + 2 moderate-level RFs/RCs, consider statin therapy	Grade B Recommend
	Children on statin therapy should be counseled and carefully monitored.	Grade A Strongly recommend
	Detailed FH and RF/RC assessment required before initiation of drug therapy.[c] High- and moderate-level RFs/RCs.[d]	Grade C Strongly recommend
	TG:	
	If average TG ≥500 mg/dL, consult lipid specialist.	Grade B Recommend
	If average TG ≥100 mg/dL in a child <10 y, ≥130 mg/dL in a child age 10–19 y, TG <500 mg/dL:	
	• Refer to dietitian for medical nutrition therapy with CHILD 1 → CHILD 2-TG × 6 mo	Grade B Strongly recommend
	Repeat FLP:	
	• → TG <100 mg/dL, continue CHILD 2-TG, monitor 6–12 mo	Grade B Strongly recommend
	• → TG >100 mg/dL, reconsult dietitian for intensified CHILD 2 TG diet counseling	Grade C Recommend
	• → TG ≥200–499 mg/dL, non–HDL ≥145 mg/dL, consider fish oil ± consult lipid specialist	Grade D Recommend
	Non–HDL-C:	
	Children ≥10 y with non–HDL-C ≥145 mg/dL after LDL-C goal achieved may be considered for additional treatment with statins, fibrates, or niacin in conjunction with a lipid specialist.	Grade D Optional

[a]Consideration of drug therapy based on the average of ≥2 FLPs, obtained at least 2 wk but no >3 mo apart.
[b]If average LDL-C ≥190 mg/dL after CHILD 2-LDL and child is age 8–9 y with + FH *or* ≥1 high-level RF/RC *or* ≥2 moderate-level RFs/RCs, statin therapy may be considered.
[c]Consideration of drug therapy based on the average of ≥2 fasting lipid profiles obtained at least 2 weeks but no more than 3 months apart.
[d]If child is obese, nutrition therapy should include calorie restriction and increased activity beyond that recommended for all children.

Source: Expert Panel on Integrated Guidelines for Cardiovascular Health and Risk Reduction in Children and Adolescents: Summary Report. *Pediatrics.* 2011;128(5):S213-S258

MEDICATIONS FOR MANAGING HYPERLIPIDEMIA

Type of Medication	Mechanism of Action	Major Effects	Examples	Adverse Reactions	FDA Approval in Youths as of This Writing
HMG CoA Reductase Inhibitors (Statins)	Inhibits cholesterol synthesis in hepatic cells, decreases cholesterol pool, resulting in upregulation of LDL receptors	Mainly lowers LDL-C; some decrease in TG and modest increase in HDL-C	Atorvastatin Fluvastatin Lovastatin Pravastatin Rosuvastatin Simvastatin	Raised hepatic enzymes, raised creatine kinase, myopathy possibly progressing to rhabdomyolysis	All statins listed approved as an adjunct to diet to lower LDL-C in adolescent boys and postmenarchal girls ages 10–18 y (8+ y for pravastatin) with heterozygous familial hypercholesterolemia (HeFH) and LDL-C ≥190 mg/dL, or ≥160 mg/dL with FH of premature CVD and 2+ CVD risk factors in the pediatric patient
Bile Acid Sequestrants	Binds intestinal bile acids interrupting enterohepatic recirculation, more cholesterol converted into bile acids, decreases hepatic cholesterol pool, upregulates LDL receptors	Lowers LDL-C; small increase in HDL; raises TG	Cholestyramine Colestipol Colesevelam	Limited to gastrointestinal tract: gas, bloating constipation, cramps	No pediatric indication listed for cholestyramine or colestipol; colesevelam indicated as monotherapy or with statin for LDL-C reduction in boys and postmenarchal girls ages 10–17 y with FH after diet trial if LDL-C ≥190 mg/dL or if LDL-C ≥160 mg/dL with family history of premature CVD or 2+ more CVD risk factors in the pediatric patient
Cholesterol Absorption Inhibitors	Inhibits intestinal absorption of cholesterol and plant sterols, decreases hepatic cholesterol pool, upregulates LDL receptors	Mainly lowers LDL-C; some decrease in TG and small increase in HDL-C	Ezetimibe	Myopathy, gastrointestinal upset, headache	No
Fibric Acid Derivatives	Agonist for peroxisome proliferator-activated receptor (PPAR) alfa nuclear receptors that upregulate lipoprotein lipase (LPL) and downregulate apolipoprotein C (apoC)-III, both increasing degradation of very-low-density lipoprotein C (VLDL-C) and TG. Hepatic synthesis of VLDL-C may also be decreased.	Mainly lowers TG and raises HDL-C, with little effect on LDL-C	Fenofibrate Gemfibrozil	Dyspepsia, constipation, myositis, anemia	No
Nicotinic Acid (Extended Release)	Inhibits release of free fatty acid (FFA) from adipose tissue; decreases VLDL-C and LDL-C production and HDL-C degradation	Lowers TG and LDL-C and raises HDL-C; can decrease Lp(a)	Niacin, extended release	Flushing, hepatic toxicity, can increase fasting blood glucose, uric acid; hyperacidity	Use not recommended in children <2 y of age
Omega-3 Fish Oil	Decreases hepatic fatty acid (FA) and TG synthesis while enhancing FA degradation/oxidation, with subsequent reduced VLDL-C release	Lowers TG, raises HDL-C, increases LDL-C and LDL-C particle size	Omega-3 acid ethyl esters	Occasional gastrointestinal side effects, but no adverse effect on glucose levels or muscle or liver enzymes or bleeding	Only 1 FDA-approved fish oil preparation for adults, but many generic fish oil capsules commercially available

Sources: Expert Panel on Integrated Guidelines for Cardiovascular Health and Risk Reduction in Children and Adolescents: Summary Report 2013 Stephen R. Daniels, MD, PhD, Irwin Benuck, MD, PhD, Dimitri A. Christakis, MD, MPH et al. *Pediatrics.* 2011;128(6):S1–S44. http://www.nhlbi.nih.gov/guidelines/cvd_ped/summary.htm#chap9

COLITIS, *CLOSTRIDIUM DIFFICILE*

Disease Management	Organization	Date	Population	Recommendations	Comments	Source
Colitis, *Clostridium difficile*	IDSA SHEA	2010	Adults	• Treatment of *C. difficile* infection. ○ Discontinue antibiotics as soon as possible. ○ Avoid antiperistaltic agents. ○ Mild–moderate *C. difficile* infection: metronidazole 500 mg PO tid × 10–14 d. ○ Severe *C. difficile* infection: vancomycin 125 mg PO QID × 10–14 d. ○ Severe complicated *C. difficile* infection taking POs: vancomycin 500 mg PO QID ± metronidazole 500 mg IV q8h. ○ Severe complicated *C. difficile* infection and NPO: 500 mg in 100 mL normal saline enema per rectum qid ± metronidazole 500 mg IV q8h. ○ Administer vancomycin as a tapered regimen for recurrent *C. difficile* infection.	• Testing for *C. difficile* or its toxins should be performed only on diarrheal stool. • Testing of stool on asymptomatic patients should be avoided. • Enzyme immunoassay (EIA) testing for *C. difficile* toxins A and B is rapid but is less sensitive than the cell cytotoxin assay. • Stool for *C. difficile* toxins by polymerase chain reaction (PCR) is rapid and very sensitive and specific.	http://www.doh.state.fl.us/disease_ctrl/epi/HAI/SHEA_IDSA_Clinical_Practice_Cdiff_Guideline.pdf
	ACG	2013	Adults and children	• Only diarrheal stools should be tested for *C. difficile*. • Nucleic acid amplification tests (NAAT) for *C. difficile* toxin genes such as polymerase chain reaction (PCR) are superior to toxins A+B enzyme immunoassay (EIA) testing as a standard diagnostic test for *C. difficile* infection (CDI). • Do not perform repeat testing. • Avoid testing for cure. • Management of mild–moderate *C. difficile* infection (CDI) ○ Stop all unnecessary antibiotics ○ Recommend empiric therapy of CDI regardless of test results if high pretest probability of CDI ○ First-line therapy ○ Metronidazole 500 mg PO tid × 10 d ○ Second-line therapy ○ Vancomycin 125 mg PO qid × 10 d ○ Indicated for intolerance of metronidazole, lack of improvement after 5–7 d on metronidazole, pregnancy, or breast-feeding ○ Avoid antiperistaltic meds • Severe or complicated CDI ○ Vancomycin 125 mg PO qid AND metronidazole 500 mg IV q8h × 10 d ○ If ileus or severe abdominal distension, use vancomycin 500 mg PO qid AND 500 mg enema PR qid AND metronidazole 500 mg IV q8h × 10 d ○ IV hydration ○ Electrolyte repletion ○ DVT prophylaxis ○ Surgical consult for all patients with complicated CDI • Recurrent CDI ○ Consider fetal microbiota transplant after third recurrence	• Limited evidence that probiotics decrease risk of recurrent CDI. • The following patients should be tested for CDI: ○ IBD patients with a flare ○ IBD patients with a surgically created pouch who develop abdominal pain • Immunosuppressed patients with an acute diarrheal illness. • Pregnant patients who develop diarrhea.	http://www.guideline.gov/content.aspx?id=45139
	EAST	2014	Adult patients with *C. difficile*–associated disease	• If surgery is indicated, recommend a subtotal or total colectomy. • For severe CDAD, patients should undergo surgery prior to the development of shock and need for vasopressors.		http://www.guideline.gov/content.aspx?id=48870

COMMON COLD

Disease Management	Organization	Date	Population	Recommendations	Comments	Source
Common Cold	Cochrane Database of Systematic Reviews	2013	Children and adults	Recommend zinc at a dose of at least 75 mg/d started within 24 h of the onset of a common cold.	Zinc at this dose reduces the duration of the common cold by about 1 d, but did not affect the severity of symptoms.	http://onlinelibrary.wiley.com/doi/10.1002/14651858.CD001364.pub4/abstract

CONCUSSIONS

Disease Management	Organization	Date	Population	Recommendations	Comments	Source
Concussions	AAN	2013	Children and young adults	• Standardized sideline assessment tools should be used to assess athletes with suspected concussions. • Teams should immediately remove from play any athlete with a suspected concussion. • Teams should not permit an athlete to return to play until he/she has been cleared to play by a licensed health care professional.		http://www.guideline.gov/content.aspx?id=43947

CONSTIPATION, IDIOPATHIC

Disease Management	Organization	Date	Population	Recommendations	Comments	Source
Constipation, Idiopathic	NICE	2010	Children age ≤18 years	1. Assess all children for fecal impaction. 2. Recommends polyethylene glycol (PEG) as first-line agent for oral disimpaction. 3. Add a stimulant laxative if PEG therapy is ineffective after 2 wk. 4. Recommends sodium citrate enemas for disimpaction only if all oral medications have failed. 5. Recommends a maintenance regimen with PEG for several months after a regular bowel pattern has been established. 6. Recommends gradually tapering maintenance dose over several months as bowel pattern allows. 7. Recommends adequate fluid intake.	Minimal fluid intake for age: Age — Volume 1–3 y — 1300 mL 4–8 y — 1700 mL 9–13 y — 2200 mL 14–18 y — 2500 mL	http://www.nice.org.uk/nicemedia/live/12993/48741/48741.pdf

	AGA	2013	Adults	• Digital examination to evaluate resting sphincter tone.
				• Discontinue all medications that can cause constipation.
				• Assess for hypercalcemia, hypothyroidism.
				• Trial of laxatives and fiber
				  ○ Bisacodyl
				  ○ Milk of Magnesia
				  ○ Polyethylene glycol
				  ○ Senna
				• Refractory constipation may require biofeedback or pelvic floor retraining.
				  ○ Severe cases of refractory slow transit constipation may require a total colectomy with ileorectal anastomosis.
						http://www.gastrojournal.org/article/S0016-5085%2812%2901545-4/fulltext

CONTRACEPTION, EMERGENCY

Disease Management	Organization	Date	Population	Recommendations	Comments	Source
Contraception, Emergency	ACOG	2010	Women of childbearing age who had unprotected or inadequately protected sexual intercourse within the last 5 d and who do not desire pregnancy	• The levonorgestrel-only regimen is more effective and is associated with less nausea and vomiting compared with the combined estrogen-progestin regimen. • The two 0.75-mg doses of the levonorgestrel-only regimen are equally effective if taken 12–24 h apart. • The single-dose 1.5-mg levonorgestrel-only regimen is as effective as the 2-dose regimen. • Recommend an antiemetic agent 1 h before the first dose of the combined estrogen-progestin regimen to reduce nausea. • Treatment with emergency contraception should be initiated as soon as possible after unprotected or inadequately protected intercourse. • Emergency contraception should be made available to patients who request it up to 5 d after unprotected intercourse.	• No clinician examination or pregnancy testing is necessary before provision or prescription of emergency contraception. • The copper intrauterine device (IUD) is appropriate for use as emergency contraception for women who desire long-acting contraception. • Information regarding effective long-term contraceptive methods should be made available whenever a woman requests emergency contraception.	http://www.guidelines.gov/content.aspx?id=15718&search=emergency+contraception

PERCENTAGE OF WOMEN EXPERIENCING AN UNINTENDED PREGNANCY DURING THE FIRST YEAR OF TYPICAL USE AND THE FIRST YEAR OF PERFECT USE OF CONTRACEPTION AND THE PERCENTAGE CONTINUING USE AT THE END OF THE FIRST YEAR—UNITED STATES

Method	Women Experiencing an Unintended Pregnancy Within the First Year of Use		Women Continuing Use at 1 Y[c]
	Typical Use[a]	Perfect Use[b]	
No method[d]	85%	85%	
Spermicides[e]	29%	18%	42%
Withdrawal	27%	4%	43%
Fertility awareness-based methods	25%		51%
Standard Days method[f]		5%	
Two Day methodTMf		4%	
Ovulation methodf		3%	
Sponge			
Parous women	32%	20%	46%
Nulliparous women	16%	9%	57%
Diaphragm[g]	16%	6%	57%
Condom[h]			
Female (Reality®)	21%	5%	49%
Male	15%	2%	53%
Combined pill and progestin-only pill	8%	0.3%	68%
Evra patch®	8%	0.3%	68%
NuvaRing®	8%	0.3%	68%
Depo-Provera®	3%	0.3%	56%
Intrauterine device			
ParaGard® (copper T)	0.8%	0.6%	78%
Mirena® (LNG-IUS)	0.2%	0.2%	80%
Implanon®	0.05%	0.05%	84%
Female sterilization	0.5%	0.5%	100%
Male sterilization	0.15%	0.10%	100%

PERCENTAGE OF WOMEN EXPERIENCING AN UNINTENDED PREGNANCY DURING THE FIRST YEAR OF TYPICAL USE AND THE FIRST YEAR OF PERFECT USE OF CONTRACEPTION AND THE PERCENTAGE CONTINUING USE AT THE END OF THE FIRST YEAR—UNITED STATES (CONTINUED)

Method	Women Experiencing an Unintended Pregnancy Within the First Year of Use		Women Continuing Use at 1 Y[c]
	Typical Use[a]	Perfect Use[b]	
Emergency contraceptive pills[i]	Not applicable	Not applicable	Not applicable
Lactational amenorrhea methods[j]	Not applicable	Not applicable	Not applicable

Adapted from Trussell J. Contraceptive efficacy. In: Hatcher RA, Trussell J, Nelson AL, Cates W, Stewart FH, Kowal D, eds. *Contraceptive Technology*. 19th rev. ed. New York, NY: Ardent Media; 2007.

[a]Among typical couples who initiate use of a method (not necessarily for the first time), the percentage who experience an unintended pregnancy during the first year if they do not stop use for any other reason. Estimates of the probability of pregnancy during the first year of typical use for spermicides, withdrawal, fertility awareness-based methods, the diaphragm, the male condom, the pill, and Depo-Provera are taken from the 1995 National Survey of Family Growth corrected for underreporting of abortion; see the text for the derivation of estimates for the other methods.

[b]Among couples who initiate use of a method (not necessarily for the first time) and who use it *perfectly* (both consistently and correctly), the percentage who experience an unintended pregnancy during the first year if they do not stop use for any other reason. See the text for the derivation of the estimate for each method.

[c]Among couples attempting to avoid pregnancy, the percentage who continue to use a method for 1 y.

[d]The percentages becoming pregnant in the typical use and perfect use columns are based on data from populations where contraception is not used and from women who cease using contraception to become pregnant. Of these, approximately 89% become pregnant within 1 y. This estimate was lowered slightly (to 85%) to represent the percentage who would become pregnant within 1 year among women now relying on reversible methods of contraception if they abandoned contraception altogether.

[e]Foams, creams, gels, vaginal suppositories, and vaginal film.

[f]The Two Day and Ovulation methods are based on evaluation of cervical mucus. The Standard Days method avoids intercourse on cycle days 8–19.

[g]With spermicidal cream or jelly.

[h]Without spermicides.

[i]Treatment initiated within 72 h after unprotected intercourse reduces the risk for pregnancy by at least 75%. The treatment schedule is 1 dose within 120 h after unprotected intercourse and a second dose 12 h after the first dose. Both doses of Plan B can be taken at the same time. Plan B (1 dose is 1 white pill) is the only dedicated product specifically marketed for emergency contraception. The Food and Drug Administration has in addition declared the following 22 brands of oral contraceptives to be safe and effective for emergency contraception: Ogestrel or Ovral (1 dose is 2 white pills); Nordette (1 dose is 4 light-orange pills); Cryselle, Levora, Low-Ogestrel, Lo/Ovral, or Quasense (1 dose is 4 white pills); Tri-Levlen or Triphasil (1 dose is 4 yellow pills); Jolessa, Portia, Seasonale, or Trivora (1 dose is 4 pink pills); Seasonique (1 dose is 4 light blue-green pills); Enpresse (1 dose is 4 orange pills); Alesse, Lessina (1 dose is 5 pink pills); Aviane (1 dose is 5 orange pills); and Lutera (1 dose is 5 white pills).

[j]Lactational amenorrhea method is a highly effective temporary method of contraception. However, to maintain effective protection against pregnancy, another method of contraception must be used as soon as menstruation resumes, the frequency or duration of breast-feeding is reduced, bottle feeds are introduced, or the baby reaches 6 mo of age. *Matern Child Health J.* 2013; 17(4): 654-660.

SUMMARY OF CHANGES IN CLASSIFICATIONS FROM WHOM MEDICAL ELIGIBILITY CRITERIA FOR CONTRACEPTIVE USE, 4TH EDITION[a,b]

Condition	COC/P/R	POP	DMPA	Implants	LNG-IUD	Cu-IUD	Clarification
Breast-feeding							The US Department of Health and Human Services recommends that infants be exclusively breast-fed during the first 4–6 mo of life, preferably for a full 6 mo. Ideally, breast-feeding should continue through the first year of life (1). {Not included in WHO MEC}
a. <1 mo postpartum {WHO: <6 wk postpartum}	3[c] {4}	2[c] {3}	2[c] {3}	2[c] {3}			
b. 1 mo to <6 mo {WHO: ≥6 wk to <6 mo postpartum}	2[c] {3}						
Postpartum (in breast-feeding or non-breast-feeding women), including postcesarean section							
a. <10 min after delivery of the placenta {WHO: <48 h, including insertion immediately after delivery of the placenta}					2 {1 if not breast-feeding and 3 if breast-feeding}	2 {3}	
b. 10 min after delivery of the placenta to <4 wk {WHO: ≥48 h to <4 wk}					2 {3}	2 {3}	
Deep venous thrombosis (DVT)/pulmonary embolism (PE)							Women on anticoagulant therapy are at risk for gynecologic complications of therapy such as hemorrhagic ovarian cysts and severe menorrhagia. Hormonal contraceptive methods can be of benefit in preventing or treating these complications. When a contraceptive method is used as a therapy, rather than solely to prevent pregnancy, the risk/benefit ratio may be different and should be considered on a case-by-case basis. {Not included in WHO MEC}
a. History of DVT/PE, not on anticoagulant therapy							
i. Lower risk for recurrent DVT/PE (no risk factors)	3 {4}						
b. Acute DVT/PE							
c. DVT/PE and established on anticoagulant therapy for at least 3 months		2 {3}	2 {3}	2 {3}	2 {3}	2 {1}	
i. Higher risk for recurrent DVT/PE (≥1 risk factors)							
• Known thrombophilia, including antiphospholipid syndrome							
• Active cancer (metastatic, on therapy, or within 6 months after clinical remission), excluding nonmelanoma skin cancer						2 {1}	
• History of recurrent DVT/PE							
ii. Lower risk for recurrent DVT/PE (no risk factors)	3[c] {4}					2 {1}	
Valvular heart disease							
a. Complicated (pulmonary hypertension, risk for atrial fibrillation, history of subacute bacterial endocarditis)						1 {2}	1 {2}
Ovarian cancer[d]						1 {Initiation = 3, Continuation = 2}	1 {Initiation = 3, Continuation = 2}
Uterine fibroids						2 {1 if no uterine distortion and 4 if uterine distortion is present}	2 {1 if no uterine distortion and 4 if uterine distortion is present}

[a]For conditions for which classification changed for ≥1 methods or the condition description underwent a major modification, WHO conditions and recommendations appear in curly brackets.

[b]Abbreviations: COC, combined oral contraceptive; Cu-IUD, copper intrauterine device; DMPA, depot medroxyprogesterone acetate; DVT, deep venous thrombosis; LNG-IUD, levonorgestrel-releasing intrauterine device; P, combined hormonal contraceptive patch; PE, pulmonary embolism; POP, progestin-only pill; R, combined hormonal vaginal ring; VTE, venous thromboembolism; WHO, World Health Organization.

[c]Consult the clarification column for this classification.

[d]Condition that exposes a women to increased risk as a result of unintended pregnancy.

SUMMARY OF RECOMMENDATIONS FOR MEDICAL CONDITIONS ADDED TO THE US MEDICAL ELIGIBILITY CRITERIA FOR CONTRACEPTIVE USE[a]

Condition	COC/P/R	POP	DMPA	Implants	LNG-IUD Initiation	LNG-IUD Continuation	Cu-IUD Initiation	Cu-IUD Continuation	Clarification
History of bariatric surgery[b]									
a. Restrictive procedures: decrease storage capacity of the stomach (vertical banded gastroplasty, laparoscopic adjustable gastric band, laparoscopic sleeve gastrectomy)	1	1	1	1	1		1		
b. Malabsorptive procedures: decrease absorption of nutrients and calories by shortening the functional length of the small intestine (Roux-en-Y gastric bypass, biliopancreatic diversion)	COCs: 3 P/R: 1	3	1	1	1		1		
Peripartum cardiomyopathy[c]									
a. Normal or mildly impaired cardiac function (New York Heart Association Functional Class I or II: patients with no limitation of activities or patients with slight, mild limitation of activity) (2)									
i. <6 mo	4	1	1	1	2		2		
ii. ≥6 mo	3	1	1	1	2		2		
b. Moderately or severely impaired cardiac function (New York Heart Association Functional Class III or IV: patients with marked limitation of activity or patients who should be at complete rest) (2)	4	2	2	2	2		2		
Rheumatoid arthritis									
a. On immunosuppressive therapy	2	1	2/3[d]	1	2	2	2	1	DMPA use among women on long-term corticosteroid therapy with a history of, or risk factors for, nontraumatic fractures is classified as Category 3. Otherwise, DMPA use for women with rheumatoid arthritis is classified as Category 2.
b. Not on immunosuppressive therapy	2	1	2	1	1	1	1	1	
Endometrial hyperplasia	1	1	1	1	1		1		
Inflammatory bowel disease (IBD) (Ulcerative colitis, Crohn disease)	2/3[d]	2	2	1	1		1		For women with mild IBD, with no other risk factors for VTE, the benefits of COC/P/R use generally outweigh the risks (Category 2). However, for women with IBD with increased risk for VTE (eg, those with active or extensive disease, surgery, immobilization, corticosteroid use, vitamin deficiencies, fluid depletion), the risks for COC/P/R use generally outweigh the benefits (Category 3).

SUMMARY OF RECOMMENDATIONS FOR MEDICAL CONDITIONS ADDED TO THE US MEDICAL ELIGIBILITY CRITERIA FOR CONTRACEPTIVE USE[a] (CONTINUED)

Condition	COC/P/R	POP	DMPA	Implants	LNG-IUD		Cu-IUD		Clarification
					Initiation	Continuation	Initiation	Continuation	
Solid organ transplantation[b]									
a. Complicated: graft failure (acute or chronic), rejection, cardiac allograft vasculopathy	4	2	2	2	3	2	3	2	Women with Budd-Chiari syndrome should not use COC/P/R because of the increased risk for thrombosis.
b. Uncomplicated	2[c]	2	2	2	2		2		

[a]Abbreviations: COC, combined oral contraceptive; Cu-IUD, copper intrauterine device; DMPA, depot medroxyprogesterone acetate; IBD, inflammatory bowel disease; LNG-IUD, levonorgestrel-releasing intrauterine device; P, combined hormonal contraceptive patch; POP, progestin-only pill; R, combined hormonal vaginal ring; VTE, venous thromboembolism.
[b]History of bariatric surgery. *Contraception.* 2010;82(1):86–94.
[c]Condition that exposes a woman to increased risk as a result of unintended pregnancy.
[d]Consult the clarification column for this classification.
[e]History of solid organ transplantation. *Transplantation.* 2013;95(10):1183–1186.

SUMMARY OF ADDITIONAL CHANGES TO THE US MEDICAL ELIGIBILITY CRITERIA FOR CONTRACEPTIVE USE	
Condition/Contraceptive Method	**Change**
Emergency contraceptive pills	History of bariatric surgery, rheumatoid arthritis, inflammatory bowel disease, and solid organ transplantation were given a Category 1.
Barrier methods	For six conditions—history of bariatric surgery, peripartum cardiomyopathy, rheumatoid arthritis, endometrial hyperplasia, IBD, and solid organ transplantation—the barrier methods are classified as Category 1.
Sterilization	In general, no medical conditions would absolutely restrict a person's eligibility for sterilization. Recommendations from the WHO Medical Eligibility Criteria for Contraceptive Use about specific settings and surgical procedures for sterilization are not included here. The guidance has been replaced with general text on sterilization.
Other deleted items	Guidance for combined injectables, levonorgestrel implants, and norethisterone enanthate has been removed because these methods are not currently available in the United States. Guidance for "blood pressure measurement unavailable" and "history of hypertension, where blood pressure *cannot* be evaluated (including hypertension in pregnancy)" has been removed.
Unintended pregnancy and increased health risk	The following conditions have been added to the WHO list of conditions that expose a woman to increased risk as a result of unintended pregnancy: history of bariatric surgery within the past 2 y, peripartum cardiomyopathy, and receiving a solid organ transplant within 2 y.

COMMON MEDICATIONS FOR THE MANAGEMENT OF COPD					
Drug	**Inhaler (µg/dose)**	**Nebulizer (mg/mL)**	**Drug**	**Inhaler (µg/dose)**	**Nebulizer (mg/mL)**
Short-acting β₂-agonists			**Combination β₂-agonist-anticholinergics**		
Albuterol	100–200[M/D]	5	Albuterol-ipratropium	100/20[SMI]	1 vial
Levalbuterol	45–90M	0.21,0.42	**Methylxanthines**		
Long-acting β₂-agonists			Aminophylline	200–600 mg pill PO	
Arformoterol		0.0075	Theophylline SR	100–600 mg pill PO	
Formoterol	4.5–12[M/D]	0.01	**Inhaled corticosteroids**		
Indacaterol	75–300[D]		Beclomethasone	50–400[M/D]	0.2–0.4
Salmeterol	25–50[M/D]		Budesonide	100,200,400[D]	0.2,0.25,0.5
Short-acting anticholinergics			Fluticasone	50–500[M/D]	
Ipratropium bromide	20, 40M	0.25–0.5	**Combination β₂-agonist-corticosteroids**		
Long-acting anticholinergics			Formoterol-Budesonide	4.5/160[M]; 9/320[D]	
Aclidinium bromide	322[D]		Formoterol-Mometasone	10/200[M] or 10/400[M]	
Tiotropium	18[D], 5[SMI]		Salmeterol-Fluticasone	50/100, 50/250, 50/500[D] 25/50, 25/125, 25/250[M]	
Phosphodiesterase-4 inhibitors			Vilanterol-Fluticasone	25/100[D]	
Roflumilast	500 µg PO daily				

Data from GOLD Guide to COPD Diagnosis, Management and Prevention. http://www.goldcopd.org/uploads/users/files/GOLD_Pocket2014_Jan30.pdf.

CHRONIC OBSTRUCTIVE PULMONARY DISEASE (COPD), EXACERBATIONS

Disease Management	Organization	Date	Population	Recommendations	Comments	Source
Chronic Obstructive Pulmonary Disease (COPD), Exacerbations	NICE GOLD	2010 2013	Adults	1. Recommends noninvasive positive pressure ventilation for moderate-severe hypercapnic respiratory failure. 2. Prednisolone 30–40 mg orally, or its equivalent IV, should be prescribed for 10–14 d. 3. Recommends antibiotics for COPD exacerbations associated with more purulent sputum or need for mechanical ventilation. 4. Bronchodilators can be delivered by either nebulizers or meter-dosed inhalers depending on the patient's ability to use the device during a COPD exacerbation. Bilevel positive airway pressure (Bi-PAP) is indicated for moderate-severe COPD exacerbations. 5. Bi-PAP decreases mortality, need for mechanical ventilation, infectious complications, and hospital length of stay.	Initial empiric antibiotics should be an aminopenicillin, macrolide, or a tetracycline and should be given for 5–10 d.	http://www.nice.org.uk/nicemedia/live/13029/49397/49397.pdf http://www.guidelines.gov/content.aspx?id=43794
	Cochrane Database of Systematic Reviews	2014		Short course corticosteroids (7 d or less) is sufficient treatment for adults with a COPD exacerbation.		http://www.cochrane.org/CD006897/AIRWAYS_are-shorter-courses-of-systemic-steroids-as-effective-as-conventional-longer-courses-in-the-treatment-of-patients-with-flare-ups-of-copd

CHRONIC OBSTRUCTIVE PULMONARY DISEASE (COPD), STABLE

Disease Management	Organization	Date	Population	Recommendations	Comments	Source

Chronic Obstructive Pulmonary Disease (COPD), Stable	NICE GOLD	2010 2013	Adults	1. Recommends confirming all suspected COPD with postbronchodilator spirometry.
				2. Recommends spirometry in all persons age >35 y who are current or ex-smokers and have a chronic cough to evaluate for early stage COPD.
				3. Recommends smoking cessation counseling.
				4. Stepwise medication approach[a]:
				  a. Short-acting β-agonist (SABA) as needed (PRN)
				  b. If persistent symptoms, add:
				    i. FEV_1 ≥50% of predicted, add either a long-acting β-agonist (LABA) or long-acting muscarinic agonist (LAMA)
				    ii. FEV_1 <50% of predicted, add either LABA + inhaled corticosteroid (ICS), or LAMA
				  c. If persistent symptoms, add:
				    i. LAMA to LABA + ICS
				5. Recommends pulmonary rehabilitation for symptomatic patients with moderate-severe COPD (FEV_1 <50% of predicted).
				6. Recommends calculating the BODE index (BMI, airflow obstruction, dyspnea, and exercise capacity on a 6-min walk test) to calculate the risk of death in severe COPD.[b]
					FEV_1/FVC <0.7 confirms the presence of airflow obstruction and COPD.
					Classification of COPD by spirometry:
					Mild COPD = FEV_1 ≥80% of predicted
					Moderate COPD = FEV_1 50–79% of predicted
					Severe COPD = FEV_1 30–49% of predicted
					Very severe COPD = FEV_1 <30% of predicted
					Can consider lung volume reduction surgery in patients with severe upper lobe emphysema and low postpulmonary rehab exercise capacity.
					Consider roflumilast, a phosphodiesterase-4 inhibitor, to reduce exacerbations for patients with severe chronic bronchitis with frequent exacerbations.
						http://www.nice.org.uk/nicemedia/live/13029/49397/49397.pdf
						http://www.guidelines.gov/content.aspx?id=43794

	ACP	2011	Adults	• Spirometry should be obtained to diagnose airflow obstruction in patients presenting with respiratory symptoms. • Bronchodilators should be prescribed for stable COPD patients with respiratory symptoms and an FEV_1 60%–80% of predicted. • Inhaled corticosteroids and long-acting anticholinergics or long-acting β-agonists should be prescribed for stable COPD patients with respiratory symptoms and an FEV_1 <60% of predicted. • Pulmonary rehabilitation should be prescribed for symptomatic COPD patients with an FEV_1 <50% of predicted. • Continuous oxygen therapy should be prescribed for COPD patients with room air hypoxemia (PaO_2 ≤55 mm Hg or SpO_2 ≤88%). • All patients should have a pneumococcal vaccine and annual influenza vaccines. • Recommend screening COPD patients for osteoporosis and depression. • No role for chronic antibiotics to prevent exacerbations. • Recommend against regular mucolytic therapy.	• No proven benefit for using spirometry to encourage smoking cessation. • No role for periodic spirometry to monitor disease status. • No role for spirometry for at-risk patients who are *asymptomatic*.	http://www.annals.org/content/155/3/179.full.pdf+html

[a]SABA: albuterol, fenoterol, levalbuterol, metaproterenol, pirbuterol, and terbutaline; LABA: arformoterol, formoterol, or salmeterol; LAMA: tiotropium; ICS: beclomethasone, budesonide, ciclesonide, flunisolide, fluticasone, mometasone, and triamcinolone.

[b]See http://www.nejm.org/doi/full/10.1056/NEJMoa021322#t=article

STABLE CORONARY DISEASE ACCF/AHA/ACP/AATS/PCNA/SCAI/STS GUIDELINES 2012, 2014

- Patients presenting with angina pectoris should be classified as *stable* or *unstable*.
- *Acute coronary syndrome* (ACS) includes high-risk unstable angina, non-ST-segment elevation myocardial infarction (NSTEMI) or ST-segment elevation myocardial infarction (STEMI).
- Resting ECG testing is recommended with all symptoms of chest pain (typical or atypical in nature).
- Exercise treadmill is the preferred initial test to be employed if the baseline is normal, the patient can exercise, and the pretest likelihood of coronary disease is intermediate (10%–90%).
- If unable to perform an exercise treadmill, then either a nuclear myocardial perfusion imaging study (MPI) or exercise echocardiogram should be employed if the pretest likelihood is >10%.
- Exercise and imaging studies should be repeated when there is a *change in clinical status* or if needed for exercise prescription.
- *Coronary computed tomography angiogram* (CTA) is a reasonable alternative in patients with an intermediate pretest probability of CAD (FRS) in whom symptoms persist despite prior normal testing, with equivocal stress tests, or in patients who cannot be studied otherwise. CTA is not indicated with known moderate or severe coronary calcification or in the presence of prior stents.
- An echocardiogram is recommended to assess resting LV function and valve disease in patients with suspected CAD, pathological Q waves, presence of heart failure, or ventricular arrhythmias.
- Patients with stable coronary disease should receive:
  - Lifestyle guidance (diet, weight loss, smoking cessation, and exercise education) *BP threshold of <140/90 mm Hg* is projected to be the new JCN 8 goal.
  - Associated risk factor assessment: Presence of *chronic kidney disease* and *psychosocial factors* such as depression, anxiety, and poor social support have been added to the classic risk factors.
  - Appropriate medicine prescription: (ASA 75–162 mg daily, moderate statin dosage, BP control and diabetic control, β-blocker therapy, and sublingual NTG).
- Coronary angiography should be considered in patients surviving sudden cardiac death, with *high-risk noninvasive test results* (large areas of silent ischemia often associated with malignant ventricular arrhythmias) and in patients in whom the *anginal symptoms cannot be controlled* with optimal medical therapy.[a]
- Coronary bypass grafting surgery (CABG) is preferred to angioplasty in diabetic patients with multivessel disease (FREEDOM Trial 2012).[b]

[a]Coronary angiography is useful in patients with presumed SIHD who have unacceptable ischemic symptoms despite GDMT (guideline determined medical therapy) and who are amenable to, and candidates for, coronary revascularization. Is reasonable to define the extent and severity of coronary artery disease (CAD) in patients with suspected SIHD whose clinical characteristics and results of noninvasive testing (exclusive of stress testing) indicate a high likelihood of severe IHD and who are amenable to, and candidates for, coronary revascularization. Is reasonable in patients with suspected symptomatic SIHD who cannot undergo diagnostic stress testing, or have indeterminate or nondiagnostic stress tests, when there is a high likelihood that the findings will result in important changes to therapy. Might be considered in patients with stress test results of acceptable quality that do not suggest the presence of CAD when clinical suspicion of CAD remains high and there is a high likelihood that the findings will result in important changes to therapy.
[b]A Heart Team approach to revascularization is recommended in patients with diabetes mellitus and complex multivessel CAD. CABG is generally recommended in preference to PCI to improve survival in patients with diabetes mellitus and multivessel CAD for which revascularization is likely to improve survival (3-vessel CAD or complex 2-vessel CAD involving the proximal LAD), particularly if a LIMA graft can be anastomosed to the LAD artery, provided the patient is a good candidate for surgery.

Source: Fihn SD, Blankenship JC, Alexander KP, et al. 2014 ACC/AHA/AATS/PCNA/SCAI/STS focused update of the guideline for the diagnosis and management of patients with stable ischemic heart disease. *J Am Coll Cardiol.* 2014. doi:10.1016/j.jacc.2014.07.017.

CORONARY ARTERY DISEASE: SEXUAL FUNCTION
AHA AND PRINCETON CONSENSUS PANEL RECOMMENDATIONS 2013

- Erectile dysfunction (ED) is associated with CAD and often precedes the diagnosis of CAD
- ED was associated with an increased risk for CV events and all-cause mortality.
- Angina pectoris during sexual activity represents <5% of all angina attacks.
- Patients with CAD with angina pectoris should undergo full medical evaluation prior to partaking in sexual activity.
- Patients should be able to perform 3–5 metabolic equivalents (METs) on a treadmill or climb 2 flights of stairs or walk briskly without angina before engaging in sexual activity.
- Post-uncomplicated MI if no symptoms on mild-to-moderate activity exist >1 wk, patient may resume sexual activity.
- Post angioplasty within 1-wk sexual activity is reasonable if the radial groin site is healed.
- Sexual activity is reasonable 6–8 wk post coronary bypass, being limited by the sterna healing or pain.
- If residual coronary lesions persist post revascularization, exercise stress testing is recommended to evaluate for significant ischemia.
- Sexual activity is contraindicated in patients with angina at low effort, refractory angina or unstable angina.
- Nitrate therapy is contraindicated with phosphodiesterase 5 (PDE5) inhibitor therapy.
- Following sildenafil (Viagra) or vardenafil (Levitra) at least 24 h must elapse before nitrates can be started; ≥48 h if tadalafil (Cialis) is used.
- Beta-blockers, calcium channel blockers and Ranolazine are not contraindicated; however, they may impair erectile dysfunction.

Source: Schwartz BG, Kloner RA. Clinical cardiology: physician update: erectile dysfunction and cardiovascular disease. *Circulation.* 2011;123:98-101. Nehra A, Jackson G, Martin Miner, et al. The Princeton III consensus recommendations for the management of erectile dysfunction and cardiovascular disease. *Mayo Clin Proc.* 2012;87:766-778. Kloner RA, Henderson L. Sexual function in patients with chronic angina pectoris. *Am J Cardiol.* 2013;111:1671-1676.

IVABRADINE					

Disease Management	Organization	Population	Recommendations	Comments	Source
CAD with Chronic Stable Angina	EMA 2014 review	Patients with chronic stable angina, with CAD, in sinus rhythm, with resting HR ≥70 bpm, that are either treated with optimal tolerated dose of β-blocker or cannot tolerate/have contraindication to β-blockers	Ivabradine (Corlentor®, Procoralan®) is used to treat symptoms of long-term stable angina.	2014 EMA review based on SIGNIFY study showed that Ivabradine has not been shown to provide benefits such as reducing the risk of heart attack or cardiovascular death, therefore the medicine should only be used to alleviate symptoms of angina. Doctors should consider stopping the treatment if there is no improvement in angina symptoms after 3 mo or if the improvement is only limited. Should not be used in combination with verapamil or diltiazem. The risk of AF is increased in the patient treated with Ivabradine and doctors should monitor patients for AF. If during treatment HR <50 bpm at rest and patients are symptomatic, the dose should be decreased to 2.5 mg 1 tab bid.	http://www.ema.europa.eu/ema/index.jsp?curl=pages/medicines/human/referrals/Corlentor_and_Procoralan/human_referral_prac_000044.jsp&mid=WC0b01ac05805c516f

CORONARY ARTERY DISEASE: THERAPY FOR UNSTABLE ANGINA/NSTEMI ACCF/AHA 2012 CLASS 1 RECOMMENDATIONS

- Aspirin (ASA) 325 mg should be administered promptly to all patients unless contraindicated.
- Clopidogrel 300–600 mg bolus or prasugrel 60 mg should be administered to all ASA-allergic patients.
- Risk stratification to initial invasive or conservative therapy is required. Early invasive treatment is indicated with refractory angina, hemodynamic or electrical instability. Most procedures are performed within 2–24 h, depending on the stability of the patient. TIMI and GRACE scores are often employed to select invasive vs conservative therapy.
- Dual antiplatelet ASA + (clopidogrel or ticagrelor) therapy is indicated upstream (before percutaneous coronary intervention) in the invasive group as well as in the conservative group.
- A *loading dose* of clopidogrel 600 mg, prasugrel 60 mg, or ticagrelor 180 mg should be given prior to PCI.
- *Maintenance therapy* of clopidogrel 75 mg daily, prasugrel 10 mg daily, or ticagrelor 90 mg twice daily should be *continued up to 12 mo.*
- If a history of gastrointestinal (GI) bleeding is noted, a PPI agent or H_2 blocker should be added to the dual antiplatelet therapy.
- PPI agents may be safely used with clopidogrel or pantoprazole. No interaction exists between PPIs and prasugrel, ticagrelor, or factor Xa inhibitors or dabigatran.
- In the conservative therapy group, if recurrent ischemia, heart failure, or serious arrhythmias occur, coronary angiogram is indicated.
- Nasal oxygen is indicated if arterial saturation is <90%, if respiratory distress is present, or other high-risk features for hypoxemia.
- Sublingual and intravenous nitroglycerin (NTG) are indicated for clinical angina.
- Oral β-blockers should be administered within the first 24 h unless contraindicated. Intravenous beta-blocker if chest pain is ongoing.
- ACE inhibitors should be administered within 24 h in patients with clinical heart failure (HF) with decreased ejection fraction (≤40%), if not contraindicated.
- Consider percutaneous coronary intervention (PCI) of the culprit coronary vessel with staged PCIs for other significant but less critical lesions. Consider CABG for significant left main lesion, double- or triple-vessel disease with decreased ejection fraction. The SYNTAX score may have predictive value in selecting PCI vs. CABG.
- *Myocardial perfusion imaging (MPI)* is indicated prior to discharge if conservative therapy is chosen.
- Dual antiplatelet (ASA 81 mg and clopidogrel 75 mg daily, prasugrel 10 mg daily, or ticagrelor 90 mg twice daily) is indicated for *at least 12 mo.* ASA should be continued lifelong.
- If warfarin is indicated postcoronary stent, see Anticoagulation with Stent section.
- Postdischarge medications include: ASA, clopidogrel 75 mg, β-blocker dose to control heart rate, statin agent, and possible ACE inhibitor if decreased ejection fraction or clinical heart failure, diabetes, or hypertension is present.

Sources: 2012 Writing Committee Members, Jneid H, Anderson JL, Wright RS, et al; American College of Cardiology Foundation; American Heart Association Task Force on Practice Guidelines. 2012 ACCF/AHA focused update of the guidelines for the management of patients with unstable angina/Non-ST elevation myocardial infarction (updated the 2007 guideline and replacing the 2011 focus update): a report of the American College of Cardiology Foundation/American Heart Association Task Force on Practice Guidelines. *Circulation.* 2012;126:875-910. ACC/AHA 2007 Guidelines *J Am Coll Cardiol.* 2007;50(7):652-726. Wright RS, Anderson JL, Adams CD, et al. 2011 ACCF/AHA focused update of the Guidelines for the Management of Patients with Unstable Angina/Non-ST-Elevation Myocardial Infarction (updating the 2007 guideline): a report of the American College of Cardiology Foundation/American Heart Association Task Force on Practice Guidelines developed in collaboration with the American College of Emergency Physicians, Society for Cardiovascular Angiography and Interventions, and Society of Thoracic Surgeons. *J Am Coll Cardiol.* 2011;57:1920-1959. ESC 2011. ECS Guidelines. http://eurheartj.oxfordjournals.org/. Palmerini T, Genereux P, Caixeta A, et al. Prognostic value of the SYNTAX score in patients with acute coronary syndromes undergoing percutaneous coronary intervention: analysis from the ACUITY (Acute Catheterization and Urgent Intervention Triage StrategY) trial. *J Am Coll Cardiol.* 2011;57:2389-2397. Patel MR, Dehmer GJ, Hirshfeld JW, Smith PK, Spertus JA. ACCF/SCAI/STS/AATS/AHA/ASNC/HFSA/SCCT 2012 Appropriate use criteria for coronary revascularization focused update: a report of the American College of Cardiology Foundation Appropriate Use Criteria Task Force, Society for Cardiovascular Angiography and Interventions, Society of Thoracic Surgeons, American Heart Association, American Society of Nuclear Cardiology, and the Society of Cardiovascular Computed Tomography. *J Am Coll Cardiol.* 2012;59:857-876.

CORONARY ARTERY DISEASE: MANAGEMENT FOR ST-ELEVATION MYOCARDIAL INFARCTION ACCF/AHA 2013. CLASS I RECOMMENDATIONS

- Patients with ST-elevation myocardial infarction with ischemic symptoms within 12 h should be treated by PCI.
- Primary PCI should be performed within **90 min** from initial medical contact by an experienced catheterization cardiologist.
- Emergency transport to PCI-capable hospital is recommended. The term "Code STEMI" is often used to confer the time urgency of the transfer. In-ambulance ECG monitoring should be used to identify ST-segment elevation.
- Emergency transfer from a non-PCI capable to a PCI-capable hospital should be considered if transfer to catheterization laboratory is capable within **120 min**.
- Fibrinolytic therapy should be considered if PCI is not capable within the optimal time frame. If fibrinolytic therapy is considered, it should be started with 30 min of hospital arrival.
- ASA 162–325 mg should be administered before primary PCI and continued indefinitely at 81 mg daily.
- $P2Y_{12}$ receptor inhibitor should be given *upstream* or *during* primary PCI and should be *continued for 1 y* with either bare metal stent or drug-eluting stents. Options include clopidogrel, prasugrel, and ticagrelor. $P2Y_{12}$ Receptor inhibitors: Clopidogrel 75 mg daily, Prasgruel 10 mg daily (5 mg daily—in patients <60 kg or ≥75 y old), Ticagrelor 90 mg bid. Prasugrel should not be administered to patients with a history of prior stroke or TIA.
- Anticoagulation therapy with unfractionated heparin and bivalirudin should be discussed with the invasive cardiologist.
- Urgent PCI of the infarct artery should be addressed urgently with stent placement. Noninfarct artery occlusions should be evaluated postinfarction to evaluate ischemia requiring subsequent PCI.
- Urgent coronary artery bypass surgery is indicated if the coronary anatomy is not amenable to PCI.
- Therapy with statin agents, β-blockers, and ACE inhibitors are indicated as with NSTEMIs.

Source: American College of Emergency Physicians; Society for Cardiovascular Angiography and Interventions, O'Gara PT, Kushner FG, Ascheim DD, et al. 2013 ACCF/AHA guideline for the management of ST-elevation myocardial infarction: executive summary: a report of the American College of Cardiology Foundation/American Heart Association Task Force on Practice Guidelines. *J Am Coll Cardiol.* 2013;61(4):485-510.

CORONARY ARTERY DISEASE: ELEVATED TROPONIN LEVELS AMERICAN COLLEGE OF CARDIOLOGY FOUNDATION TASK FORCE 2012

- Elevated troponin levels are an *imperfect diagnostic test* and are dependent upon the probability of underlying CAD. New high-sensitivity troponin assays require further testing.
- Establishing **high pretest probability** and **global risk scores** (TIMI, GRACE, PERSUIT) are often needed to determine the significance of elevated troponin levels.
- Clinical factors that establish a high pretest probability include: a history of typical angina, typical ECG changes consistent with ischemia (ST-segment changes), history of established coronary risk factors, or the history of known CAD.
- Elevated troponin levels in patients with *high pretest probability of CAD* (typical chest pain and ECG changes of ischemia) have a predictive accuracy of ≥95% to establish acute coronary syndrome.
- Elevated troponin levels in patients with *low pretest probability of CAD* (atypical chest pain and nonspecific ECG changes) have a predictive accuracy of only 50% to establish ACS.
- *Global risk scores* should be employed to further establish the role of early conservative vs early invasive therapy in patients with elevated troponin levels and a high pretest probability.
- Cardiac causes for elevated troponin levels are: ACS, coronary spasm or embolism, cocaine or methamphetamine use, stress cardiomyopathy, congestive heart failure, myocarditis or pericarditis, trauma, infiltrative diseases, postprocedure (ablation, electric shock, coronary bypass surgery, and post-coronary angioplasty).
- Noncardiac causes for elevated troponin levels are: pulmonary embolus, renal failure, stroke, sepsis, drug toxicity (anthracycline), and hypoxia.

Source: Newby LK, Jesse RL, Babb JD, et al. ACCF 2012 expert consensus document of practical clinical considerations in the interpretation of troponin elevations: a report of the American College of Cardiology Foundation task force on Clinical Expert Consensus Documents. *J Am Coll Cardiol.* 2012;60:2427-2463.

CORONARY ARTERY DISEASE: LONG-TERM ANTIPLATELET THERAPY AMERICAN COLLEGE OF CHEST PHYSICIANS 2012

- ASA is recommended for persons ≥50 y old *without symptomatic* CVD at 75–100 mg daily.
- Mono antiplatelet therapy with ASA 75–100 mg or clopidogrel 75 mg is recommended with *established CAD*.
- Dual antiplatelet therapy (ticagrelor 90 mg twice daily plus ASA 81 mg or clopidogrel 75 mg plus ASA 75–100 mg daily) for 1-y post-ACS with PCI with or without stent placement.
- Dual antiplatelet therapy with *elective PCI without stent* should receive clopidogrel 75 mg or ASA 75–100 mg daily for 1 mo, then long-term ASA therapy is recommended.
- Dual antiplatelet therapy with *elective PCI and bare metal stent (BMS) or drug eluting stent (DES)* is recommended for 1 y. The minimum duration of dual therapy is 4–6 wk for BMS, 3 mo for –limus stents and 6 mo for –taxel stents.
- No antiplatelet or OAC is recommended with systolic dysfunction without thrombus. If LV thrombus is present, OAC is recommended for 3 mo.

Source: Vandvik PO, Lincoff AM, Gore JM, et al; American College of Chest Physicians. Primary and secondary prevention of cardiovascular disease: Antithrombotic Therapy and Prevention of Thrombosis, 9th ed: American College of Chest Physician Evidence-Based Clinical Practice Guidelines. *Chest.* 2012;141:e637S-e668S.

CORONARY ARTERY DISEASE: STENT THERAPY USE OF TRIPLE ANTICOAGULATION TREATMENT
Sources: AMERICAN COLLEGE OF CARDIOLOGY/AMERICAN HEART ASSOCIATION/EUROPEAN SOCIETY OF CARDIOLOGY

The prudent use of triple anticoagulation therapy with aspirin, clopidogrel, and warfarin in AF patients at high risk of thromboembolism and recent coronary stent placement remains a *matter of clinical judgment,* balancing the risk of thrombotic vs. bleeding events.

Facts:

- Bare-metal stents are the stents of choice if TAT is required.
- Drug-eluting stents should be reserved for high-risk clinical or anatomic situations (diabetic patients or if the coronary lesions are unusually long, totally occlusive, or in small blood vessels) if TAT is required.
- Dual antiplatelet therapy with clopidogrel (75 mg/d) and ASA (81 mg/d) is the most effective therapy to *prevent coronary stent thrombosis.*
- Warfarin anticoagulation is the most effective therapy to *prevent thromboembolism* in high-risk AF patients as defined by the $CHA_2DS_2\text{-}VAS_c$ risk score (≥ 2).
- In nonvalvular AF ok to consider NOACs. Following coronary revascularization, in high-risk patients with AF may be reasonable to use Clopidogrel 75 mg daily concurrently with OAC but without ASA.
- TAT is the most effective therapy to *prevent* both *coronary stent thrombosis* and the *occurrence* of embolic strokes in high-risk patients.
- However, the addition of DAPT to warfarin increases the bleeding risk by 3.7-fold.
- Therefore, awaiting a definitive clinical trial (WOEST Trial), risk stratification of patients to evaluate the *thromboembolic potential of AF* vs the *bleeding potential* should be performed.
- The HAS-BLED (see box below) bleeding risk score is the best measure of bleeding risk. A high risk of bleeding is defined by a score >3.

Source: January CT, Wann LS, Alpert JS, et al. 2014 AHA/ACC/HRS Guideline for the Management of Patients With Atrial Fibrillation. *Circulation.* 2014. http://circ.ahajournals.org/content/early/2014/04/10/CIR.0000000000000041.

Hypertension (≥ 160 mm Hg), **a**bnormal kidney function (creatinine ≥ 2, chronic dialysis, transplant), **a**bnormal liver function (cirrhosis, bilirubin >2×, AST >3×), **s**troke, **b**leeding history or anemia, labile INR (<60% within range), **e**lderly (age ≥ 65 y), **d**rugs/ alcohol (use of ASA or clopidogrel) or alcohol (≥ 8 alcoholic drinks/wk). *Each risk factor is assigned 1 point for a total of 9 points.*

- If DAPT or TAT is required, *prophylactic GI therapy* with an H_2 blocker (except cimetidine) or PPI agent should be maintained. If omeprazole (Prilosec) is considered, the risk-to-benefit ratio needs to be considered because of its possible interference with clopidogrel function.
- In patients with a high risk of bleeding, TAT should be reserved for AF patients with a high thromboembolic risk. If the bleeding risk is high but the AF thromboembolic risk is low, DAPT therapy is suggested.

AF, atrial fibrillation; ASA, aspirin; AST, aspartate transaminase; DAPT, dual antiplatelet therapy; INR, international normalized ratio; GI, gastrointestinal; PPI, proton pump inhibitor; TAT, triple anticoagulation therapy.

Sources: Adopted from European Heart Rhythm Association, European Association for Cardio-Thoracic Surgery, Camm AJ, Kirchhof P, Lip GY, et al. Guidelines for the management of atrial fibrillation: the Task Force for the Management of Atrial Fibrillation of the European Society of Cardiology (ESC). *Eur Heart J.* 2010;31:2369-2429. Lip GY. Managing the anticoagulated patient with atrial fibrillation at high risk of stroke who needs coronary intervention. *BMJ.* 2008;337:a840. Rubboli A, Kovacic JC, Mehran R, Lip GY. Coronary stent implantation in patients committed to long-term oral anticoagulation: successfully navigating the treatment options. *Chest.* 2011;139:981-987. King SB 3rd, Smith SC Jr, Hirshfeld JW Jr, et al. 2007 focused update of the ACC/AHA/SCAI 2005 guideline update for percutaneous coronary intervention: a report of the American College of Cardiology/American Heart Association Task Force on Practice guidelines. *J Am Coll Cardiol.* 2008;51:172-208. Wright RS, Anderson JL, Adams CD, et al. 2011 ACCF/AHA focused update of the Guidelines for the Management of Patients with Unstable Angina/ Non-ST-Elevation Myocardial Infarction (updating the 2007 guideline): a report of the American College of Cardiology Foundation/American Heart Association Task Force on Practice Guidelines developed in collaboration with the American College of Emergency Physicians, Society for Cardiovascular Angiography and Interventions, and Society of Thoracic Surgeons. *J Am Coll Cardiol.* 2011;57:1920-1959. Abraham NS, Hlatky MA, Antman EM, et al; ACCF/ACG/AHA. ACCF/ACG/AHA 2010 expert consensus document on the concomitant use of proton pump inhibitors and thienopyridines: a focused update of the ACCF/ACG/AHA 2008 expert consensus document on reducing the gastrointestinal risks of antiplatelet therapy and NSAID use. A Report of the American College of Cardiology Foundation Task Force on Expert Consensus Documents. *J Am Coll Cardiol.* 2010;56:2051-2066. Holmes DR Jr, Kereiakes DJ, Kleiman NS, Moliterno DJ, Patti G, Grines CL. Combining antiplatelet and anticoagulation therapies. *J Am Coll Cardiol.* 2009;54:95-109. January CT, Wann LS, Alpert JS, et al. 2014 AHA/ACC/HRS Guideline for the Management of Patients With Atrial Fibrillation. *Circulation.* 2014. http://circ.ahajournals.org/content/early/2014/04/10/CIR.0000000000000041.

CORONARY ARTERY DISEASE: STENT THERAPY USE OF TRIPLE ANTICOAGULATION TREATMENT

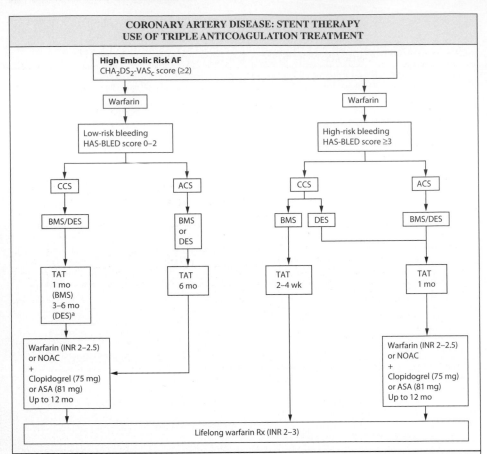

ACS, acute coronary syndrome; AF, atrial fibrillation; ASA, aspirin; BMS, bare metal stent; CCS, patient with chronic coronary syndrome (stable coronary artery disease); DES, drug eluting stent; INR, international normalized ratio; Rx, therapy [warfarin (INR 2–2.5) + aspirin (81 mg daily) + clopidogrel (75 mg daily)]; TAT, triple anticoagulation therapy.
[a]DES stents if sirolimus, everolimus, or tacrolimus require 3-month dual platelet therapy (ASA plus clopidogrel). If DES stent is paclitaxel, 6-mo dual therapy is required.

Sources: European Heart Rhythm Association; European Association for Cardio-Thoracic Surgery, Camm AJ, Kirchhof P, Lip GY, et al. Guidelines for the management of atrial fibrillation: the Task Force for the Management of Atrial Fibrillation of the European Society of Cardiology (ESC). *Eur Heart J.* 2010;31:2369-2429. Lip GY. Managing the anticoagulated patient with atrial fibrillation at high risk of stroke who needs coronary intervention. *BMJ.* 2008;337:a840. Rubboli A, Kovacic JC, Mehran R, Lip GY. Coronary stent implantation in patients committed to long-term oral anticoagulation: successfully navigating the treatment options. *Chest.* 2011;139:981-987. King SB 3rd, Smith SC Jr, Hirshfeld JW Jr, et al. 2007 focused update of the ACC/AHA/SCAI 2005 guideline update for percutaneous coronary intervention: a report of the American College of Cardiology/American Heart Association Task Force on Practice guidelines. *J Am Coll Cardiol.* 2008;51:172-208.

2014 AHA/ACC/HRS Guideline for the Management of Patients With Atrial Fibrillation. CT January, LS Wann, JS Alpert et al. *Circulation.* 2014. http://circ.ahajournals.org/content/early/2014/04/10/CIR.0000000000000041. Wright RS, Anderson JL, Adams CD, et al. 2011 ACCF/AHA focused update of the Guidelines for the Management of Patients with Unstable Angina/Non-ST-Elevation Myocardial Infarction (updating the 2007 guideline): a report of the American College of Cardiology Foundation/American Heart Association Task Force on Practice Guidelines developed in collaboration with the American College of Emergency Physicians, Society for Cardiovascular Angiography and Interventions, and Society of Thoracic Surgeons. *J Am Coll Cardiol.* 2011;57:1920-1959. Abraham NS, Hlatky MA, Antman EM, et al; ACCF/ACG/AHA. ACCF/ACG/AHA 2010 expert consensus document on the concomitant use of proton pump inhibitors and thienopyridines: a focused update of the ACCF/ACG/AHA 2008 expert consensus document on reducing the gastrointestinal risks of antiplatelet therapy and NSAID use. A Report of the American College of Cardiology Foundation Task Force on Expert Consensus Documents. *J Am Coll Cardiol.* 2010;56:2051-2066. Holmes DR Jr, Kereiakes DJ, Kleiman NS, Moliterno DJ, Patti G, Grines CL. Combining antiplatelet and anticoagulation therapies. *J Am Coll Cardiol.* 2009;54:95-109.

CAD IN WOMEN

- CVD is the leading cause of mortality in women.
- AHA recommends the risk assessment of CVD in women should begin at age 20 y, identifying women at higher risk.
- There are racial/ethnic differences in risk factors, with black and Hispanic women having a higher prevalence of hypertension and diabetes. The highest CVD morbidity and mortality occurs in black women.
- Autoimmune diseases (systemic lupus erythematosus, rheumatoid arthritis) and preeclampsia are significant risk factors for CVD in women.
- Psychological stress (anxiety, depression) and socioeconomic disadvantages are associated with a higher CVD risk in women.
- *Microvascular disease with endothelial dysfunction*, also known as *female pattern disease*, is the etiology of ischemia in more women than men.
- Women are more likely to have atypical cardiovascular symptoms such as: sudden or extreme fatigue, dyspnea, sleep disturbances, anxiety, nausea, vomiting, indigestion.
- *ACC/AHA guidelines recommend a routine exercise stress test* as the initial evaluation in symptomatic women who have a good exercise capacity and a normal baseline ECG. Exercise stress perfusion study (myocardial perfusion scintigraphy [MPS]) or exercise echo should be reserved for symptomatic women with higher pretest likelihood for CAD or indeterminate routine testing.
- Women often receive less medical therapy and lifestyle counseling than men.
- After PCI procedure, women experience higher rate of complications and mortality than men.
- Management of stable CAD should be the same as in men which include ASA, β-blocker, statin, ACE inhibitor (ejection fraction [EF] <40%), nitrate/calcium channel blocker (CCB) for angina management.
- In microvascular disease, β-blockers have shown to be superior to CCB for angina management. Statins, ACE inhibitors, ranolazine, and exercise can improve angina scores and endothelial dysfunction in female pattern disease.

Sources: Moasca L, Benjamin EJ, Berra K, et al. Effectiveness-based guidelines for the prevention of cardiovascular disease in women—2011 update: a guideline from the American Heart Association. *Circulation.* 2011;123:1243-1262. Gulati M, Shaw LJ, Bairey Merz CN. Myocardial ischemia in women: lessons from the NHLBI WISE study. *Clin Cardiol.* 2012;35:141-148.

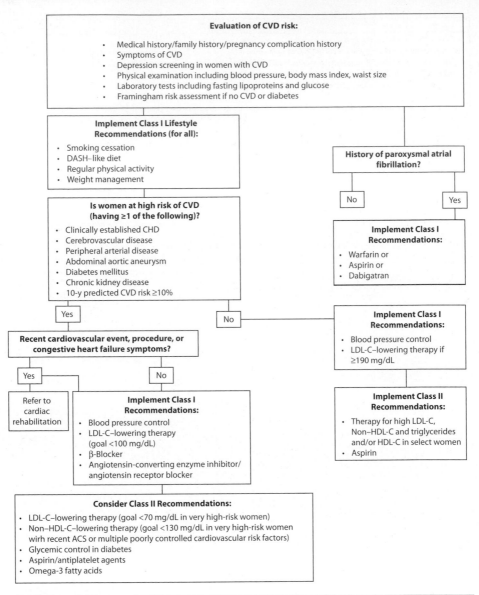

Figure: Flow diagram for CVD preventive care in women.

ACS, acute coronary syndrome; CHD, coronary heart disease; CVD, cardiovascular disease; DASH, dietary approaches to stop hypertension; HDL-C, high-density lipoprotein cholesterol; LDL-C, low-density lipoprotein cholesterol.

Source: Moasca L, Benjamin EJ, Berra K et al. Effectiveness-based guidelines for the prevention of cardiovascular disease in women—2011 update: a guideline from the American Heart Association. *Circulation.* 2011;123:1243-1262.

DELIRIUM

Disease Management	Organization	Date	Population	Recommendations	Comments	Source
Delirium	NICE	2010	Adults age ≥18 y in the hospital or in long-term care facilities	1. Perform a short Confusion Assessment Method (CAM) screen to confirm the diagnosis of delirium. 2. Recommended approach to the management of delirium: a. Treat the underlying cause b. Provide frequent reorientation and reassurance to patients and their families c. Provide cognitively stimulating activities d. Ensure adequate hydration e. Prevent constipation f. Early mobilization g. Treat pain if present h. Provide hearing aids or corrective lenses if sensory impairment is present i. Promote good sleep hygiene j. Consider short-term antipsychotic use (<1 wk) for patients who are distressed or considered at risk to themselves or others	Recommended antipsychotics are haloperidol or olanzapine given at the lowest effective dose.	http://www.nice.org.uk/nicemedia/live/13060/49909/49909.pdf
	American Geriatrics Society	2015		Do not use physical restraints for behavioral control in elderly patients with delirium.		http://www.choosingwisely.org/societies/american-geriatrics-society/

DEMENTIA

Disease Management	Organization	Date	Population	Recommendations	Comments	Source
Dementia	ACP AAFP	2008 2008	Adults with dementia	1. Recommend a trial of therapy with a cholinesterase inhibitor or memantine based on individual assessment of relative risks vs benefits. 2. The choice of medication is based on tolerability, side effect profile, ease of use, and medication cost. 3. The evidence is insufficient to compare the relative efficacy of different medications for dementia. 4. Evidence is insufficient to determine the optimal duration of therapy.	1. A beneficial effect of cholinesterase inhibitors or memantine is generally observed within 3 mo. 2. Good-quality data in mild-to-moderate Alzheimer disease and vascular dementia show that cholinesterase inhibitors provide a modest improvement in global assessment, but no clinically important cognitive improvement. Subsets of patients may have significant cognitive improvement. 3. Five high-quality studies evaluated memantine use in moderate-to-severe Alzheimer disease and vascular dementia and show statistically significant improvement in global assessment, but no clinically important cognitive improvement.	http://www.annals.org/content/148/5/370.full.pdf

DEMENTIA, ALZHEIMER DISEASE					
Disease Management	Organization	Date	Population	Recommendations	Comments	Source
Dementia, Alzheimer Disease	NICE	2011	Adults	• Donepezil, galantamine, and rivastigmine are recommended as options for mild-to-moderate Alzheimer disease. • Memantine is recommended as an option for managing moderate Alzheimer disease in patients who cannot tolerate acetylcholinesterase inhibitors.	• Common adverse effects of acetylcholinesterase inhibitors include diarrhea, nausea, vomiting, muscle cramps, and insomnia. • Common adverse effects of memantine are dizziness, headache, constipation, somnolence, and hypertension.	http://www.nice.org.uk/nicemedia/live/13419/53619/53619.pdf
Dementia, Feeding Tubes	American Geriatrics Society	2013	Patients with advanced dementia	• Percutaneous feeding tubes are not recommended for older adults with advanced dementia. • Careful hand-feeding should be offered.	• Careful hand-feedings and tube feedings have identical outcomes of death, aspiration pneumonia, functional status, and patient comfort. In addition, tube feeding is associated with agitation, increased use of physical and chemical restraints, and worsening pressure ulcers.	http://americangeriatrics.org/health_care_professionals/clinical_practice/clinical_guidelines_recommendations/

DEPRESSION

Disease Management	Organization	Date	Population	Recommendations	Comments	Source
Depression	USPSTF	2009	Children and adolescents	• Adequate evidence showed that SSRIs, psychotherapy, and combined therapy will decrease symptoms of major depressive disorder in adolescents age 12–18 y. • Insufficient evidence to support screening and treatment of depression in children age 7–11 y.	• Good evidence showed that SSRIs may increase absolute risk of suicidality in adolescents by 1%–2%. Therefore, SSRIs should be used only if close clinical monitoring is possible. • Fluoxetine and citalopram yielded statistically significant higher response rates than did other SSRIs.	http://www.uspreventiveservicestaskforce.org/uspstf/uspschdepr.htm

Disease Management	Organization	Date	Population	Recommendations	Comments	Source
Diabetes Mellitus, Gestational (GDM)	ACOG	2013	Pregnant women	• Women with gestational diabetes should be treated with nutrition therapy. • For pharmacologic therapy of GDM, oral medications and insulin are equivalent in efficacy. • Women with GDM and estimated fetal weight of 4500 g or more should be counseled regarding option of scheduled cesarean delivery vs vaginal trial of labor. • Women with GDM should follow fasting and one hour postprandial glucose levels.		http://www.guideline.gov/content.aspx?id=47014

DIABETES MELLITUS, GESTATIONAL (GDM)

DIABETES MELLITUS (DM), TYPE 1

Disease Management	Organization	Date	Population	Recommendations	Comments	Source

Diabetes Mellitus (DM), Type 1	ADA	2013	Adults and children	1. Recommends intensive insulin therapy with >3 injections daily using both basal and prandial insulin or an insulin pump.
				2. Self-monitoring blood glucose >3 times daily in all patients using multiple insulin injections or an insulin pump.
				3. Recommends assessment of psychological and social situation as part of diabetic evaluation.
				4. Recommends glucose (15–20 g) for all conscious patients with hypoglycemia.
				5. Advise all patients not to smoke.
				6. Recommends beginning these screening tests after 5 y with type 1 DM
				  a. Urine albumin-to-creatinine ratio and serum creatinine annually
				  b. Dilated funduscopic exam annually
				  c. Monofilament screening for diabetic neuropathy annually
				  d. Comprehensive foot examination at least annually
				7. Recommends screening at diagnosis for other autoimmune conditions:
				  a. Tissue transglutaminase IgA antibodies
				  b. Thyroperoxidase and thyroglobulin antibodies
				  c. TSH
				8. Fasting lipid panel at age 10 y or at puberty (consider as early as age 2 y for a strong family history of hyperlipidemia).
				  a. Repeat annually if results abnormal or every 5 y if results acceptable.
				9. Consider statin therapy if age ≥10 y and LDL >160 mg/dL despite good glycemic control and lifestyle modification.
				10. Aspirin 75–162 mg/d if:
				  a. Primary prevention of CVD if 10-year risk of coronary artery disease (CAD) >10%
				  b. Secondary prevention of CVD
					1. Glycemic control recommendations for **toddlers (age 0–6 y):**
					  a. Before meals, capillary blood gas (CPG) 100–180 mg/dL
					  b. Bedtime, CPG 110–200 mg/dL
					  c. HgbA1c <8.5%
					2. Glycemic control recommendations for **school-age (age 6–12 y):**
					  a. Before meals, CPG 90–180 mg/dL
					  b. Bedtime, CPG 100–180 mg/dL
					  c. HgbA1c <8%
					3. Glycemic control recommendations for **adolescents (age 13–19 y):**
					  a. Before meals, CPG 90–130 mg/dL
					  b. Bedtime, CPG 90–150 mg/dL
					  c. HgbA1c <7.5%
						http://care.diabetesjournals.org/content/36/Supplement_1/S11.full

Disease Management	Organization	Date	Population	Recommendations	Comments	Source
DIABETES MELLITUS (DM), TYPE 2						
Diabetes Mellitus (DM), Type 2	AACE	2010	Nonpregnant adults	1. Endorsed the use of HgbA1c ≥6.5% as a means of diagnosing type 2 DM. 2. HgbA1c is not recommended for diagnosing type 1 DM or gestational diabetes.		http://www.aace.com/pub/pdf/guidelines/AACEposition A1cfeb2010.pdf
	NICE	2009	Adults	1. Consider adding a DPP-4 (dipeptidyl peptidase-4) inhibitor[a] or pioglitazone to metformin as a second-line agent if glycemic control is inadequate and a significant risk of hypoglycemia or sulfonylurea contraindication exists. 2. Consider adding a DPP-4 inhibitor[a] or pioglitazone to a sulfonylurea as a second-line agent if glycemic control is inadequate and a metformin contraindication exists. 3. Consider a glucagon-like peptide-1 (GLP-1) mimetic (eg, exenatide) as a third-line agent when glycemic control is inadequate (HgbA1c >7.5%) with metformin and a sulfonylurea. 4. Consider adding insulin when glycemic control is inadequate (HgbA1c >7.5%) with oral agents alone.	1. Avoid pioglitazone in people with heart failure or who have a higher risk of fracture. 2. Avoid metformin if the glomerular filtration rate (GFR) is <45 mL/min/1.73 m².	http://www.nice.org.uk/nicemedia/live/12165/44318/44318.pdf
	ADA	2013	Adults and children	1. Self-monitoring blood glucose ≥3 times daily in all patients using multiple insulin injections or an insulin pump. 2. Recommends HgbA1c every 3 mo if therapy has changed or if blood glucose control is inadequate. 3. Provide diabetes self-management education, including education about hypoglycemia management and adjustments during illness. 4. Provide family planning for women of reproductive age. 5. Provide medical nutrition therapy. 6. Weight loss is recommended for all overweight or obese diabetic patients. 7. Keep saturated fat intake <7% of total calories. 8. Reduction of protein intake to 0.8–1 g/kg/d for early stages of CKD and 0.8 g/kg/d for later stages of CKD. 9. Recommends at least 150 min/wk of moderate physical activity. 10. The glucose range for critically ill patients is 140–180 mg/dL (7.8–10 mmol/L). 11. The glucose range for noncritically ill patients in the hospital is <140 mg/dL premeal (<7.8 mmol/L) and random blood glucose <180 mg/dL (<10 mmol/L). 12. Recommends the following: a. Immunizations: annual influenza vaccination if age ≥6 mo, pneumococcal polysaccharide vaccine if age ≥2 y, and 1× revaccination if age ≥65 y, and hepatitis B vaccination if unvaccinated and ages 19–59 y b. Target BP <130/80 mm Hg	1. Glycemic control recommendations: a. Preprandial CPG 70–130 mg/dL b. Postprandial CPG <180 mg/dL (1–2 h postmeals) c. HgbA1c <7% 2. Consider bariatric surgery if BMI >35 kg/m² and if diabetes is difficult to control with lifestyle modification and medications. 3. Angiotensin-converting enzyme inhibitors (ACEIs) or ARBs are first-line antihypertensives. 4. Second-line antihypertensives are a thiazide diuretic if GFR ≥30 mL/min/1.73 m² or a loop diuretic if GFR <30 mL/min/1.73 m². 5. Clopidogrel 75 mg/d is an alternative for persons ASA intolerant. 6. Nephrology referral indicated if GFR <60 mL/min/1.73 m², or if heavy proteinuria or structural kidney disease present. 7. Consider a serum TSH in women age >50 y.	http://care.diabetesjournals.org/content/36/Supplement_1/S11.full

DIABETES MELLITUS (DM), TYPE 2

Disease Management	Organization	Date	Population	Recommendations	Comments	Source

Diabetes Mellitus (DM), Type 2 (continued)				c. Statin therapy if:
				  i. Overt CVD present
				  ii. Age >40 years and ≥1 CV risk factor[b]
				  iii. LDL >100 mg/dL despite lifestyle modification
				  iv. LDL >70 mg/dL if DM2 and overt cardiovascular disease
				d. ASA 75–162 mg/d if:
				  i. Primary prevention of CVD if 10-year risk of CAD >10%
				  ii. Secondary prevention of CVD
				e. Annual check of urine albumin-to-creatinine ratio and serum creatinine
				f. Annual serum creatinine and fasting lipid profile
				g. Annual dilated funduscopic exam
				h. Annual monofilament screening for diabetic neuropathy
				i. At minimum, annual comprehensive foot exam
					8. Consider assessing patients for the following comorbidities that are increased with DM:
					a. Hearing impairment
					b. Obstructive sleep apnea
					c. Fatty liver disease
					d. Low testosterone in men
					e. Periodontal disease
					f. Cognitive impairment	

	ACP	2012	Adults older than 18 y	• Oral pharmacologic therapy should be added for treatment of type 2 DM when lifestyle modifications, including diet, exercise, and weight loss, have failed to adequately control hyperglycemia. • Recommends metformin as the initial pharmacologic agent to treat most patients with type 2 DM. • Recommend adding another oral agent to metformin if patients have persistent hyperglycemia despite metformin and lifestyle modifications.	• All dual-regimens were more effective than monotherapy and decreased the HbA1c levels by an average of 1% more. • Most monotherapy regimens had similar efficacy and reduced HbA1c levels by an average of 1%. • Studies suggest that metformin decreases all-cause mortality slightly more than sulfonylureas with a much lower rate of hypoglycemia.	http://www.annals.org/content/156/3/I-36.full.pdf+html
		2011	Hospitalized adults older than 18 y	• Avoid intensive insulin therapy in hospitalized patients (even if in SICU/MICU). • Recommends a target blood glucose level of 140–200 mg/dL if insulin therapy is used in SICU/MICU patients.	• Intensive insulin therapy (targeting blood glucose levels of 80–110 mg/dL) in SICU/MICU patients does not improve mortality, but has a 5-fold increased risk of hypoglycemia.	http://www.annals.org/content/154/4/260.full.pdf+html

	AAP	2013	Children and adolescents with newly diagnosed DM 2	• Insulin therapy should be initiated for children with:
				  ◦ Diabetic ketoacidosis
				  ◦ HbA1c >9%
				  ◦ Random glucose >250 mg/dL
				• Diet, exercise, and metformin are initial therapy for other situations.
				• Recommend moderate-to-vigorous exercise for 60 min daily.
				• Limit nonacademic screen time t <2 h/d.
				• Monitor HbA1c every 3 mo.
				• Desire HbA1c <7%.
						pediatrics.**aap**publications.org/content/131/2/364.full.pdf

[a]Sitagliptin or vildagliptin.
[b]Cardiovascular risk factors: hypertension, smoking, positive family history, men age ≥45 y and women age ≥55 y, or hyperlipidemia.

Lifestyle modification: diet, exercise, and medically or surgically-assisted weight loss if BMI>35 (see box below)

HgbA1c <7.5%

Monotherapy*
- Metformin 1st choice
  >If metformin CI or not tolerated use:
- GLP-1RA¥
- DPP4-I¥
- SGLT-2
- AG-I

If HgbA1c <7.0%# in 3 mo add second agent

HgbA1c <7.5%–8.9%

Dual therapy*
- Metformin
  PLUS
- GLP-1 RA¥
- DPP4-I¥
- SGLT-2
- Basal insulin
- TZD
- AG-I
- Sulfonylurea
- Colsevelam

If HgbA1c <7.0%# in 3 mo add second agent

Triple therapy*
- Metformin
- Second-line agent from dual therapy list
  PLUS
- GLP-1 RA¥
- SGLT-2
- Basal insulin
- DPP4-I¥
- TZD
- Sulfonylurea
- Colsevelam

HgbA1c <9.0%

Asymptomatic
Dual therapy
OR
Triple therapy

Symptomatic
Treat with insulin +/– other agents

If HgbA1c >7.0%# in 3 mo intensify or add insulin therapy

Medical weight loss
- Phentermine; orlistat; lorcaserin

Surgical weight loss
- Lap band; gastric sleeve; gastric bypass

Adapted from *Endocrine Practice*, 2013; 19: 327 **and** *Diabetes Care* 2012;35:1364-1379.
GLP-1 RA=glucagon-like peptide-1 receptor antagonist; DPP-4 I=dipeptidyl peptidase-4 inhibitor; SGLT-2 = sodium glucose cotransporter 2; TZD = thiazolidinediones; AG-I-alpha-glucosidase inhibitors
* - suggested order of usage
¥ -do not use DPP4-I and GLP-1 RA simultaneously
-Consider goal HgbA1c ≤6.5% if young, no hypoglycemia, and no cardiovascular disease

BLOOD-GLUCOSE-LOWERING THERAPY: NICE, 2009

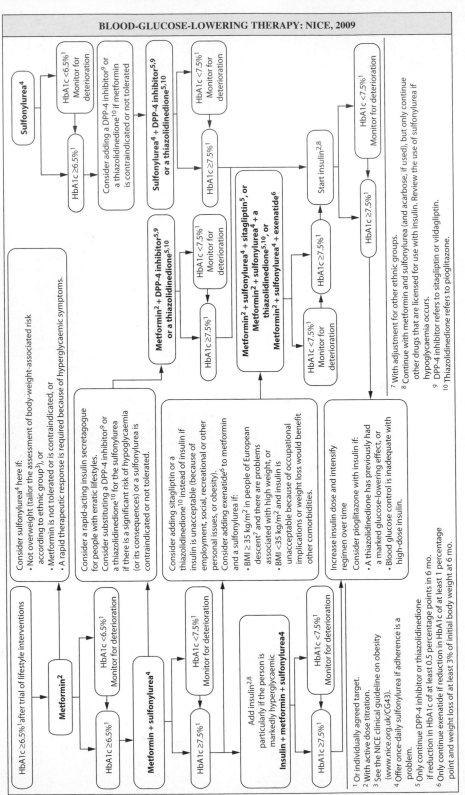

DIABETIC FOOT PROBLEMS, INPATIENT MANAGEMENT

Disease Management	Organization	Date	Population	Recommendations	Comments	Source
Diabetic Foot Problems, Inpatient Management	NICE	2011	Hospitalized adults older than 18 y with diabetic foot problems	• Every hospital should have a multidisciplinary foot care team to assess and treat any diabetic patient with foot problems. • Every patient with a diabetic foot problem should undergo an assessment for: 　○ Need for debridement, pressure off-loading 　○ Vascular inflow 　○ Infection of the foot 　○ Glycemic control 　○ Neuropathy • If osteomyelitis is suspected, obtain an x-ray, and if x-ray is normal, obtain an MRI. • Provide off-loading for diabetic foot ulcers. • For mild diabetic foot infections, treat with empiric antibiotics that provide good gram-positive organisms coverage. • For moderate-to-severe diabetic foot infections, treat with empiric antibiotics that provide coverage of gram-positive, gram-negative, and anaerobic bacteria.	• The diabetic foot care team should include: 　○ Diabetologist 　○ Surgeon with expertise managing DM foot problems 　○ DM nurse specialist 　○ Podiatrist 　○ Tissue viability nurse	http://www.nice.org.uk/nicemedia/live/13416/53556/53556.pdf

	DYSPEPSIA		

Disease Management	Organization	Date	Population	Recommendations	Comments	Source

Dyspepsia	NICE	2014	Adults	1. Recommend smoking cessation and weight reduction.
				2. Consider discontinuation of offending medications (calcium channel blockers, nitrates, theophylline, bisphosphonates, steroids, and NSAIDs.
				3. Consider testing for *H. pylori* after a 2-wk washout of proton pump inhibitors.
				4. Empiric trial of proton pump inhibitor therapy.
				5. Consider laparoscopic fundoplication for patients who do not wish to continue with acid suppressive therapy long term.
				6. Consider specialist referral for:
				  a. Dyspepsia refractory to meds
				  b. Consideration of surgery
				  c. Refractory *H. pylori* infection
				  d. Barrett esophagus
						http://www.guideline.gov/content.aspx?id=48563

Disease Management	Organization	Date	Population	Recommendations	Comments	Source
Dysphagia	ASGE	2014	Adults	1. Recommend endoscopic dilation for benign esophageal strictures or eosinophilic esophagitis. 2. Recommend through-the-scope balloon dilation for complex esophageal strictures. 3. Concomitant antisecretory therapy with dilation for peptic strictures. 4. Reserve esophageal stents for refractory esophageal strictures. 5. Options for endoscopic management of achalasia include pneumatic dilatation or botulinum toxin injections.		http://www.guideline.gov/content.aspx?id=47786

DYSPHAGIA

EATING DISORDERS

Disease Management	Organization	Date	Population	Recommendations	Comments	Source

Eating Disorders	APA	2013	Adults and children with eating disorders	• Psychiatric management begins with the establishment of a therapeutic alliance.
				• Recommend a multidisciplinary approach with a psychiatrist, dietician, social worker, and physician.
				• Components of the initial evaluation include:
				  ○ A thorough history and physical examination
				  ○ Assessment of the social history
				  ○ An evaluation of the height and weight history
				  ○ Any family history of eating disorders or mental health disorders?
				  ○ Assess attitude of eating, exercising, and appearance
				  ○ Assess for suicidality
				  ○ Assess for substance abuse
				  ○ Recommend nutritional rehab for seriously underweight patients
				  ○ Recommend nasogastric tube feeding over parenteral nutrition for patients not meeting caloric requirements with oral feeds alone
				  ○ Psychosocial rehab for patients with both anorexia nervosa and bulimia nervosa.
				  ○ Prozac is preferred agent to prevent relapse during maintenance phase of bulimia nervosa
				  ○ Labs
				    ○ CBC
				    ○ Chemistry panel
				    ○ TSH
				  ○ Additional testing
				    ○ Bone mineral densitometry if amenorrhea for more than 6 months
				    ○ Dental evaluation for history of purging
						http://www.guideline.gov/content.aspx?id=9318

ECTOPIC PREGNANCY

Disease Management	Organization	Date	Population	Recommendations	Comments	Source

Ectopic Pregnancy	NICE	2012	Pregnant women	• Recommended evaluation for stable women with an early pregnancy
				  ○ Transvaginal ultrasound (TVUS) with a crown-rump length ≥7 mm but no cardiac activity
				    – Repeat ultrasound in 7 d
				    – Quantitative β-hCG q48h × 2 levels
				  ○ TVUS with gestational sac ≥25 mm and no fetal pole
				    – Repeat ultrasound in 7 d
				    – Quantitative β-hCG q48h × 2 levels
				• Management of ectopic pregnancies
				  ○ Methotrexate candidates
				    – No significant pain
				    – Adnexal mass <3.5 cm
				    – No cardiac activity on TVUS
				    – β-hCG <5000 IU/L
				    – Dose is 50 mg/m² IM
				  ○ Laparoscopy if:
				    – Unstable patient
				    – Severe pain
				    – Adnexal mass >3.5 cm
				    – Cardiac activity seen
				    – β-hCG >5000 IU/L
				  ○ Rhogam 250 IU to all Rh-negative women who undergo surgery for an ectopic
					• Ectopic pregnancy can present with:
					  ○ Abdominal or pelvic pain
					  ○ Vaginal bleeding
					  ○ Amenorrhea
					  ○ Breast tenderness
					  ○ GI symptoms
					  ○ Dizziness
					  ○ Urinary symptoms
					  ○ Rectal pressure
					  ○ Dyschezia
					• Most normal intrauterine pregnancies will show an increase in β-hCG level by at least 63% in 48 h.
					• Intrauterine pregnancies are usually apparent by TVUS if β-hCG >1500 IU/L.
						www.guidelines.gov/
						content.aspx?id=39274

EPILEPSY

Disease Management	Organization	Date	Population	Recommendations	Comments	Source

Epilepsy	NICE	2012	Children and adults	• Educate adults about all aspects of epilepsy.
				• Diagnosis of epilepsy should be made by a specialist in epilepsy.
				• Evaluation of epilepsy
				  ○ Electroencephalogram
				  ○ Sleep-deprived EEG if standard EEG is inconclusive
				  ○ Neuroimaging to evaluate for any structural brain abnormalities
				    – MRI is preferred for children <2 y, adults, refractory seizures, and focal seizures
				  ○ Measurement of prolactin is not recommended
				  ○ Chemistry panel
				  ○ ECG in adults
				  ○ Urine toxicology screen
				• Antiepileptic drugs (AED)
				  ○ Start AED only after the diagnosis of epilepsy is made
				  ○ Focal seizures
				    – Carbamazepine
				    – Lamotrigine
				    – Adjunctive AED: levetiracetam, oxcarbazepine, or sodium valproate
				  ○ Generalized tonic–clonic seizures
				    – Sodium valproate
				    – Lamotrigine
				    – Carbamazepine
				    – Oxcarbazepine
				    – Adjunctive AED: levetiracetam or topiramate
				  ○ Absence seizures
				    – Ethosuximide
				    – Sodium valproate
				    – Alternative: lamotrigine
				  ○ Myoclonic seizures
				    – Sodium valproate
				    – Alternatives: levetiracetam or topiramate
					• AED can decrease the efficacy of combined oral contraceptive pills.	http://www.guidelines.gov/content.aspx?id=36082

ERECTILE DYSFUNCTION (ED)

Disease Management	Organization	Date	Population	Recommendations	Comments	Source

Erectile Dysfunction (ED)	EAU	2009	Adult men	1. Recommends a medical and psychosexual history on all patients.
				2. Recommends a focused physical examination to assess CV status, neurologic status, prostate disease, penile abnormalities, and signs of hypogonadism.
				3. Recommends checking a fasting glucose, lipid profile, and total testosterone levels.
				4. Recommends psychosexual therapy for psychogenic ED.
				5. Recommends testosterone therapy for androgen deficiency if no contraindications present.[a]
				6. Selective phosphodiesterase 5 (PDE5) inhibitors are first-line therapy for idiopathic ED.
					1. Selective PDE5 inhibitors:
					  a. Sildenafil
					  b. Tadalafil
					  c. Vardenafil
					2. Avoid nitrates and use α-blockers with caution when prescribing a selective PDE5 inhibitor.
						http://www.uroweb.org/gls/EU/2010%20Male%20Sex%20Dysfunction.pdf

[a]Prostate CA, breast CA, or signs of prostatism.

FRACTURES

Disease Management	Organization	Date	Population	Recommendations	Comments	Source
Hip Fractures	AAOS	2014	Elderly patients with hip fractures	1. Recommend preop pain control in patients with hip fractures. 2. Insufficient evidence to support preop traction in hip fractures. 3. Recommend hip fracture surgery within 48 hours of admissions. 4. Do not delay hip fracture surgery for patients on aspirin +/– clopidogrel. 5. Recommend operative fixation for non-displaced femoral neck fractures. 6. Recommend unipolar or bipolar hemiarthroplasty for displaced femoral neck fractures. 7. Recommend prolonged thromboprophylaxis to prevent venous thromboembolism after hip fracture surgery. 8. Recommend intensive physical therapy post-discharge to improve functional outcomes. 9. Recommend evaluation for osteoporosis in all patients who have sustained a hip fracture.		http://www.guideline.gov/content.aspx?id=48518

GALLSTONES

Disease Management	Organization	Date	Population	Recommendations	Comments	Source

Gallstones	NICE	2014	Adults with or suspected of having gallstones	1. Obtain liver function tests and ultrasound if suspected gallstone disease.
				2. Consider magnetic resonance cholangiopancreatography (MRCP) if ultrasound has not detected common bile duct stones but the:
				  a. Common bile duct is dilated
				  b. Liver function tests are abnormal
				3. Offer cholecystectomy for symptomatic gallstones or acute cholecystitis.
				4. Offer percutaneous cholecystostomy for acute cholecystitis or gallbladder empyema if surgery is contraindicated.
				5. Options for choledocholithiasis:
				  a. Cholecystectomy and intraoperative clearance of CBD stones.
				  b. ERCP prior to cholecystectomy
						http://www.guideline.gov/content.aspx?id=49014

GASTROINTESTINAL BLEEDING, UPPER (UGIB)

Disease Management	Organization	Date	Population	Recommendations	Comments	Source

Gastrointestinal Bleeding, Upper (UGIB)	NICE	2012	Adults	• Recommend a formal risk assessment for patients with an UGIB.
				  ○ Blatchford score at first assessment
				  ○ Rockall score after endoscopy
				• Avoid platelet transfusions in patients who are not actively bleeding and are hemodynamically stable.
				• For UGIB, give FFP if:
				  ○ Fibrinogen <100 mg/dL
				  ○ Partial thromboplastin time >1.5 × normal
				• Prothrombin complex concentrate (PCC) indicated for UGIB on warfarin.
				• Timing of endoscopy
				  ○ Immediately for unstable patients
				  ○ Within 24 h for stable patients
				• Management of nonvariceal bleeding
				  ○ Surgical clips
				  ○ Thermal coagulation
				  ○ Epinephrine injection
				  ○ Fibrin or thrombin glue
				  ○ Proton pump inhibitors
				• Recurrent bleeding can be assessed by repeat endoscopy or by interventional radiology angioembolization
				• Management of variceal bleeding
				  ○ Esophageal variceal band ligation
				  ○ Terlipressin or octreotide infusions
				  ○ Prophylactic third-generation cephalosporin
				  ○ Transjugular intrahepatic portosystemic shunt for recurrent esophageal variceal bleeding or gastric variceal bleeding
					• Patients should stop NSAIDs.
					• Alcohol cessation if a factor.
					• Low-dose aspirin can be resumed if needed for secondary prevention of vascular events once hemostasis has been achieved.
					• Ongoing use of thienopyridine agents (eg, clopidogrel, ticagrelor, or prasugrel) should be only after discussion with appropriate specialist.
						http://www.guidelines.gov/content.aspx?id=37563

GLAUCOMA, CHRONIC OPEN ANGLE

Disease Management	Organization	Date	Population	Recommendations	Comments	Source
Glaucoma, Chronic Open Angle	NICE	2009	Adults	1. All persons with known or suspected chronic open-angle glaucoma (COAG) or ocular hypertension (OHT) should undergo the following: a. Intraocular pressure monitoring using tonometry b. Central corneal thickness measure'ment c. Peripheral anterior chamber depth assessments using gonioscopy d. Visual field testing e. Optic nerve assessment using slit-lamp exam. 2. Recommends monitoring patients with OHT at least annually for COAG (every 6 mo for high-risk patients). 3. Recommends monitoring patients with COAG every 6–12 mo based on disease progression. 4. Recommends prostaglandin analogue therapy for early-to-moderate COAG patients at risk of visual loss. 5. Consider surgery with pharmacologic augmentation for advanced COAG. 6. Recommends β-blocker drops for mild OHT until age 60 y. 7. Recommends prostaglandin analogue drops for any degree of OHT. 8. Recommends additional medication therapy for uncontrolled OHT despite single-agent therapy.	1. Alternative pharmacologic treatments for OHT or suspected COAG in patients whose intraocular pressures remain elevated on monotherapy include: a. Prostaglandin analogues b. β-blockers c. Carbonic anhydrase inhibitors d. Sympathomimetics	http://www.guidelines.gov/content.aspx?id=14444

GOUT, ACUTE ATTACKS

Disease Management	Organization	Date	Population	Recommendations	Comments	Source

Gout, Acute Attacks	ACR	2012	Adults	• Therapy options for acute gout attacks
				  ○ Mild-moderate attacks involving 1–2 joints
				    – NSAIDs: full-dose naproxen, sulindac, or indomethacin is preferred.
				    – Colchicine 1.2 mg PO × 1 then 0.6 mg 1 h later then 0.6 mg daily-bid.
				    – Corticosteroids: prednisone or prednisolone 0.5 mg/kg PO daily for 5–10 d.
				  ○ Severe attacks or polyarticular gout
				    – Colchicine + NSAIDs
				    – Colchicine + steroids
				  ○ Expert opinion to continue urate-lowering therapy (eg, allopurinol) during acute attacks
				  ○ Ice applied to affected joints can help
				• Pharmacologic urate-lowering therapy
				  ○ Allopurinol
				    – Starting dose should not exceed 100 mg/d
				    – Uptitrate dose every 2–4 wk to max of 800 mg/d, unless renal impairment exists.
				    – Desire uric acid level of <6 mg/dL
				  ○ Consider adding a uricosuric agent (eg, probenecid) for refractory hyperuricemia despite urate-lowering therapy
				  ○ Initiate allopurinol after an acute gout attack has resolved and continue prophylactic anti-inflammatory agents for 3 mo beyond achieving urate level <6 mg/dL
				    – Colchicine 0.6 mg daily-bid
				    – Naproxen 250 mg PO bid
					• Consider HLAB*5801 testing prior to the initiation of allopurinol for patients at particularly high risk of allopurinol hypersensitivity reaction.
					  ○ Highest risk group are those of Korean, Han Chinese, or Thai descent, especially if Stage 3 or higher CKD is present.
						www.guideline.gov/content.aspx?id=38624
						www.guideline.gov/content.aspx?id=38625

HEADACHE

Disease Management	Organization	Date	Population	Recommendations	Comments	Source
Headache	ACR	2012		Do not do imaging for uncomplicated headaches.		http://www.choosingwisely.org/societies/american-college-of-radiology/

Headache, Migraine Prophylaxis	AAN	2012	Adults	• The following medications have **established efficacy** for migraine prophylaxis:
				  ○ Divalproex sodium
				  ○ Sodium valproate
				  ○ Topiramate
				  ○ Metoprolol
				  ○ Propranolol
				  ○ Timolol
				• Frovatriptan is effective for menstrual migraine prophylaxis.
				• The following medications are **probably effective** for migraine prophylaxis:
				  ○ Amitriptyline
				  ○ Venlafaxine
				  ○ Atenolol
				  ○ Nadolol
					• Lamotrigine and clomipramine are ineffective for migraine prevention.	http://www.neurology.org/content/78/17/1337.full.pdf+html

HEADACHE DIAGNOSIS ALGORITHM: ICSI, 2011

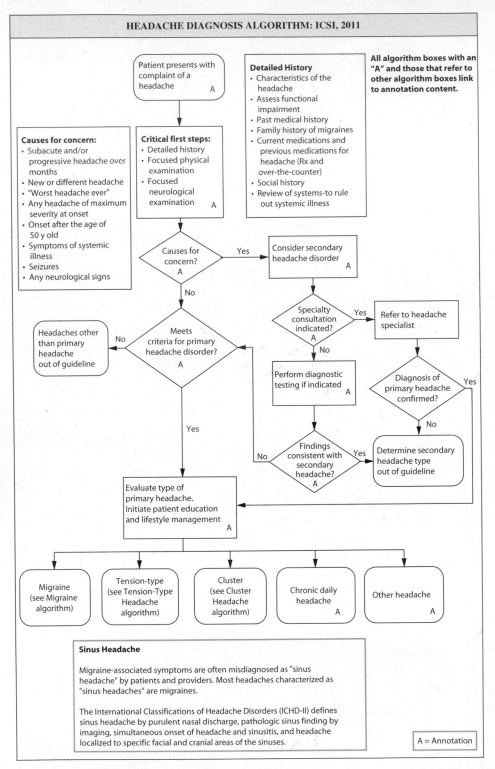

Patient presents with complaint of a headache A

Detailed History
- Characteristics of the headache
- Assess functional impairment
- Past medical history
- Family history of migraines
- Current medications and previous medications for headache (Rx and over-the-counter)
- Social history
- Review of systems-to rule out systemic illness

All algorithm boxes with an "A" and those that refer to other algorithm boxes link to annotation content.

Causes for concern:
- Subacute and/or progressive headache over months
- New or different headache
- "Worst headache ever"
- Any headache of maximum severity at onset
- Onset after the age of 50 y old
- Symptoms of systemic illness
- Seizures
- Any neurological signs

Critical first steps:
- Detailed history
- Focused physical examination
- Focused neurological examination A

Causes for concern? A — Yes → **Consider secondary headache disorder** A

No

Specialty consultation indicated? A — Yes → **Refer to headache specialist**

No

Meets criteria for primary headache disorder? A — No → **Headaches other than primary headache out of guideline**

Perform diagnostic testing if indicated A

Diagnosis of primary headache confirmed? — Yes →

No

Yes

Findings consistent with secondary headache? A — Yes → **Determine secondary headache type out of guideline**

No

Evaluate type of primary headache. Initiate patient education and lifestyle management A

- **Migraine** (see Migraine algorithm)
- **Tension-type** (see Tension-Type Headache algorithm)
- **Cluster** (see Cluster Headache algorithm)
- **Chronic daily headache** A
- **Other headache** A

Sinus Headache

Migraine-associated symptoms are often misdiagnosed as "sinus headache" by patients and providers. Most headaches characterized as "sinus headaches" are migraines.

The International Classifications of Headache Disorders (ICHD-II) defines sinus headache by purulent nasal discharge, pathologic sinus finding by imaging, simultaneous onset of headache and sinusitis, and headache localized to specific facial and cranial areas of the sinuses.

A = Annotation

MIGRAINE TREATMENT ALGORITHM: ICSI, 2011

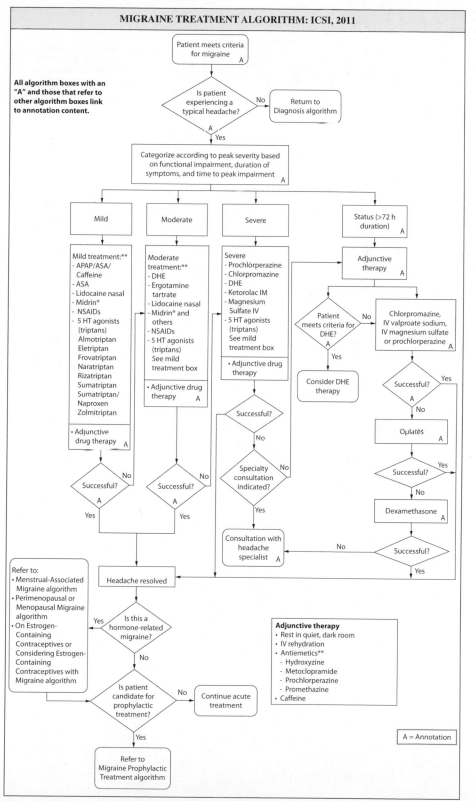

All algorithm boxes with an "A" and those that refer to other algorithm boxes link to annotation content.

Patient meets criteria for migraine
A

Is patient experiencing a typical headache? — No → Return to Diagnosis algorithm

A ↓ Yes

Categorize according to peak severity based on functional impairment, duration of symptoms, and time to peak impairment
A

Mild | Moderate | Severe | Status (>72 h duration) A

Mild treatment:**
- APAP/ASA/ Caffeine
- ASA
- Lidocaine nasal
- Midrin*
- NSAIDs
- 5 HT agonists (triptans)
  Almotriptan
  Eletriptan
  Frovatriptan
  Naratriptan
  Rizatriptan
  Sumatriptan
  Sumatriptan/ Naproxen
  Zolmitriptan

• Adjunctive drug therapy A

Moderate treatment:**
- DHE
- Ergotamine tartrate
- Lidocaine nasal
- Midrin* and others
- NSAIDs
- 5 HT agonists (triptans)
  See mild treatment box

• Adjunctive drug therapy A

Severe
- Prochlorperazine
- Chlorpromazine
- DHE
- Ketorolac IM
- Magnesium Sulfate IV
- 5 HT agonists (triptans)
  See mild treatment box

• Adjunctive drug therapy

Adjunctive therapy A

Patient meets criteria for DHE? A — No → Chlorpromazine, IV valproate sodium, IV magnesium sulfate or prochlorperazine A

Yes ↓

Consider DHE therapy

Successful? A — Yes →

No ↓

Opiates A

Successful? A — Yes →

No ↓

Dexamethasone A

Successful? — No → Consultation with headache specialist A

Yes ↓

Successful? A — No → Specialty consultation indicated? — No

Yes ↓

Consultation with headache specialist A

Successful? A — Yes → Headache resolved

No ↓

Refer to:
• Menstrual-Associated Migraine algorithm
• Perimenopausal or Menopausal Migraine algorithm
• On Estrogen-Containing Contraceptives or Considering Estrogen-Containing Contraceptives with Migraine algorithm

Headache resolved

Is this a hormone-related migraine? — Yes →

No ↓

Is patient candidate for prophylactic treatment? — No → Continue acute treatment

Yes ↓

Refer to Migraine Prophylactic Treatment algorithm

Adjunctive therapy
• Rest in quiet, dark room
• IV rehydration
• Antiemetics**
  - Hydroxyzine
  - Metoclopramide
  - Prochlorperazine
  - Promethazine
• Caffeine

A = Annotation

TENSION-TYPE HEADACHE ALGORITHM: ICSI, 2011

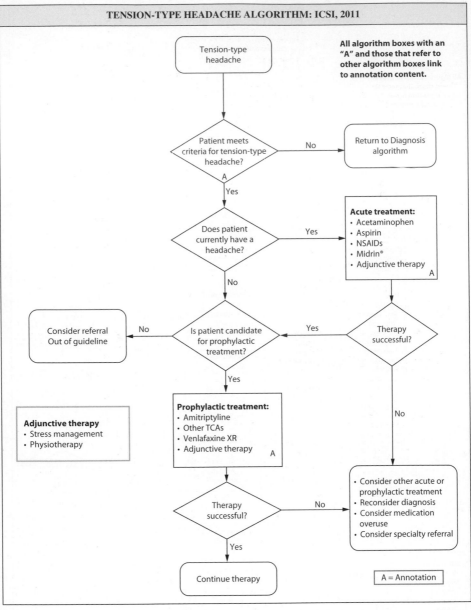

CLUSTER HEADACHE ALGORITHM: ICSI, 2011

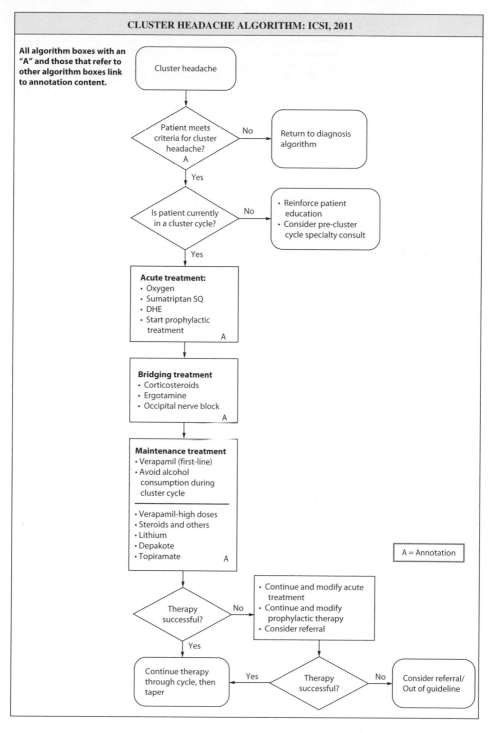

All algorithm boxes with an "A" and those that refer to other algorithm boxes link to annotation content.

Cluster headache

Patient meets criteria for cluster headache?
A

No → Return to diagnosis algorithm

Yes

Is patient currently in a cluster cycle?

No →
• Reinforce patient education
• Consider pre-cluster cycle specialty consult

Yes

Acute treatment:
• Oxygen
• Sumatriptan SQ
• DHE
• Start prophylactic treatment
A

Bridging treatment
• Corticosteroids
• Ergotamine
• Occipital nerve block
A

Maintenance treatment
• Verapamil (first-line)
• Avoid alcohol consumption during cluster cycle

• Verapamil-high doses
• Steroids and others
• Lithium
• Depakote
• Topiramate
A

A = Annotation

Therapy successful?

No →
• Continue and modify acute treatment
• Continue and modify prophylactic therapy
• Consider referral

Yes

Therapy successful?

Yes → Continue therapy through cycle, then taper

No → Consider referral/ Out of guideline

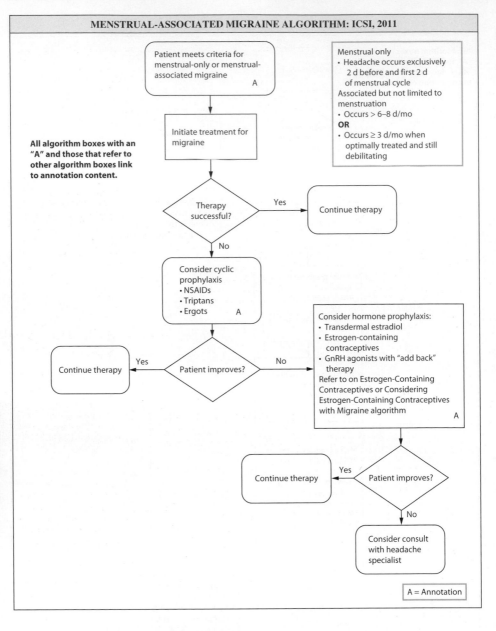

MENSTRUAL-ASSOCIATED MIGRAINE ALGORITHM: ICSI, 2011

Patient meets criteria for menstrual-only or menstrual-associated migraine   A

Menstrual only
• Headache occurs exclusively 2 d before and first 2 d of menstrual cycle
Associated but not limited to menstruation
• Occurs > 6–8 d/mo
OR
• Occurs ≥ 3 d/mo when optimally treated and still debilitating

All algorithm boxes with an "A" and those that refer to other algorithm boxes link to annotation content.

Initiate treatment for migraine

Therapy successful? — Yes → Continue therapy

No

Consider cyclic prophylaxis
• NSAIDs
• Triptans
• Ergots   A

Continue therapy ← Yes — Patient improves? — No →

Consider hormone prophylaxis:
• Transdermal estradiol
• Estrogen-containing contraceptives
• GnRH agonists with "add back" therapy
Refer to on Estrogen-Containing Contraceptives or Considering Estrogen-Containing Contraceptives with Migraine algorithm   A

Continue therapy ← Yes — Patient improves?

No

Consider consult with headache specialist

A = Annotation

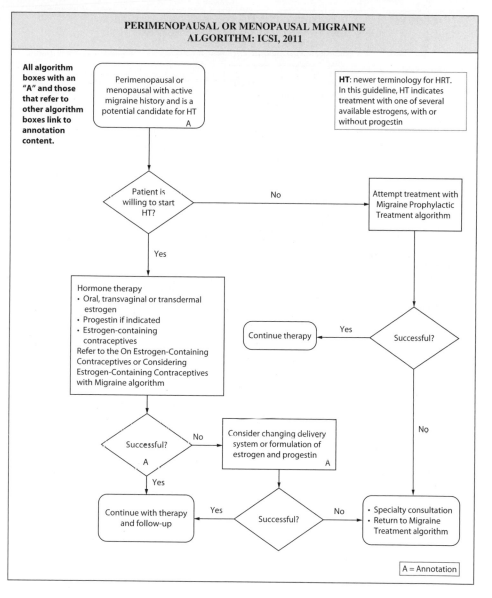

PERIMENOPAUSAL OR MENOPAUSAL MIGRAINE ALGORITHM: ICSI, 2011

All algorithm boxes with an "A" and those that refer to other algorithm boxes link to annotation content.

Perimenopausal or menopausal with active migraine history and is a potential candidate for HT — A

HT: newer terminology for HRT. In this guideline, HT indicates treatment with one of several available estrogens, with or without progestin

Patient is willing to start HT?

No → Attempt treatment with Migraine Prophylactic Treatment algorithm

Yes

Hormone therapy
- Oral, transvaginal or transdermal estrogen
- Progestin if indicated
- Estrogen-containing contraceptives

Refer to the On Estrogen-Containing Contraceptives or Considering Estrogen-Containing Contraceptives with Migraine algorithm

Successful? — A

No → Consider changing delivery system or formulation of estrogen and progestin — A

Yes → Continue therapy

Successful?

Yes → Continue therapy

No

Successful?

Yes → Continue with therapy and follow-up

No →
- Specialty consultation
- Return to Migraine Treatment algorithm

A = Annotation

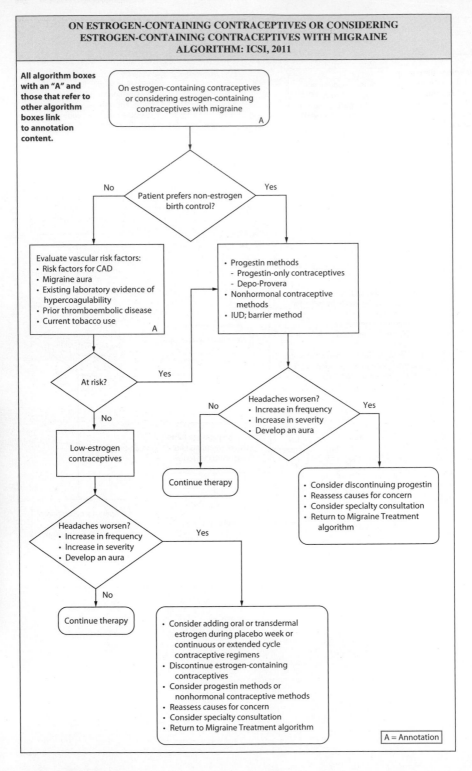

ON ESTROGEN-CONTAINING CONTRACEPTIVES OR CONSIDERING ESTROGEN-CONTAINING CONTRACEPTIVES WITH MIGRAINE ALGORITHM: ICSI, 2011

All algorithm boxes with an "A" and those that refer to other algorithm boxes link to annotation content.

On estrogen-containing contraceptives or considering estrogen-containing contraceptives with migraine — A

Patient prefers non-estrogen birth control?

No → Evaluate vascular risk factors:
- Risk factors for CAD
- Migraine aura
- Existing laboratory evidence of hypercoagulability
- Prior thromboembolic disease
- Current tobacco use — A

Yes → Progestin methods
- Progestin-only contraceptives
- Depo-Provera
- Nonhormonal contraceptive methods
- IUD; barrier method

At risk?

Yes → (to Progestin methods)

No → Low-estrogen contraceptives

Headaches worsen?
- Increase in frequency
- Increase in severity
- Develop an aura

No → Continue therapy

Yes → Consider discontinuing progestin
- Reassess causes for concern
- Consider specialty consultation
- Return to Migraine Treatment algorithm

Headaches worsen?
- Increase in frequency
- Increase in severity
- Develop an aura

No → Continue therapy

Yes → Consider adding oral or transdermal estrogen during placebo week or continuous or extended cycle contraceptive regimens
- Discontinue estrogen-containing contraceptives
- Consider progestin methods or nonhormonal contraceptive methods
- Reassess causes for concern
- Consider specialty consultation
- Return to Migraine Treatment algorithm

A = Annotation

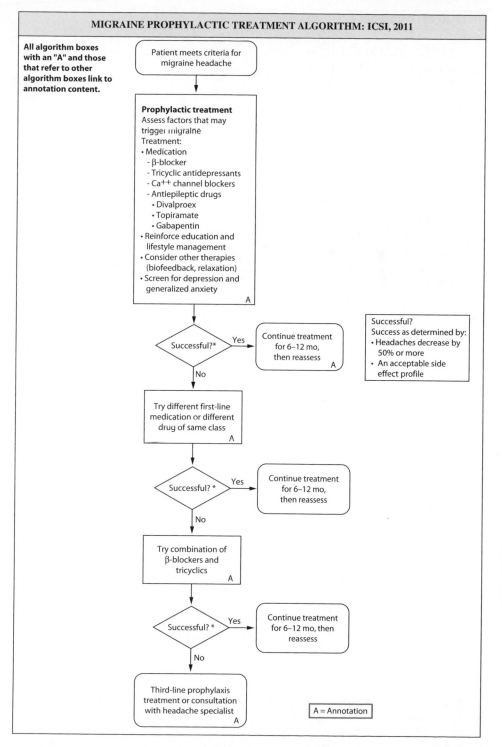

MIGRAINE PROPHYLACTIC TREATMENT ALGORITHM: ICSI, 2011

All algorithm boxes with an "A" and those that refer to other algorithm boxes link to annotation content.

Patient meets criteria for migraine headache

Prophylactic treatment
Assess factors that may trigger migraine
Treatment:
• Medication
  - β-blocker
  - Tricyclic antidepressants
  - Ca++ channel blockers
  - Antiepileptic drugs
    • Divalproex
    • Topiramate
    • Gabapentin
• Reinforce education and lifestyle management
• Consider other therapies (biofeedback, relaxation)
• Screen for depression and generalized anxiety
A

Successful?* — Yes → Continue treatment for 6–12 mo, then reassess A

No

Successful?
Success as determined by:
• Headaches decrease by 50% or more
• An acceptable side effect profile

Try different first-line medication or different drug of same class A

Successful? * — Yes → Continue treatment for 6–12 mo, then reassess

No

Try combination of β-blockers and tricyclics A

Successful? * — Yes → Continue treatment for 6–12 mo, then reassess

No

Third-line prophylaxis treatment or consultation with headache specialist A

A = Annotation

HEARING LOSS, SUDDEN

Disease Management	Organization	Date	Population	Recommendations	Comments	Source
Hearing Loss, Sudden	AAO-HNS	2012	Adults age 18 y and older	• Distinguish hearing loss into sensorineural or conductive hearing loss. • Counsel patients with incomplete recovery of hearing about the benefits of hearing aids. • Evaluate patients with idiopathic sudden sensorineural hearing loss (ISSNHL) for retrocochlear pathology by obtaining an MRI of the internal auditory canal, auditory brainstem responses, and an audiology exam. • Consider treatment of ISSNHL with incomplete hearing recovery with systemic or intratympanic steroids or hyperbaric oxygen therapy. • In patients with ISSNHL, recommend against antivirals, thrombolytics, vasodilators, or antioxidants for treatment and against CT scanning of the head or routine lab testing.		http://oto.sagepub.com/content/146/3_suppl/S1.full.pdf+html

HEART FAILURE
Source: ADAPTED FROM ACC/AHA, 2005

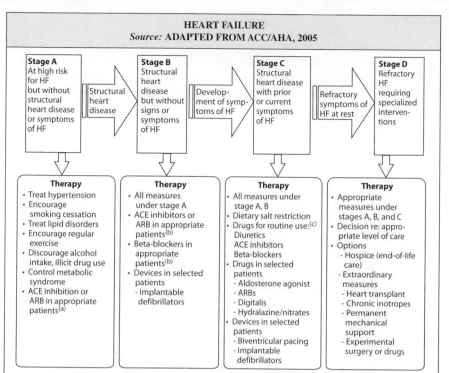

Stage A: Patients with hypertension, atherosclerotic disease, diabetes mellitus, metabolic syndrome, *or* those using cardiotoxins or having a family history of cardiomyopathy

Stage B: Patients with previous MI, LV remodeling including LVH and low EF, or asymptomatic valvular disease

Stage C: Patients with known structural heart disease; shortness of breath and fatigue, reduced exercise tolerance

Stage D: Patients who have marked symptoms at rest despite maximal medical therapy (eg, those who are recurrently hospitalized or cannot be safely discharged from the hospital without specialized interventions)

(a) History of atherosclerotic vascular disease, diabetes mellitus, or hypertension and associated cardiovascular risk factors.

(b) Recent or remote MI, regardless of ejection fraction; or reduced ejection fraction regardless of MI Hx. Use ARB in patients post-MI who cannot tolerate ACE inhibitors.

(c) Evidence suggests that isosorbide dinitrate plus hydralazine reduces mortality in blacks with advanced heart failure. (*NEJM.* 2004;351:2049)

Comments: Exercise training in patients with HF seems to be safe and beneficial overall in improving exercise capacity, quality of life, muscle structure, and physiologic responses to exercise. (*Circulation.* 2003;107:1210-1225)

HF, heart failure; LV, left ventricle

Source: Adapted from the American College of Cardiology, American Heart Association, Inc. *J Am Coll Cardiol.* 2005;46:1-82 and *Circulation.* 2005;112:154-235. 2009 ACCF/AHA Guidelines. *J Am Coll Cardiol.* 2009;53(150): 1334-1378.

HEART FAILURE
Source: ADAPTED FROM ACCF/AHA 2013
CLASSIFICATION, CLINICAL ASSESSMENT IN HEART FAILURE
CLASS I RECOMMENDATIONS

1. Classification:
   - I. Heart failure with reduced ejection fraction (HFrEF) referred to as *systolic heart failure* when LVEF ≤40%
   - II. Heart failure with preserved ejection fraction (HFpEF) referred to as diastolic dysfunction
     - HFpEF when LVEF >40%
2. Lifetime risk of developing HF for Americans ≥40 y old is 20%.
3. Overall mortality is 50% in 5 y; varies with HF stage with
   - Stage B having a 5-y mortality of 4%
   - Stage C having a 5-y mortality of 25%
   - Stage D having a 5-y mortality of 80%
4. Patients with idiopathic dilated cardiomyopathy should have a 3-generational family history obtained to exclude familial disease.
5. Risk Score evaluation should be considered to help predict the ultimate outcome; chronic heart failure—Seattle Heart Failure Model (http://depts.washington.edu/shfm/)
6. Identify prior cardiac or noncardiac disease that may lead to HF.
7. Obtain history to include diet or medicine nonadherence; current or past use of alcohol, illicit drugs, and chemotherapy; or recent viral illness.
8. Identify the patient's present activity level and desired post-treatment level.
9. Assess the patient's volume status, orthostatic BP changes, height and weight, and body mass index.
10. Hypertension and lipid disorders should be controlled in accordance with contemporary guideline to lower the risk of HF. Other risk factors should be controlled or avoided.
11. Initial blood work should measure N-terminal pro-brain natriuretic peptide (NT-proBNP) or BNP levels to support clinical judgment for diagnosis, especially in the setting of uncertainty for the diagnosis. Other labs to include CBC, chemistry panel, lipid profile, troponin I level, and TSH level.
12. 12-lead ECG should be obtained.
13. 2D echocardiogram is indicated to determine the systolic function, diastolic function, valvular function, and pulmonary artery pressure.
14. Coronary arteriography to be performed in patients with angina or significant ischemia with HF unless the patient is not eligible for surgery.
15. Initiate diuretic therapy and salt restriction if volume overloaded. Diuretics do not improve long-term survival, but improve symptoms and short-term survival. Once euvolemic and symptoms have resolved, carefully start to wean dosage as an outpatient to lowest dose possible to prevent electrolyte disorders and activation of the renin angiotensin system.
16. ACE inhibitor or ARB, which reduces morbidity and mortality, should be considered early in the initial course to decrease afterload unless contraindicated if decreased ejection fraction noted (systolic dysfunction). Both agents improve long-term survival but are seldom employed together because of marginal benefit. Titrate dosage to that employed in clinical studies as BP allows.
17. Specific beta-blockers (carvedilol, sustained release metoprolol succinate, bisoprolol) should be added to reduce morbidity and mortality. These specific β-blockers improve survival the most in systolic heart failure. Titrate dosage to heart rate 65–70 beats/min.
18. Start aldosterone antagonist in patients with moderate or severe symptoms (NYHA II-IV) and reduced ejection fraction. Creatinine should be <2.5 mg/dL in men and <2 mg/dL in women, and the potassium should be <5 mEq/L.
19. The combination of hydralazine and nitrates should be employed to improve outcome in African Americans with moderate-to-severe HF with decreased ejection fraction in addition to optimal therapy. If ACE inhibitor or ARB agent is contraindicated, hydralazine and nitrates may be used as alternative therapy.
20. Statins are not beneficial as adjunctive therapy when prescribed solely for the diagnosis of HF. In all patients with a recent or remote hx of CAD, CVA, PAD, or hyperlipidemia, statins should be used according to guidelines.
21. Discontinue anti-inflammatory agents, diltiazem, and verapamil.
22. Nutritional supplements as treatment for HF are not recommended in patients with current or prior symptoms of systolic dysfunction (HFrEF).
23. Calcium channel blockers are not recommended as routine treatment for patients with HFrEF.
24. Remember that exercise training is beneficial in HF patients with decreased ejection fraction (systolic dysfunction) or preserved ejection fraction (diastolic dysfunction) once therapy is optimized.
25. Intracardiac cardiac defibrillator is indicated for secondary survival benefit in patients who survive cardiac arrest, ventricular fibrillation, or hemodynamically significant ventricular tachycardia.
26. Intracardiac cardiac defibrillator is indicated for primary survival benefit in patients with ischemic or nonischemic cardiomyopathy with EF ≤35% with New York Heart Association (NYHA) class II or III. The patient should be stable on GDMT (guideline determined medical therapy) optimal chronic medical HF therapy and at least 40 days post-MI.
27. Biventricular heart pacemaker (CRT) should be considered in refractory HF with ejection fraction equal to or less than 35% with NYHA class II, III or ambulatory class IV on GDMT. The rhythm should be sinus, with a QRS ≥150 ms, ± LBBB.
28. Long-term anticoagulation therapy is not recommended in patients with chronic systolic function while in sinus rhythm in the absence of AF, a prior thromboembolic event or cardioembolic source.
29. In patient with AF and HFrEF anticoagulation with Warfarin is recommended. Alternative therapy with NOAC is reasonable when non-valvular AF.

HEART FAILURE
Source: **ADAPTED FROM ACCF/AHA 2013**
CLASSIFICATION, CLINICAL ASSESSMENT IN HEART FAILURE
CLASS I RECOMMENDATIONS (CONTINUED)

30. In HF patients with preserved systolic function (diastolic dysfunction), randomized data on therapy are lacking. The goal is to control blood volume (diuretic), control systolic blood pressure (β-blocker, ACE inhibitor, ARB agent, or diuretic), slow heart rate (β-blocker), and treat coronary artery ischemia. Whether β-blockers, ACE inhibitors, ARB agents, or aldosterone antagonists improve survival independently is yet to be proven.

31. Comprehensive written discharge instruction should be given to all patients. Diet, weight monitoring, medicine, and salt adherence should be emphasized. Activity should be discussed along with education of symptoms of worsening HF.

32. Post-discharge appointment with physician and healthcare team with attention to information on discharge medications.

Source: Adapted from: ACCF/AHA 2009 Guidelines. *J Am Coll Cardiol.* 2009;53(15):1333-1378; *N Engl J Med.* 2012;WARCET Trial; American Academy of Family Physicians; American Academy of Hospice and Palliative Medicine; American Nurses Association; American Society of Health-System Pharmacists; Heart Rhythm Society; Society of Hospital Medicine, Bonow RO, Ganiats TG, Beam CT, et al. ACCF/AHA/AMA-PCPI 2011 performance measures for adults with heart failure: a report of the American College of Cardiology Foundation/American Heart Association Task Force on Performance Measures and the American Medical Association-Physician Consortium for Performance Improvement. *J Am CollCardiol.* 2012;59(20):1812-1832. Yancy CW, Jessup M, Bozkurt B, et al. 2013 ACCF/AHA Guideline for the management of heart failure: a report of the American College of Cardiology Foundation/American Heart Association Task Force on practice guidelines. *Circulation.* 2013;128:e240-e327

HEART FAILURE

Disease Management	Organization	Population	Recommendations	Comments	Source
Heart Failure	FDA 2015	Patients with stable, symptomatic, chronic HF, in sinus rhythm, with LVEF ≤35%, who are in sinus rhythm with a resting HR ≥70 bpm, and either are on maximally tolerated doses of β-blocker or have a contraindication to β-blocker use.	Ivabradine (Corlanor®) was approved to reduce hospitalization from worsening HF. *Starting dose:* 5 mg 1 tab bid. Maximum dose 7.5 mg bid (dose can be increased after 1 mo as needed based on resting HR and tolerability). *Contraindications:* acute decompensated HF; BP <90/50 mm Hg, SSS, sinoatrial block, third degree AV block (unless a functioning demand pacemaker is present), resting HR <60 bpm prior to treatment, severe hepatic impairment, pacemaker dependent, concomitant use of strong cytochrome P450 3A4 (CYPRA4) inhibitors.	SHIFT study showed that Ivabradine reduced the time to first occurrence of hospitalization for worsening heart failure compared to placebo.	http://www.fda.gov/NewsEvents/Newsroom/PressAnnouncements/ucm442978.htm http://pi.amgen.com/united_states/corlanor/corlanor_pi_hcp.pdf
	EMA 2012	Patients with chronic heart failure NYHA II-IV, with systolic dysfunction, in sinus rhythm, with resting HR ≥75 bpm, in combination with standard therapy including β-blocker therapy or when β-blocker therapy is contraindicated or not tolerated.	Ivabradine was approved in treatment for HF.	2014 EMA review based on SIGNIFY study showed: Ivabradine should not be used in combination with verapamil or diltiazem. The risk of AF is increased in patient treated with Ivabradine and doctors should monitor patients for AF.	http://www.ema.europa.eu/ema/index.jsp?curl=pages/medicines/human/medicines/000598/human_med_000727.jsp&mid=WC0b01ac058001d124

HELICOBACTER PYLORI INFECTIONS

Disease Management	Organization	Date	Population	Recommendations	Comments	Source
Helicobacter pylori Infection	Cochrane Database Systematic Reviews	2013	Adults	Recommend using longer duration therapy for PPI-based *H. pylori* therapy.	75 studies analyzing PPI + two antibiotics, PPI bismuth-based quadruple therapy, or PPI + three antibiotics were studied. The relative risk of *H. pylori* persistence was 0.65–0.69 for different regimens using longer course therapies vs shorter duration therapies.	http://www.cochrane.org/CD008337/UPPERGI_ideal-length-of-treatment-for-helicobacter-pylori-h.-pylori-eradication

HEMOCHROMOSTOSIS

Disease Management	Organization	Recommendations	Comments	Source
Hereditary Hemochromostosis (HH)	**Hemochromatosis (HH)** 2011 practice guidelines *Hepatology*;54:328–343	**Clinical Features** 1. Asymptomatic patients with abnormal iron studies should be evaluated for hemochromatosis. 2. All patients with liver disease should be evaluated for hemochromatosis. **Diagnosis** 3. Combination of transferrin saturation (TS) and ferritin should be done—if either abnormal (TS > 45% or ferritin > upper limit of normal) the HFE mutation analysis indicated. 4. Screening (iron studies and HFE mutation studies) recommended for first-degree relatives. 5. Liver biopsy is recommended for diagnosis and prognosis in patients with phenotypic markers of iron overload who are not C282Y homozygotes or compound heterozygotes (C282Y, H63D). 6. Liver biopsy to stage the degree of liver disease in C282Y homozygote or compound heterozygotes if liver enzymes elevated or ferritin >1000 μg/L. **Treatment of Hemochromatosis** 7. Therapeutic phlebotomy weekly until ferritin level 50–100 μg/L. 8. C282Y homozygotes who have an elevated ferritin (but <1000 μg/L) should proceed to phlebotomy without liver biopsy. 9. Patients with end-organ damage due to iron overload should undergo regular phlebotomy to keep ferritin between 50–100 μg/L. 10. Vitamin C and iron supplements should be avoided but other dietary adjustments not necessary. 11. Patients should be monitored on a regular basis for reaccumulation of iron and undergo maintenance with targeted ferritin levels of 50–100 μg/L. 12. Iron chelation with deferoxamine or deferasirox not recommended in hemochromatosis. (*Blood.* 2010;116: 317–325. *Blood.* 2008; 111:3373–3376.)	1. Symptoms besides liver function abnormalities include skin pigmentation, pancreatic dysfunction with diabetes, arthralgias, impotence, and cardiac involvement with ECG changes and heart failure. 2. Other rare mutations causing phenotypic hemochromatosis include transferrin receptor 2 mutation, ferroportin mutations and H ferritin mutation. 3. The most devastating complication of hemochromatosis is a 20-fold increase in the risk of hepatocellular carcinoma (HCC). Less than 1% of patients whose ferritin has never been >1000 μg/L develop HCC while the risk rises considerably in patients with cirrhosis and ferritin level >1000 μg/L. These patients should be screened with hepatic ultrasound every 6 mo. Alfa fetoprotein (AFP) is elevated in only 60% of patients with HCC and should not be used as a single screening test. 4. Patients with hemochromatosis are at increased risk for certain bacterial infections whose virulence is increased in the pretence of iron. These include Listeria monocytogenes (most common in renal dialysis patients), Yersinia enterocolitica and Vibrio vulniticus (uncooked seafood is a common source). Infections are made more virulent by iron overload of macrophages impairing their anti-bacterial activity. Secondary iron overload (most commonly secondary to a transfusion requirement due to blood or bone marrow disease) is best managed by iron chelation beginning when the ferritin rises above 1000 μg/L. In contrast to HH excess iron is deposited primarily in the reticuloendothelial system although visceral iron overload does occur overtime.	

Disease Management	Organization	Date	Population	Recommendations	Comments	Source
Hepatitis B Virus (HBV)	NIH AASLD	2009 2009	Adults and children with HBV infection	1. Recommend HBV immunoglobulin and HBV vaccine to all infants born to HbsAg-positive women. 2. Recommend antiviral therapy for adults and alanine transaminase (ALT) >2× normal, moderate-severe hepatitis on biopsy, compensated cirrhosis or advanced fibrosis and HBV DNA >20,000 IU/mL; or for reactivation of chronic HBV after chemotherapy or immunosuppression. 3. Recommend antiviral therapy in children for ALT >2× normal and HBV DNA >20,000 IU/mL for at least 6 mo. 4. Optimal monitoring practices have not been defined.	1. The most important predictors of cirrhosis or hepatocellular carcinoma (HCC) in chronic HBV infection are persistently elevated HBV DNA and serum ALT levels, HBV genotype C infection, male gender, older age, and coinfection with hepatitis C virus or human immunodeficiency virus (HIV). a. Persons at risk for HCC should be screened by ultrasound every 6–12 mo 2. No randomized controlled trials have demonstrated a decrease in overall mortality, liver-specific mortality, or the rate of HCC with anti-HBV therapies. 3. Consider lamivudine or interferon-α for initial anti-HBV therapy.	http://www.guidelines.gov/content.aspx?id=14240 http://www.guidelines.gov/content.aspx?id=15475

HEPATITIS B VIRUS INFECTION

Disease Management	Organization	Date	Population	Recommendations	Comments	Source
Hepatitis B Virus Infection	NICE	2013	Adults	• Offer antiviral therapy to adults if: 　○ Without a liver biopsy to adults with a transient elastography score ≥11 kPa 　○ HBV DNA>2000 IU/mL and ALT>30 IU/mL (males) or >19 IU/mL (females) 　○ Cirrhosis and detectable HBV DNA • Initial antiviral options for HBV infection 　○ Peginterferon α-2a 　○ Entecavir 　○ Tenofovir disoproxil • Coinfection with HBV and HCV 　○ Peginterferon alfa-2a and ribavirin	• Consider a liver biopsy to confirm fibrosis for a transient elastography score 6–10 kPa. • Monitor CBC, liver panel and renal panel at 2, 4, 12, 24, 36, and 48 wk while on interferon therapy. • Monitor CBC, liver panel and renal panel at 4 wk and every 3 mo while on tenofovir therapy.	http://www.guideline.gov/content.aspx?id=46933
			Children and young adults	• Consider liver biopsy if HBV DNA >2000 IU/mL and ALT >30 IU/mL (males) or >19 IU/mL (females) • Initial antiviral options 　○ Peginterferon α-2a		
			Pregnant women	• Consider tenofovir disoproxil if HBV DNA >10^7 IU/mL in third trimester	• Reduces risk of HBV transmission to baby	

HEPATITIS C VIRUS (HCV)

Disease Management	Organization	Date	Population	Recommendations	Comments	Source

Hepatitis C Virus (HCV)	AASLD	2009	Adults with HCV infection	1. Recommends education on methods to avoid transmission to others.
				2. Recommends antiviral treatment for:
				  a. Bridging fibrosis or compensated cirrhosis
				  b. Consideration of acute HCV infection
				3. Test quantitative HCV RNA before treatment and at 12 wk of therapy.
				4. Patients who lack antibodies for hepatitis A and B viruses should receive vaccination.
				5. Recommend abstaining from alcohol consumption.
				6. Insufficient evidence to recommend herbal therapy.
					1. Optimal therapy is the combination of peginterferon-α and ribavirin.
					  a. Duration of therapy is 48 wk for HCV genotypes 1 and 4
					  b. Duration of therapy is 24 wk for HCV genotypes 2 and 3
						http://www.guidelines.gov/content.aspx?id=14708

	WHO	2014		1. Recommend pegylated interferon with ribavirin for adults and children with chronic HCV infection 2. Recommend telaprevir or boceprevir in combination with pegylated interferon with ribavirin for genotype 1 chronic HCV infection 3. Sofosbuvir in combination with ribavirin +/– pegylated interferon for genotypes 1, 2, 3, or 4 HCV infection		http://www.guideline.gov/content.aspx?id=48895

HOARSENESS

Disease Management	Organization	Date	Population	Recommendations	Comments	Source
Hoarseness	AAO-HNS	2009	Persons with hoarseness	1. Recommends against the routine use of antibiotics to treat hoarseness. 2. Recommends voice therapy for all patients with hoarseness and a decreased voice quality of life. 3. All patients with chronic hoarseness >3 mo should undergo laryngoscopy. 4. Recommends against routine use of antireflux medications unless the patient exhibits signs or symptoms of gastroesophageal reflux disease. 5. Recommends against the routine use of corticosteroids to treat hoarseness. 6. Recommends against screening neck imaging (CT or MRI scanning) for chronic hoarseness prior to laryngoscopy. 7. Consider surgery for possible laryngeal CA, benign laryngeal soft-tissue lesions, or glottis insufficiency. 8. Consider botulinum toxin injections for spasmodic dysphonia.	Nearly one-third of Americans will have hoarseness at some point in their lives.	http://www.guidelines.gov/content.aspx?id=15203

HUMAN IMMUNODEFICIENCY VIRUS (HIV)

Disease Management	Organization	Date	Population	Recommendations	Comments	Source

Human Immunodeficiency Virus (HIV)	IDSA	2009	HIV-infected adults and children	1. Recommends education to avoid high-risk behaviors to minimize risk of HIV transmission.
				2. Assess for the presence of depression, substance abuse, or domestic violence.
				3. Baseline labs: CD4 count; quantitative HIV RNA by PCR (viral load); HIV genotyping; CBCD, chemistry panel, G6PD testing; fasting lipid profile; HLA B5701 test (if abacavir is used); urinalysis; PPD; *Toxoplasma* antibodies; HBsAg, HBsAb, and HCV antibodies; VDRL; urine NAAT for gonorrhea; and urine NAAT for chlamydia (except in men age <25 y); Pap smear in women.[a]
				4. Monitoring labs:
				  a. CD4 counts and HIV viral load every 3–4 mo.
				  b. Frequency of repeat sexually transmitted disease (STD) screening is undefined.
				  c. Annual PPD test.
				  d. Persons starting antiretroviral medications should have a repeat fasting glucose and lipid panel 4–6 wk after initiation of therapy.
				5. Vaccination for pneumococcal infection, influenza, varicella, hepatitis A, and HBV according to standard immunization charts.
				6. All HIV-infected women of childbearing age should be counseled regarding contraception.
				7. Pap smear in women every 6 mo.
				8. Consider annual mammography in all women age ≥40 y.
				9. Hormone replacement therapy is not recommended.
				10. All women age ≥65 y should have a dual-energy x-ray absorptiometry (DXA) test of spine/hips.
					1. Homosexual men and women with abnormal cervical Pap smear results and persons with a history of genital warts should undergo anogenital human papilloma virus (HPV) screening and anal Pap testing.
					2. Serum testosterone level should be considered in men complaining of fatigue, ED, or decreased libido.
					3. Chest x-ray should be obtained in persons with pulmonary symptoms or who have a positive PPD test result.
						http://www.guidelines.gov/content.aspx?id=15440

[a]CBCD, complete blood count with differential; G6PD, glucose-6-phosphate dehydrogenase; HBsAb, hepatitis B surface antibody; HBsAg, hepatitis B surface antigen; HLA, human leukocyte antigen; NAAT, nucleic acid amplification test; PCR, polymerase chain reaction; PPD, purified protein derivative; RNA, ribonucleic acid; VDRL, Venereal Disease Research Laboratory.

HUMAN IMMUNODEFICIENCY VIRUS, ANTIRETROVIRAL THERAPY (ART)

Disease Management	Organization	Date	Population	Recommendations	Comments	Source

Human Immunodeficiency Virus (HIV), Antiretroviral Therapy (ART)	HHS	2010	HIV-infected children	1. ART is recommended for all children with symptomatic HIV disease.
				2. Recommends ART for:
				  a. Infants age <12 mo
				  b. Asymptomatic children with HIV RNA ≥100,000 copies/mL
				  c. Children age 1–5 y with CD4 <25%
				  d. Children age ≥5 y with CD4 <350 cells/mm^3
				  e. Children age ≥1 y with acquired immunodeficiency syndrome (AIDS) or symptomatic HIV infection
				3. HIV genotype testing is recommended:
				  a. Prior to initiation of therapy in all treatment-naïve children
				  b. Prior to changing therapy for treatment failure
				4. Recommends evaluating all children 4–8 wk after initiation of ART for possible side effects and to evaluate response to therapy.
				  a. Reevaluate children every 3–4 mo thereafter
					Specific ART recommendations are beyond the scope of this book.	http://www.guideline.gov/content.aspx?id=38702

HUMAN IMMUNODEFICIENCY VIRUS-1 (HIV-1), ANTIRETROVIRAL USE

Disease Management	Organization	Date	Population	Recommendations	Comments	Source

Human Immunodeficiency Virus-1 (HIV-1), Antiretroviral Use	HHS	2013	Adults and adolescents	• Antiretroviral-naïve patients should start:
				  ○ Efavirenz/tenofovir/emtricitabine
				  ○ Ritonavir-boosted atazanavir/tenofovir/emtricitabine
				  ○ Ritonavir-boosted darunavir/tenofovir/emtricitabine
				  ○ Raltegravir/tenofovir/emtricitabine
				  ○ Rilpivirine-based regimens are an alternative
				  ○ Selection of a regimen should be individualized
				    – Efavirenz is teratogenic
				    – Tenofovir should be used cautiously with renal insufficiency
				    – Ritonavir-boosted atazanavir and rilpivirine should not be used with high-dose proton pump inhibitors
				• Coreceptor tropism assay is recommended whenever a CCR5 coreceptor antagonist is considered.
				• HLA-B*5701 screening before starting abacavir.
				• Interruption of HAART is recommended for drug toxicity, intercurrent illness, or operations that precludes oral intake.
				Management of a treatment—experienced patient is complex and should be managed by an HIV specialist.
					• This guideline focuses on antiretroviral management in HIV-1-infected individuals.
					• Baseline evaluation should include:
					  ○ CD4 T-cell count
					  ○ HIV-1 antibody testing
					  ○ HIV RNA viral load
					  ○ CBC, chemistry panel, liver panel, urinalysis
					  ○ Serologies for HAV, HBV, and HCV
					  ○ Fasting glucose and lipid panel
					  ○ HIV-1 genotypic resistance testing
					  ○ STD screening
					  ○ Psychosocial assessment
					  ○ Substance abuse screening
					  ○ HIV risk behavior screening
					  ○ CD_4 <350 cells/mm^3
					  ○ Consider for CD_4 350–500 cells/mm^3
					  ○ Pregnant women as soon as possible to prevent perinatal transmission
					  ○ Consider for preventing heterosexual transmission
					  ○ Patients must commit to strict adherence to HAART therapy
						http://aidsinfo.nih.gov/guidelines/html/1/adult-and-adolescent-arv-guidelines/0

HUMAN IMMUNODEFICIENCY VIRUS (HIV), PREGNANCY

Disease Management	Organization	Date	Population	Recommendations	Comments	Source

Human Immunodeficiency Virus (HIV), Pregnancy	CDC	2010	HIV-infected pregnant women	1. Recommends combination ART regimens during the antepartum period.
				2. Women who were taking ART prior to conception should have their regimen reviewed (ie, teratogenic potential of drugs), but continue combination ART throughout the pregnancy.
				3. Initial prenatal labs should include a CD4 count, HIV viral load, and HCV antibody.
				  a. If HIV RNA is detectable (>500–1000 copies/mL), perform HIV genotypic resistance testing to help guide antepartum therapy.
				4. Women who do not require ART for their own health should initiate combination ART between 14 and 28 gestational weeks and continue until delivery.
				  a. Zidovudine should be a component of the regimen when feasible.
				  b. Recommend against single-dose intrapartum/newborn nevirapine in addition to antepartum ART.
				5. Antepartum monitoring:
				  a. Monitor CD4 count every 3 mo.
				  b. HIV viral load should be assessed 2–4 wk after initiating or changing ART, monthly until undetectable, and then at 34–36 wk.
				  c. Recommend a first-trimester ultrasound to confirm dating.
				  d. Screen for gestational diabetes at 24–28 wk.
				6. Scheduled cesarean delivery is recommended for HIV-infected women who have HIV RNA levels >1000 copies/mL and intact membranes near term.
				7. Intrapartum IV zidovudine is recommended for all HIV-infected pregnant women.
				8. Avoid artificial rupture of membranes.
				9. Avoid routine use of fetal scalp electrodes.
				10. Breast-feeding is not recommended.
					1. Avoid Methergine for postpartum hemorrhage in women receiving a protease inhibitor or efavirenz.
					2. If women do not receive antepartum/ intrapartum ART prophylaxis, infants should receive zidovudine for 6 wk.
					3. Infants born to HIV-infected women should have an HIV viral load checked at 14 d, at 1–2 mo, and at 4–6 mo.
						http://www.guideline.gov/content.aspx?id=38253

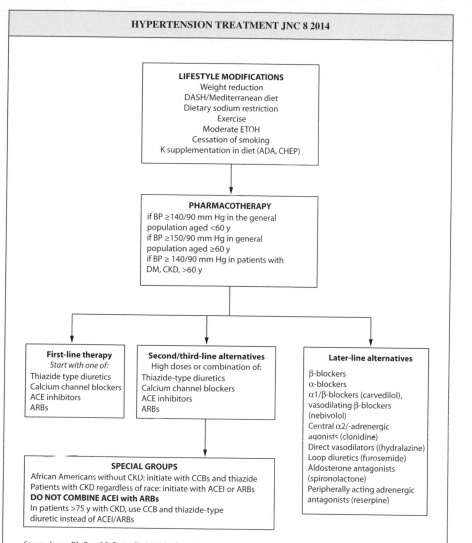

HYPERTENSION TREATMENT JNC 8 2014

LIFESTYLE MODIFICATIONS
Weight reduction
DASH/Mediterranean diet
Dietary sodium restriction
Exercise
Moderate ETOH
Cessation of smoking
K supplementation in diet (ADA, CHEP)

PHARMACOTHERAPY
if BP ≥140/90 mm Hg in the general
population aged <60 y
if BP ≥150/90 mm Hg in general
population aged ≥60 y
if BP ≥ 140/90 mm Hg in patients with
DM, CKD, >60 y

First-line therapy
Start with one of:
Thiazide type diuretics
Calcium channel blockers
ACE inhibitors
ARBs

Second/third-line alternatives
High doses or combination of:
Thiazide-type diuretics
Calcium channel blockers
ACE inhibitors
ARBs

Later-line alternatives
β-blockers
α-blockers
α1/β-blockers (carvedilol),
vasodilating β-blockers
(nebivolol)
Central α2-/adrenergic
agonists (clonidine)
Direct vasodilators ((hydralazine)
Loop diuretics (furosemide)
Aldosterone antagonists
(spironolactone)
Peripherally acting adrenergic
antagonists (reserpine)

SPECIAL GROUPS
African Americans without CKD: initiate with CCBs and thiazide
Patients with CKD regardless of race: initiate with ACEI or ARBs
DO NOT COMBINE ACEI with ARBs
In patients >75 y with CKD, use CCB and thiazide-type
diuretic instead of ACEI/ARBs

Source: James PA, Oparil S, Carter BL. 2014 Evidence-based guideline for the management of high blood
pressure in adults. Report from the panel members appointed to the Eighth Joint National Committee (JNC8).
JAMA. 2014;311(5):507-520. doi:10.1001/jama.2013.284427.

JNC 8 2014
ANTIHYPERTENSIVE THERAPY

Initiate therapy:
- BP ≥140/90 mm Hg in the general population aged <60 y old
- BP ≥150/90 mm Hg in general population aged ≥60 y old

Goal therapy:
- BP <140/90 mm Hg in patients <60 y old
- BP <150/90 mm Hg in patients ≥60 y old
- BP <140/90 mm Hg in patients with DM, CKD who are <60 y old

Antihypertensive therapy:
- In the general nonblack population, including those with DM, initial treatment should include a thiazide-type diuretic, CCB, ACEI, or ARB
- In the general black population, including those with DM, initial treatment should include a thiazide-type diuretic or CCB
- In all population aged ≥18 y old with CKD (+/-DM), treatment should include an ACEI/ARB to improve kidney outcomes
- Patients with CKD regardless of race: initiate with ACEI or ARBs
- In patients >75 y old with CKD, use CCB and thiazide-type diuretic instead of ACEI/ARBs
- If BP cannot be reached within 1 mo increase the dose of the initial drug or add a second and then third drug from the recommended classes
- **Do not use an ACEI and ARB together!**
- β-blockers, α-blockers, central α-2-adrenergic agonists (eg, clonidine), direct vasodilators (eg, hydralazine), aldosterone receptor antagonists (eg, spironolactone), peripherally acting adrenergic antagonists (eg, reserpine), and loop diuretics (eg, furosemide) are not recommended as a first-line therapy.

Source: James PA, Oparil S, Carter BL. 2014 Evidence-based guideline for the management of high blood pressure in adults. Report from the panel members appointed to the Eighth Joint National Committee (JNC8) *JAMA*. 2014;311(5):507-520. doi:10.1001/jama.2013.284427.

ACC/AHA/ASH 2015
ANTIHYPERTENSIVE THERAPY FOR PATIENTS WITH CAD

1. *Patients with HTN and chronic stable angina*
   - Goal therapy: <140/90 mm Hg for secondary prevention of CV events on patients with HTN and CAD.
     <130/80 mm Hg may be appropriate for patients with CAD, previous MI, stroke or TIA, or CAD equivalents (CAD, PAD, AAA).
   - Treatment should include:
     1. β-blocker in patients with a history of prior MI.
     2. ACEI/ARB if prior MI, LV systolic dysfunction, DM, or CKD.
     3. A thiazide or thiazide-like diuretic.
   - If β-blocker is contraindicated or produce intolerable side effects, a nondihydropyridine CCB may be substituted but NOT if there is LV dysfunction.
   - If either angina or HTN remains uncontrolled, a long-acting dihydropyridine CCB can be added to the basic regimen of β-blocker, ACEI/ARB, and thiazide/thiazide-like diuretic. Combination of β-blocker and either of the nondihydropyridine CCB should be used with caution in patients with symptomatic CAD and HTN because of the increased risk of significant bradyarrhythmias and HF.
   - There are no special contraindications in HTN patients for the use of antiplatelet or anticoagulant drugs, except that in patients with uncontrolled severe HTN who are taking antiplatelet or anticoagulant drugs, the BP should be lowered without delay to reduce the risk of hemorrhagic stroke.
2. *Patients with HTN and ACS*
   - BP target <140/90 mm Hg in patients with HTN and ACS that are hemodynamically stable. BP target <130/80 mm Hg at the time of hospital discharge is reasonable. BP should be lowered slowly and caution is advised to avoid decreases in DBP to <60 mm Hg because this may reduce coronary artery perfusion and worsen ischemia.
   - If no contraindication to β-blockers, the initial therapy of HTN should include a short-acting $β_1$-selective β-blocker without intrinsic sympathomimetic activity (metoprolol tartrate or bisoprolol). β-Blocker therapy should typically be initiated orally within 24 h of presentation. For patients with severe HTN or ongoing ischemia, an intravenous β-blocker (esmolol) can be considered. For hemodynamically unstable patients or when decompensated HF exists, the initiation of β-blocker therapy should be delayed until stabilization has been achieved.
   - Nitrates should be considered to lower BP or relieve ongoing ischemia or pulmonary congestion. Nitrates should be avoided in patients with suspected RV infarction and in those with hemodynamic instability. Sublingual or IV nitroglycerin therapy is preferred for initial treatment and can be transitioned later to a longer-acting form if needed.
   - If contraindication/intolerance/side effects to β-blocker and no presence of LV dysfunction or HF, ok to substitute with nondihydropyridine CCB (verapamil, diltiazem). If the angina or HTN is not controlled on β-blocker alone, a longer-acting dihydropyridine CCB may be added after optimal use of ACEI.
   - ACEI/ARB should be added if anterior MI, persistent HTN, LV dysfunction, HF, or DM. For lower-risk ACS patients with preserved LV function and no DM, ACEI can be considered a first-line agent for BP control.
   - Aldosterone antagonists are indicated for patients who are already receiving a β-blocker and ACEI after MI and have LV dysfunction and either HF or DM. Serum K levels must be monitored. These agents should be avoided in patients with elevated serum creatinine levels (≥2.5mg/dL in men, ≥2.0 mg/dL in women) or elevated K levels (≥5.0 mEq/L).
   - Loop diuretics are preferred over thiazide/thiazide-type diuretics for patients with ACS who have HF (NYHA III or IV) or for patients with CKD and estimated glomerular filtration rate <39 mL/min. If HTN remains uncontrolled despite a β-blocker, an ACEI, and an aldosterone antagonist, a thiazide/thiazide-type diuretic may be added in selected patients for BP control.

ACC/AHA/ASH 2015
ANTIHYPERTENSIVE THERAPY FOR PATIENTS WITH CAD (CONTINUED)

3. *Patients with HTN and HF of ischemic origin*

- BP target is <140/90 mm Hg, but consideration can be given to lowering the BP even further, to <130/80 mm Hg. In patients with an elevated DBP who have CAD and HF with evidence of myocardial ischemia, the BP should be lowered slowly. In older hypertensive individuals with wide pulse pressures, lowering SBP may cause very low DBP values (<60 mm Hg). This should alert the clinician to assess carefully any untoward signs or symptoms, especially those caused by myocardial ischemia and worsening HF. Octogenarians should be checked for orthostatic changes with standing, and an SBP <130 mm Hg and a DBP <65 mm Hg should be avoided.

- Treatment should include management of risk factors (dyslipidemia, obesity, DM, smoking, dietary sodium, and closely monitored exercise program).

- The patient should be treated with ACEI/ARB, β-blocker (carvedilol, metoprolol succinate, bisoprolol, or nebivolol) and aldosterone receptor antagonists. These drugs have shown to improve outcomes for patients with HF and reduced EF.

- Thiazide/thiazide-type diuretic should be used for BP control and to reverse volume overload and associated symptoms. In patients with severe HF (NYHA III or IV), or those with severe renal impairment (eGFR <30 mL/min), loop diuretics should be used for volume control, but they are less effective than thiazide/thiazide-type diuretics in lowering BP. Diuretics should be used together with an ACE/ARB and a β-blocker.

- Studies have shown equivalence of benefit of ACEI and ARB (candesartan or valsartan) in HF with reduced EF. Either class of agents is effective in lowering BP.

- The aldosterone receptor antagonists spironolactone and eplerenone have been shown to be beneficial in HF and should be included in the regimen if there is HF (NYHA III or IV) with reduced EF <40%. One or the other may be substituted for a thiazide diuretic in patients requiring a K-sparing agent. If an aldosterone receptor antagonist is administered with an ACEI/ARB in the presence of renal insufficiency, serum K level should be monitored frequently. Should not be used if creatinine level ≥2.5 mg/dL in men or ≥2.0 mg/dL in women, or if serum K level ≥5mEq/L. Spironolactone or eplerenone may be used with a thiazide/thiazide-type diuretic in resistant HTN.

- Hydralazine plus isosorbide dinitrate should be added to the regimen of diuretic, ACE inhibitor, or ARB, and β-blocker in African American patients with NYHA class III or IV HF with reduced ejection fraction. Others may benefit similarly, but this has not yet been tested.

- In patients who have hypertension and HF with preserved ejection fraction, the recommendations are to control systolic and diastolic hypertension, ventricular rate in the presence of atrial fibrillation, and pulmonary congestion and peripheral edema.

- Use of β-adrenergic blocking agents, ACEI/ARBs, or CCB in patients with HF with preserved ejection fraction and hypertension may be effective to minimize symptoms of HF.

- In IHD, the principles of therapy for acute hypertension with pulmonary edema are similar to those for STEMI and NSTEMI, as described above. If the patient is hemodynamically unstable, the initiation of these therapies should be delayed until stabilization of HF has been achieved.

- Drugs to avoid in patients with hypertension and HF with reduced ejection fraction are nondihydropyridine CCBs (such as verapamil and diltiazem), clonidine, moxonidine, and hydralazine without a nitrate. α-Adrenergic blockers such as doxazosin should be used only if other drugs for the management of hypertension and HF are inadequate to achieve BP control at maximum tolerated doses. Nonsteroidal anti-inflammatory drugs should also be used with caution in this group, given their effects on BP, volume status, and renal function.

Source: Rosendorff C, Lackland DT, Allison M, et al. Treatment of hypertension in patients with coronary artery disease: a scientific statement from the American Heart Association, American College of Cardiology, and American Society of Hypertension. *JACC.* 2015. 65(18):1998-2038.

AMERICAN SOCIETY OF HYPERTENSION (ASH) 2013 ANTIHYPERTENSIVE THERAPY

Goal therapy:
- BP<150/90 mm Hg in patients ≥80 y old
- BP<140/90 mm Hg in patients 60–79 y old
- BP <140/90 mm Hg or <130/80 mm Hg (if tolerated), in patients <50 y old

In patients with CKD or diabetes:
- BP <140/90 mm Hg (without proteinuria)
- BP <130/80 mm Hg (with proteinuria)—no consensus

Antihypertensive therapy:
- Start lifestyle changes
- In stage I (140–159/90–99) in patients without CV risks, some months of regularly monitored lifestyle management without drugs can be considered.
- In black patients: initiate with CCB or thiazide. If unable to control BP, add ACEI/ARB. If needed add Spironolactone, centrally acting agents, β-blockers.
- In nonblack patients <60 y old initiate with ACEI/ARB. If uncontrolled, add CCB, thiazide. If needed add Spironolactone, centrally acting agents, β-blockers. In nonblack patients ≥60 y old initiate with CCB or thiazide. If needed add Spironolactone, centrally acting agents, β-blockers.

Source: Clinical practice guidelines for the management of hypertension in the community: a statement by the American Society of Hypertension and the International Society of Hypertension. *J Clin Hypertens.* 2014. doi: 10.1111/jch.12237.

AMERICAN DIABETES ASSOCIATION ADA 2013—ANTIHYPERTENSIVE THERAPY

Goal therapy:
- BP <140/80 mm Hg in patients with diabetes and HTN
- BP <130/80 mm Hg in young patients, if no side effects
- BP 110–129/65–79 in pregnant patients with diabetes and chronic HTN (lower than this may be associated with impaired fetal growth)

Antihypertensive therapy:
- Start lifestyle changes
- Initiate with ACEI or ARB
- Administer one or more antihypertensive medications at bedtime. Closely monitor eGFR, serum K levels if any ACEI/ARB/ diuretic is used
- Safe in pregnancy: methyldopa, labetalol, diltiazem, clonidine, and prazosin

Source: Standards of Medical Care in Diabetes. *Diabetes Care.* January 2014;37(suppl 1). www.care.diabetesjournals.org.

CANADIAN HYPERTENSION EDUCATION PROGRAM
CHEP 2014/2015—ANTIHYPERTENSIVE THERAPY

- The diagnosis of HTN should be based on out-of-office measurements (home or ambulatory). Electronic (oscillometric) measurement methods are preferred to manual measurements. HBPM[a] and ABPM[b] identify white coat hypertension (as well as diagnose masked hypertension). (10% may have marked hypertension.)
- Risk factors cluster, therefore the management of HTN is combining global cardiovascular risk management and vascular protection including advice and treatment for smoking cessation.
- Structured exercise prescription as lifestyle modification.
- Resistance or weight training does not adversely affect BP in normotensive or mildly hypertensive individuals.
- Stress management should be considered as an intervention in hypertensive patients in whom stress may be contributing to BP elevation.

Initiate therapy:
- BP ≥160/100 mm Hg in patients without macrovascular target organ damage or other CV risk factors
- BP ≥140/90 mm Hg in patients with macrovascular target organ damage or other independent CV risk factors
- BP >130/80 mm Hg in patients with diabetes
- SBP >160 mm Hg in very elderly (≥80 y)

Goal therapy:
- BP <140/90 mm Hg in the general population, including those with CKD
- BP <130/80 mm Hg in patients with DM
- SBP <150 mm Hg in the very elderly (≥80 y)
- Caution in elderly patients who are frail and in patients with CAD and have low DBP <60 mm Hg

Antihypertensive agents:
- Combination of both lifestyle modifications and antihypertensive medicines are generally necessary to achieve target blood pressures. Adopting health behaviors is integral to the management of hypertension.
- Optimum management of the hypertensive patient requires assessment and communication of overall cardiovascular risk.
- Initial therapy should be monotherapy with a thiazide diuretic, a beta-blocker in patients <60 y, an ACEI in non-black patients, a long-acting CCB or an ARB.
- First-line combinations: thiazide diuretic or CCB with either an ACEI, ARB, or β-blocker. **Combination of ACEI and ARB is not recommended!** Caution in combination of nondihydropyridine and a β-blocker.
- In patients with diabetes, the combination preferred: ACEI with dihydropyridine rather than ACEI with HCTZ.
- Single pill combination therapies improve achieving optimal BP control.
- **ISH**: initial monotherapy with a thiazide diuretic, a long-acting dihydropyridine CCB, or an ARB. Combination of 2 or more first-line agents or other classes like α-blockers, ACEI, centrally acting agents, or nondihydropyridine CCBs
- β-blockers are not recommended as first-line therapy for uncomplicated hypertension/uncomplicated ISH in patients ≥60 y. ACEIs are not recommended as first-line therapy for uncomplicated hypertension in black patients. α-blockers are not recommended as first line agents for uncomplicated hypertension/uncomplicated ISH.
- The patient with hypertension attributable to atherosclerotic renal artery stenosis should be primarily medically managed, because renal angioplasty and stenting offer no benefits over optimal medical therapy alone. Renal artery angioplasty and stenting for atherosclerotic hemodynamically significant renal artery stenosis *could be considered* for patients with uncontrolled HTN resistant to maximally tolerated pharmacotherapy, progressive renal function loss, and acute PE.
- Global cardiovascular risk should be assessed in all hypertensive patients. Informing patients of their global risk improves the effectiveness of risk factor modification.
- Statin therapy is recommended in high-risk hypertensive patients based on having established atherosclerotic disease or at least 3 of the following: male, ≥55 y, smoking, type 2 diabetes, total-C/HDL-C ratio ≥6, premature family history of CV disease, previous stroke or TIA, LVH, ECG abnormalities, microalbuminuria or proteinuria, peripheral vascular disease.
- Low-dose ASA should be started in hypertensive patients ≥50 y for vascular protection. Caution should be exercised if BP is not controlled.
- Advice in combination with pharmacotherapy (eg, varenicline, bupropion, nicotine replacement therapy) should be offered to all smokers with a goal of smoking cessation.

[a]HBPM = home BP measurement
[b]ABPM = ambulatory BP measurement
Sources: https://www.hypertension.ca/en/chep.
Padwal R, Poirier L, Quinn R, et al. The 2013 Canadian Hypertension Education Program Recommendations.

IMPACT OF HEALTH BEHAVIOR MANAGEMENT ON BLOOD PRESSURE

Intervention	Systolic BP (mm Hg)	Diastolic BP (mm Hg)
Diet and weight control	−6.0	−4.8
Reduced salt/sodium intake <2000 mg sodium (Na)a	−5.4	−2.8
Reduced alcohol intake (<2 drinks/day)	−3.4	−3,4
DASH diet	−11.4	−5.5
Physical activity (30–40 min 5–7 × week)	−3.1	−1.8
Relaxation therapies	−5.5	−3.5

a2000 mg sodium (Na) = 87 mmol sodium (Na) = 5 g of salt (NaCl) ~1 teaspoon of table salt
Source: Adapted from Canadian Hypertension Education Program (CHEP) Recommendations. 2015. www.hypertension.ca/en/chep.

LIFESTYLE MODIFICATIONS FOR TREATMENT OF HYPERTENSION[a,b]

Modification	Recommendation	Approximate SBP Reduction (Range)
Weight reduction	Maintain normal body weight (BMI 18.5–24.9 kg/m^2).	5–20 mm Hg per 10-kg weight loss
Adopt DASH eating plan	Consume diet rich in fruits, vegetables, and low-fat dairy products with a reduced content of saturated and total fat.	8–14 mm Hg
Dietary sodium reduction	Reduce dietary sodium intake to less than 100 mmol/d (2.4 g sodium or 6 g sodium chloride).	2–8 mm Hg
Physical activity	Engage in regular aerobic physical activity such as brisk walking (at least 30 min/d, most days of the week).	4–9 mm Hg
Moderation of alcohol consumption	Limit consumption to no more than 2 drinks (1 oz or 30 mL ethanol; eg, 24 oz beer, 10 oz wine, or 3 oz 80-proof whiskey) per day in most men and to no more than 1 drink per day in women and lighter-weight persons.	2–4 mm Hg

DASH, Dietary Approaches to Stop Hypertension.
[a]For overall cardiovascular risk reduction, stop smoking.
[b]The effects of implementing these modifications are dose- and time-dependent and could be greater for some individuals.
DASH diet found to be effective in lowering SBP in adolescents.
Source: Couch SC, Saelens BE, Levin L, Dart K, Falciglia G, Daniels SR. The efficacy of a clinic-based behavioral nutrition intervention emphasizing a DASH-type diet for adolescents with elevated blood pressure. *J Pediatr.* 2008;152:494-501. Aronow WS, Fleg JL, Pepine CJ, et al. ACCF/AHA 2011 expert consensus document on hypertension in the elderly: a report of the American College of Cardiology Foundation Task Force on Clinical Expert Consensus documents developed in collaboration with the American Academy of Neurology, American Geriatrics Society, American Society for Preventive Cardiology, American Society of Hypertension, American Society of Nephrology, Association of Black Cardiologists, and European Society of Hypertension. *J Am Coll Cardiol.* 2011;57:2037-2110.

RECOMMENDED MEDICATIONS FOR COMPELLING INDICATIONS

Compelling Indication[a]	Diuretic	BB	ACEI	ARB	CCB	AldoANT
Heart failure	X	X	X	X		X
Post-MI		X	X			X
High coronary disease risk	X	X	X		X	
Diabetes	X	X	X	X	X	
Chronic kidney disease[b]			X	X		
Recurrent stroke prevention	X		X			

ACEI, ACE inhibitor; AldoANT, aldosterone antagonist; ARB, angiotensin receptor blocker; BB, beta-blocker; CCB, calcium channel blocker.
[a]Compelling indications for antihypertensive drugs are based on benefits from outcome studies or existing clinical guidelines; the compelling indication is managed in parallel with the BP.
[b]ALLHAT: Patients with hypertension and reduced GFR: no difference in renal outcomes (development of end-stage renal disease [ESRD] and/or decrement in GFR of ≥50% from baseline) comparing amlodipine, lisinopril, and chlorthalidone. (*Arch Intern Med.* 2005;165:936-946) Data do *not* support preference for CCB, alfa-blockers, or ACEI compared with thiazide diuretics in patients with metabolic syndrome. (*Arch Intern Med.* 2008;168:207-217; *J Am Coll Cardiol.* 2011;57:2037-2110; 2012 CHEP Recommendations, http://www.hypertension.ca)

COMPLICATED HYPERTENSION CHEP 2014

- **HTN and documented CAD**
  - ACEI is recommended for patients with HTN and documented CAD.
  - For patients with stable angina, β-blockers are preferred as initial therapy.
  - Combination of ACEI with ARB is not recommended, in HTN patients with CAD but absence of LV systolic dysfunction.
  - In high-risk patients, combination of ACEI and a dihydropyridine CCB is preferable to an ACEI and a thiazide/thiazide-like diuretic in selected patients.
  - Myocardial ischemia may be exacerbated when DBP ≤60 mm Hg—caution in lowering DBP too much. (grade D)
- **HTN and recent STEMI/NSTEMI**
  - Initial therapy should include β-blocker and an ACEI or ARB. CCB may be used if β-blockers are contraindicated. Should not use nondihydropyridine CCBs with heart failure.
- **HTN with heart failure**
  - When LVEF <40% ACEI/ARBs and β-blockers are recommended as initial therapy.
  - Aldosterone antagonists may be added for patients with a recent CV hospitalization, acute MI, elevated BNP/NT-proBNP levels, or symptomatic cardiomyopathy NYHA class II-IV. Diuretics can be used if needed: thiazide/thiazide-like diuretic for BP control, loop diuretics for volume control.
  - If ACEI/ARB contraindicated or not tolerated, a combination of hydralazine and isosorbide dinitrate is recommended.
  - For HTN patients whose BP is not controlled, and ARB may be added to an ACEI and other antihypertensive drug treatment. (grade A) (Watch for hypotension, hyperkalemia, worsening renal function.)
- **HTN with stroke/TIA**
  Acute stroke (72 h)
  - For patients eligible for thrombolytic therapy very high BP >185/110 mm Hg should be treated concurrently in patient receiving thrombolytic therapy for acute ischemic stroke to reduce the risk of intracranial hemorrhage.
  - For patients not eligible for thrombolytic therapy extreme SBP elevation >220 or DBP>120 mm Hg may be treated to reduce BP by 15% and not more than 25% over the first 24 h.
  After acute stroke
  - Strong consideration should be given to the initiation of antihypertensive therapy after the acute phase of a stroke or TIA.
- **HTN with LVH**
  - Initial therapy with ACEI/ARB, long-acting CCB, or thiazide/thiazide-like diuretics. Hydralazine, minoxidil should not be used.
- **HTN with nondiabetic CKD**
  - Goal BP <140/90 mm Hg.
  - If proteinuric CKD initiate with ACEI or ARB.
  - ACEI in combination with ARB is not recommended for patients with nonproteinuric CKD.
- **HTN with diabetes**
  - Goal BP 130/80 mm Hg.
  - Initiate with ACEI, dihydropyridine CCBS, thiazide/thiazide-like diuretic, or ARB.
  - If additional CVD, CKD, microalbuminuria, or CV risk factors, initiate with an ACEI or ARB.
  - Combination preferred: ACEI with dihydropyridine rather than ACEI with HCTZ.

Source: http://www.hypertension.ca/en/chep

REFRACTORY HYPERTENSION
Source: AMERICAN COLLEGE OF CARDIOLOGY/AMERICAN HEART ASSOCIATION/EUROPEAN SOCIETY OF CARDIOLOGY

Definition:
Failure to reach BP goal (<140/90 mm Hg, or 130/80 mm Hg in patients with diabetes, heart disease, or chronic kidney disease) using three different antihypertensive drug classes.

Incidence: 20%–30% of HTN patients

Common Causes:
1. Nonadherence to drugs/diet
2. Suboptimal therapy/BP measurement (fluid retention, inadequate dosage)
3. Diet/drug interactions (caffeine, cocaine, alcohol, nicotine, NSAIDs, steroids, BCP, erythropoietin, natural licorice, herbs)
4. Common secondary causes:
   Obstructive sleep apnea
   Diabetes
   Chronic kidney disease
   Renal artery stenosis
   Obesity
   Endocrine disorders (primary hyperaldosteronism, hyperthyroidism, hyperparathyroidism, Cushing syndrome), pheochromocytoma

Therapy:
- Exclude nonadherence and incorrect BP measurement
- Review drug and diet history
- Screen for secondary causes:
  History of sleep disorders/daytime sleepiness/tachycardias/BPs in both arms
  Routine labs: sodium, potassium, creatinine, CBC, ECG, urinalysis, blood glucose, cholesterol
  Additional evaluation: aldosterone: renin ratio, renal ultrasound with Doppler flow study, serum or urine catecholamine levels, morning cortisol level
- Lifestyle therapy:
  Weight loss (10-kg weight loss results in a 5–20 mm Hg decrease in SBP); diet consult for low sodium (2.3 g daily), high fiber, and high potassium (DASH diet results in an 8–14 mm Hg decrease in SBP); exercise aerobic training results in a 4–9 mm Hg decrease in SBP; and restriction of excess alcohol (1 oz in men and 0.5 oz in women) results in a 2–4 mm Hg decrease in SBP
- Pharmacologic therapy:
  Consider volume overload
- Switch from HCTZ to chlorthalidone (especially if GFR <40 mL/min)
- Switch to loop diuretic if GFR <30 mL/min (eg, furosemide 40 mg bid)
- Use CCB (amlodipine or nifedipine) + ACE inhibitor or ARB
  Consider catecholamine excess
- Switch to vasodilating β-blocker (carvedilol, labetalol, nebivolol)
  Consider aldosterone excess (even with normal serum K+ level)
- Spironolactone or eplerenone
  Finally, consider hydralazine or minoxidil
  If already on β-blocker, clonidine adds little BP benefit

- Nonpharmacologic therapy: still under investigation
  Carotid baroreceptor stimulation (*Hypertension*. 2010;55:1-8)
    May lower BP 33/22 mm Hg
  Renal artery nerve denervation (SYMPLICITY HTN-3) did not show a significant reduction of SBP in patients with resistant hypertension, 6 mo after the procedure.
  Source: Bhatt DL, Kandzari DE, O'Neill WW, et. al. A controlled trial of renal denervation for resistant hypertension. *N Engl J Med.* 2014;370:1393-1401

ACE, angiotensin-converting enzyme; ARB, angiotensin receptor blocker; BCP, birth control pill; bid, twice a day; BP, blood pressure; CBC, complete blood count; CCB, calcium channel blocker; DASH diet, Dietary Approaches to Stop Hypertension diet; ECG, electrocardiogram; GFR, glomerular filtration rate; HCTZ, hydrochlorothiazide; HTN, hypertension; NSAIDs, nonsteroidal antiinflammatory drugs; SBP, systolic blood pressure.
Sources: Calhoun DA, Jones D, Textor S, et al; American Heart Association Professional Education Committee. Resistant hypertension: diagnosis, evaluation, and treatment: a scientific statement from the American Heart Association Professional Education Committee of the Council for High Blood Pressure Research. *Circulation.* 2008;117:e510–e526. JNC VII. *Arch Intern Med.* 2003;289:2560-2572; *European* 2007 Guidelines. 2007;28:1462-1536.

HYPERTENSION: CHILDREN AND ADOLESCENTS

Indications for Antihypertensive Drug Therapy in Children and Adolescents

- Symptomatic hypertension
- Secondary hypertension
- Hypertensive target organ damage
- Diabetes (types 1 and 2)
- Persistent hypertension despite nonpharmacologic measures (weight management counseling if overweight; physical activity; diet management)

Sources: Pediatrics. 2011;128(5):S213-S258. Kavey RE, Allada V, Daniels SR, et al; American Heart Association Expert Panel on Population and Prevention Science; American Heart Association Council on Cardiovascular Disease in the Young; American Heart Association Council on Epidemiology and Prevention, et al. Cardiovascular risk reduction in high-risk pediatric patients: a scientific statement from the American Heart Association Expert Panel on Population and Prevention Science; the Councils on Cardiovascular Disease in the Young, Epidemiology and Prevention, Nutrition, Physical Activity and Metabolism, High Blood Pressure Research, Cardiovascular Nursing, and the Kidney in Heart Disease; and the Interdisciplinary Working Group on Quality of Care and Outcomes Research: endorsed by the American Academy of Pediatrics. *Circulation.* 2006;114:2710-2738.

HYPERTENSION: TREATMENT IN SPECIAL POPULATIONS
ESH/ESC GUIDELINES 2013

- *White-coat HTN* is defined as elevated BP in doctor's office with normal home BPs
  - White-coat hypertension at low risk (unassociated with additional risk factors) should receive lifestyle intervention and close follow-up
  - White-coat hypertension at higher risk (associated with additional risk factors, metabolic disorders, or organ damage) should receive lifestyle intervention and drug therapy
- *Masked HTN* is defined as normal BP in the doctor's office with elevated BPs at home.
  - Masked hypertension at low risk (with or without additional risk factors) should receive lifestyle intervention and drug therapy due to the higher CV risk
- *Elderly HTN occurs in patients ≥65 y old*
  - In all elderly hypertensive patients SBP >160 mm Hg should be reduced to SBP between 140 and 150 mm Hg based upon good evidence
  - In *fit* elderly hypertensive patients <80 y old, SBP >160 mm Hg may be reduced to <140 mm Hg, if therapy is well tolerated
  - Diuretics and calcium antagonist may be preferred in isolated systolic hypertension, although all medications have been used with success
- *Very elderly HTN* occurs in patients ≥80 y old
  - In *fit* very elderly patients >80 y old, SBP should be reduced to 140–150 mm Hg
  - In *frail* very elderly patients >80 y old, SBP goal needs to be individualized
- Hypertensive therapy during *pregnancy*
  - Drug therapy should be started with persistent BP ≥150/95 mm Hg and BP ≥140/90 mm Hg if associated with gestational hypertension, subclinical organ damage or if associated with symptoms
  - Women with hypertension with childbearing potential should not receive renin-angiotensin system (RAS) blockers
  - Methyldopa and nifedipine should be initial therapy for hypertension. Labetalol and nitroprusside are the intravenous drugs of choice
- Hypertension goal with CAD, diabetes, and nephropathy
  - SBP goal <140 mm Hg should be considered

Source: Adapted from Mancia G, Fagard R, Narkiewicz K, et al. 2013 ESH/ESC guidelines for the management of arterial hypertension: the Task Force for the management of arterial hypertension of the European Society of Hypertension (ESH) and the European Society of Cardiology (ESC). *Eur Heart J.* 2013;34:2159-2219.

HYPERTENSIVE TREATMENT IN PREGNANCY AHA/ASA 2014 GUIDELINES

- Risk factors of pregnancy-induced hypertension: obesity, age >40 y old, chronic HTN, personal or family history of preeclampsia, gestational HTN, nulliparity, multiple pregnancy, preexisting vascular disease, collagen vascular disease, diabetes, renal disease.
- Severe hypertension per JNC VII: BP ≥160/110 mm Hg (high risk of stroke and eclampsia).
- BP goal during pregnancy: 130–155/80–105 mm Hg.
- **Prevention of eclampsia recommendations**:
  - Women with chronic primary or secondary hypertension, or previous pregnancy-related hypertension, should take low dose aspirin from the 12th week of gestation until delivery.
  - Calcium supplementation (of at least 1 g/d, orally) should be considered for women with low dietary intake of calcium (<600 mg/d) to prevent preeclampsia.
- **Treatment of hypertension in pregnancy and postpartum recommendations**:
  - Severe hypertension in pregnancy should be treated with safe and effective antihypertensive medications such as methyldopa, labetalol, and nifedipine, with consideration of maternal and fetal side effects.
  - Atenolol, ARBs, and direct renin inhibitors are contraindicated in pregnancy and should not be used.
  - Because of the increased risk of future hypertension and stroke 1 to 30 y after delivery in women with a history of preeclampsia it is reasonable to:
    - Consider evaluating all women starting 6 mo to the 1 y postpartum, as well as those who are past childbearing age, for a history of preeclampsia/eclampsia, and document their history of preeclampsia/eclampsia as a risk factor
    - Evaluate and treat for cardiovascular risk factors including hypertension, obesity, smoking, and dyslipidemia
  - After giving birth, women with chronic hypertension should be continued on their antihypertensive regime, with dosage adjustments to reflect the decrease in volume of distribution and glomerular filtration rate that occurs following delivery. They should also be monitored carefully for the development of postpartum preeclampsia.

Source: Bushnell C, McCullough LD, Awad IA, et al. Guidelines for the *Prevention of Stroke in Women A Statement for Healthcare Professionals From the American Heart Association/American Stroke Association*. *Stroke*. 2014;45. doi: 10.1161/01.str.0000442009.06663.48.

HYPOGONADISM, MALE

Disease Management	Organization	Date	Population	Recommendations	Comments	Source

Hypogonadism, Male	EAU	2012	Adults	• Testosterone testing should be done in:
				  ○ Pituitary masses
				  ○ ESRD
				  ○ Moderate-to-severe COPD
				  ○ Infertility
				  ○ Osteoporosis
				  ○ HIV infection
				  ○ DM type 2
				  ○ Signs and symptoms of hypogonadism
				• Indications for testosterone treatment are patients with low testosterone and:
				  ○ Hypogonadism
				  ○ Delayed puberty
				  ○ Klinefelter syndrome
				  ○ Sexual dysfunction
				  ○ Low bone mass
				  ○ Hypopituitarism
				• Contraindications to testosterone use:
				  ○ Prostate CA
				  ○ PSA >4 ng/mL
				  ○ Male breast CA
				  ○ Severe sleep apnea
				  ○ Male infertility
				  ○ Hematocrit >50%
				  ○ Symptomatic BPH
				• Monitor response to therapy, PSA and hematocrit 3, 6, and 12 mo after starting therapy.
					• Caused by androgen deficiency.
					• Primary hypogonadism
					  ○ Klinefelter syndrome
					  ○ Cryptorchidism
					  ○ Congenital anorchia
					  ○ Testicular CA
					  ○ Orchitis
					  ○ Chemotherapy
					• Secondary hypogonadism
					  ○ Kallmann syndrome
					  ○ Pituitary tumor
					  ○ Renal failure
					  ○ Hemochromatosis
					  ○ Hypothyroidism
					  ○ Anabolic steroid abuse
					  ○ Morbid obesity
					  ○ Radiotherapy
					  ○ Idiopathic hypogonadotrophic hypogonadism
					  ○ Androgen insensitivity syndrome
						http://www.uroweb.org/gls/pdf/16_Male_Hypogonadism_LR%20II.pdf

Disease Management	Organization/Population	Recommendations	Comments	Source
Iron Deficiency Anemia	British Society of Gastroenterology Adult. *Gut.* 2011; 60:1309–1316	**A. Scope of Problem** Iron deficiency anemia (IDA) is the most common cause of anemia and occurs in 2%–5% of adult men and postmenopausal women in the developed world. More than 25% of the world's population is anemic with one-half attributed to iron deficiency. (*N Engl J Med.* 2015:372:1832) **B. Diagnosis** Serum ferritin <30, iron transferrin saturation <10%, and hypochromic, microcytic RBCs on peripheral smear. MCV Usually >80 until hemoglobin drops to <10 g/dL. (*N Eng J Med.* 2005; 352:1741–1744. *N Eng J Med.* 1999; 341:1986–1995). **C. Clinical evaluation** Upper and lower gastrointestinal investigations (esophagogastroduodenoscopy and colonoscopy preferred) should be done in all post menopausal females and all male patients unless there is a history of recent non-GI significant blood loss. (*Am J Med.* 2001:111:439–445) Gastrointestinal evaluation should proceed whether or not fecal occult blood testing is positive. Iron deficiency without significant anemia should also be evaluated with GI evaluation in postmenopausal women and men >50 y old. (*N Engl J Med.* 1993;329:1691–1695) If the patient is postgastrectomy upper and lower GI investigation is indicated in those >50 y old. If upper and lower GI tracts are normal, small bowel visualization is indicated if the patient has symptoms of small bowel disease and/or fecal occult positive stools. (*Best Pract Res Clin Haematol.* 2005:18:319–322)	1. Symptoms of IDA include weakness, headache, irritability, fatigue, exercise intolerance, and restless leg syndrome. Symptoms may occur without anemia in patients with iron depletion (Ferritin <30 ng/mL). As many as 40% of patients with IDA will experience pica (appetite for clay, starch, and paper products) and/or pagophagia (craving for ice) which resolves rapidly with iron repletion. 2. Rarely, in severe iron deficiency, dysphagia and esophageal webs (Plummer-Vinson syndrome) occur as well as koilonychias (spoon nails), glossitis with decreased salivary flow and alopecia also occurs with severe prolonged IDA. 3. Besides GI and genitourinary blood loss other infrequent causes of iron deficiency include intravascular hemolysis (especially paroxysmal nocturnal hemoglobinuria and microangiopathic hemolytic anemia) pulmonary hemosiderosis, and congenital IDA (germline mutation in the TMPRSS6 gene) which leads to a reduction in iron absorption and mobilization. 4. Optimal absorption of oral iron occurs when iron is taken 15–30 min before a meal with 500 mg of vitamin C or a glass of orange juice. 20%–25% of patients will have GI side effects including abdominal pain, nausea, constipation, and diarrhea. Side effects are related to the amount of elemental iron delivered with each dose. The most commonly used iron preparation is ferrous sulfate that contains 65 mg of elemental iron. If patients have intolerable GI problems, lowering the elemental iron intake by giving ferrous gluconate (28–36 mg of elemental iron) or titrating liquid ferrous sulfate (44 mg iron per 5 mL) can be successful although duration of therapy will be extended. Patients who continue to be intolerant of oral iron can be successfully treated with IV iron preparations (iron sucrose preferred). (*Blood.* 2014: 123:326–333. *Transfusion.* 2008:48:988–995.) 5. A simple iron absorption test can determine whether or not a patient has iron malabsorption. Check a baseline iron level and then a second iron level 2–4 h after ingesting a single 325 mg ferrous sulfate tablet with water. An increase in the iron level of at least 100 µg/dL indicates adequate absorption.	www.guideline.gov/search/search.aspx?term=iron + deficiency+ management. *N Engl J Med.* 2015:372: 1832.

		IDA	

Disease Management	Organization/Population	Recommendations	Comments	Source
Iron Deficiency Anemia (continued)		**D. Iron replacement therapy** Ferrous sulfate (65mg elemental iron) should be administered 2–3 times a day depending on tolerance. Taking iron 15–30 min before a meal with orange juice or 500 mg. of vitamin C will enhance absorption. Treatment should be continued for 4–8 mo to fully replete iron stores. 20%–25% of patients on iron therapy will have GI side effects (abdominal bloating, pain, nausea, vomiting, diarrhea/constipation). Reducing the elemental iron concentration of each dose may avoid side effects. In patients who continue to be intolerant of iron, non-compliant or have diminished iron absorption intravenous iron (iron sucrose—Venofer®—preferred) should be given to replete iron stores and correct the anemia. **E. Refractory Iron Deficiency** In patients who have been compliant but do not correct their iron deficiency with oral iron must have further evaluation. Many gastric bypass patients have reduced iron absorption due to bypass of the duodenum where the majority of iron absorption takes place. Occasionally patients have significant continued blood loss for which oral iron is insufficient to maintain iron stores. Other possible causes such as celiac sprue, *H. pylori* infection, and autoimmune gastritis must be evaluated and treated. (*Haematologica.* 2005; 90:585-595). Antacids and protein pump inhibitors will also reduce iron absorption. Hereditary iron-refractory iron deficiency syndrome is an autosomal recessive disorder caused by mutations affecting iron transport. Only 50 patients with this syndrome have been reported. Patients with refractory iron deficiency anemia are treated successfully with intravenous iron preparations.	6. Other hypochromic, microcytic anemias should be ruled out (see Table 1). Diagnosing iron deficiency in patients who also have anemia of chronic disease (ACD) is difficult. Circulating transferrin receptor (sTFR) is elevated when iron deficiency is present and a high sTFR/ferritin index is consistent with concurrent IDA and ACD. A bone marrow examination with absent stainable iron stores, although invasive, will also confirm a diagnosis of IDA in the presence of ACD. Recombinant erythropoietin is not effective in treating anemia in patients who are iron deficient. (*N Engl J Med.* 2014;371:324) 7. Indications for IV iron therapy includes refractory noncompliance, gastric bypass, iron malabsorption, and continued blood loss with IDA and inadequate iron repletion with oral therapy. IV iron causes a modest early increase in reticulocytes compared to oral iron but it still takes 8–10 wk for hemoglobin levels to normalize. Iron dextran was the first IV preparation of iron used but problems with anaphylaxis were significant. Iron sucrose (Venofer®) is effective and has a 15-fold reduction in the risk of anaphylaxis compared to iron dextran. This can be dosed at 150–200 mg once or twice a week until the calculated iron deficit is administered. Ferric gluconate complex (Ferrlecit®) is similar to iron sucrose. Ferumoxytol (Feraheme®) is composed of iron oxide nanoparticle and is approved for use only in patients with renal failure. Ferric carboxymaltose (Ferinject®) is the newest IV iron option with 1000 mg elemental iron weekly with more rapid infusion times. Low phosphate levels have been reported with this drug. It has been shown to be helpful in patients with iron deficiency and heart failure. (*Ann Int Med.* 2010;152:4-5) 8. In patients who malabsorb iron, further diagnostic studies should be done to look for celiac disease (IgA anti-tissue transglutamine antibody, duodenal biopsy). *Helicobacter pylori* infection of the stomach (dx by serology, stool antigen, urea breath test, gastric biopsy) autoimmune gastritis (gastrin level, intrinsic factor, and parietal cell antibodies, gastric biopsy) and congenital iron deficiency (recessive germ line mutation in TMPR556). (*N Engl J Med.* 2012; 366:376-377. *Arch Int Med.* 2000; 160:1229-1230. *Blood.* 2014; 123:326-333. *Am Fam Physician.* 2013;87:98)	

THE COMMON CAUSES OF MICROCYTIC HYPOCHROMIC ANEMIA

Microcytic, hypochromic anemia	Ferritin Level	RDW	Hgb Electrophoresis	Iron/TIBC	Mentzer Index[a]
Iron deficiency	<30	High	Normal	<10%	>13
Beta thalassemia	Normal	Normal	↑A₂F	~20%	<13
Alfa thalassemia	Normal	Normal	Normal	~20%	<13
Anemia of chronic disease	High	High	Normal	10%–15% Low transferrin	>13
Hemoglobin E (mutation in beta-globin gene-common in Asia)	Normal	Normal	↑HgbE (30% if trait 90% if homozygote)	~20%	<13

[a]Menzer index, MCV-Hed cell number in millions. Iron def >13. Thalassemia minor <13. RDW, random distribution of width.

IDENTIFYING RISK OF SERIOUS ILLNESS IN CHILDREN UNDER 5 y

Category	Green—Low Risk	Yellow—Intermediate risk	Red—High Risk
Color of skin, lips, or tongue	Normal color	Pallor	Mottled, ashen, or blue
Activity	• Responds normally to social cues • Smiles • Awakens easily • Strong cry	• Abnormal response to social cues • No smile • Wakes only with prolonged stimulation • Decreased activity	• No response to social cues • Appears toxic • Stuporous • Weak, high-pitched cry

Respiratory	• Normal breathing	• Nasal flaring
		• Tachypnea
		  ○ >50 breaths/min (6–12 mo)
		  ○ >40 breaths/min (>1 y)
		• SpO₂ ≤95%
		• Pulmonary rales
			• Grunting
			• Marked tachypnea
			  ○ >60 breaths/min
			• Moderate to severe chest retractions

Circulation	• Normal skin and eyes
	• Moist mucous membranes
		• Tachycardia
		  ○ >160 beats/min (<12 mo)
		  ○ >150 beats/min (12–24 mo)
		  ○ >140 beats/min (2–5 y)
		• Capillary refill ≥3 s
		• Dry mucous membranes
		• Poor feeding
		• Decreased urine output
			• Findings in yellow zone PLUS
			• Reduced skin turgor

Other	• Nontoxic appearance	• Temperature ≥39°C (age 3–6 mo) • Fever ≥5 d • Rigors • Swelling of a limb or joint • Nonweight bearing on one extremity	• Temperature ≥38°C (<3 mo) • Nonblanching rash • Bulging fontanelle • Neck stiffness • Status epilepticus • Focal neurological signs • Focal seizures

Traffic Light System for Identifying Risk of Serious Illness in Children Under 5 y
Adapted from National Institute for Health and Care Excellence (NICE) Guideline on Feverish Illness in children: assessment and initial management in children younger than 5 years; 2013 May (Clinical Guideline no. 160)

INFERTILITY, MALE

Disease Management	Organization	Date	Population	Recommendations	Comments	Source
Infertility, Male	EAU	2012	Adults	• Assessment of male infertility includes: 　○ Semen analysis 　○ Check FSH, LH, and testosterone levels 　○ Screen for gonorrhea and *Chlamydia* 　○ *Substance abuse screening* • Refer patients with abnormal screens to a specialist in male infertility for potential treatments that may include clomiphene citrate, tamoxifen, human chorionic gonadotropin (hCG), dopamine agonists, or surgical treatments depending on the underlying etiology.	• Infertility is defined as the inability of a sexually active couple not using contraception to conceive in 1 year.	http://www.uroweb.org/gls/pdf/15_Male_Infertility_LR%20II.pdf

INFLAMMATORY BOWEL DISEASE, CROHNS DISEASE

Disease Management	Organization	Date	Population	Recommendations	Comments	Source

Inflammatory Bowel Disease, Crohn Disease	NICE	2012	Children, young adults, and adults with Crohn disease	• Inducing remission in Crohn disease
				  ◦ Glucocorticoids are recommended for a single exacerbation in a 12-mo period
				    – Prednisolone, methylprednisolone, or IV hydrocortisone
				  ◦ Add azathioprine or mercaptopurine to steroids if steroids cannot be tapered or ≥2 exacerbations in last 12 mo
				  ◦ Infliximab or adalimumab are indicated with active fistulizing refractory to conventional therapy
				• Maintaining remission
				  ◦ Azathioprine
				  ◦ Mercaptopurine
				• Managing strictures
				  ◦ Balloon dilatation is an option for single stricture that is short, straight, and accessible by colonoscopy
				• Recommend routine surveillance for osteopenia or osteoporosis.
						www.guideline.gov/content.aspx?id=38574

INFLAMMATORY BOWEL DISEASE, ULCERATIVE COLITIS

Disease Management	Organization	Date	Population	Recommendations	Comments	Source

Inflammatory Bowel Disease, Ulcerative Colitis	NICE	2013	Children, young adults, and adults	• Mild-moderate proctitis and proctosigmoiditis to achieve and maintain remission
				 ○ Aminosalicylate suppository or enemas
				 ○ Oral aminosalicylate
				 ○ Topical corticosteroid
				• Mild-moderate extensive left-sided colitis
				 ○ Induction dose oral aminosalicylate
				 ○ Consider adding oral tacrolimus to oral prednisolone if remission not achieved after 4 wks of prednisolone therapy
				• Maintain remission with low-dose aminosalicylate
				• Severe acute ulcerative colitis
				 ○ IV methylprednisolone
				 ○ Consider IV cyclosporine for those in whom steroids cannot be used or have not improved after 72 h of steroid therapy
				 ○ Consider a colectomy for:
				  ○ Persistent diarrhea >8 bowel movements/day
				  ○ Fevers
				  ○ Hemodynamic instability
				  ○ Toxic megacolon
				  ○ CRP >4.5 mg/dL
					• Oral prednisolone is an adjunct to aminosalicylates for proctitis or colitis if remission is not attained within 4 weeks.
					• Consider adding oral azathioprine or oral mercaptopurine to maintain remission if not maintained by aminosalicylates alone.
					• Monitor bone health in children and young adults with chronic active disease or who require frequent steroid therapy.
						http://www.guideline.gov/content.aspx?id=46936

INFLUENZA

Disease Management	Organization	Date	Population	Recommendations	Comments	Source

Influenza	IDSA	2009	Adults and children	1. Antiviral treatment is recommended for:
				  a. Lab-confirmed cases of influenza within 48 h of symptom onset
				  b. Strongly suspected influenza within 48 h of symptom onset
				  c. Hospitalized patients with severe, complicated, or progressive lab-confirmed influenza or influenza-like illness with high likelihood of complications even if >48 h from symptom onset
				2. Antiviral options include oseltamivir and zanamivir.
				  a. Oseltamivir for influenza A or B:
				    75 mg by mouth (PO) twice daily (bid) (adults); 30 mg PO bid (≤15 kg); 45 mg PO bid (16–23 kg); 60 mg PO bid (24–40 kg); 75 mg PO bid (>40 kg or age ≥13 y) × 5 d. Avoid in children age <1 y
				  b. Zanamivir for influenza A or B: 2 puffs bid × 5 d (children age ≥7 y and adults); avoid in asthmatic patients
					1. Consider an influenza nasal swab for diagnosis during influenza season in:
					  a. Persons with acute onset of fever and respiratory illness
					  b. Persons with fever and acute exacerbation of chronic lung disease
					  c. Infants and children with fever of unclear etiology
					  d. Severely ill persons with fever or hypothermia
					2. Rapid influenza antigen tests have a 70%–90% sensitivity in children and a 40%–60% sensitivity in adults.
					3. Direct or indirect fluorescent antibody staining is useful screening tests.
					4. Influenza PCR may be used as a confirmatory test.
						http://www.guidelines.gov/content.aspx?id=14173

	AAP	2013	Children aged 6 months and older	• Oseltamivir remains the antiviral drug of choice for the management of influenza infections.
				• Treatment indicated if symptom onset within 48 h and:
				  ○ Any child hospitalized with presumed influenza or with severe, complicated, or progressive illness attributable to influenza, regardless of influenza immunization status
				  ○ Influenza infection of any severity in children at high risk of complications of influenza infection
						http://www.guideline.gov/content.aspx?id=47372

Disease Management (AKI)	Organization	Date	Population	Recommendations	Comments	Source
ACUTE KIDNEY INJURY (AKI)						
Acute kidney Injury (AKI)	NICE	2013	Children and adults	• Perform a urinalysis in all patients with AKI. • Do not routinely obtain a renal ultrasound when the cause of the AKI has been identified. • Detect AKI with any of the following criteria: ○ Rise in serum creatinine ≥0.3 mg/dL in 48 h ○ 50% or more rise in creatinine in last 7 d ○ Urine output <0.5 mL/kg/h • Refer for renal replacement therapy patients with any of the following refractory to medical management: ○ Hyperkalemia ○ Metabolic acidosis ○ Uremia ○ Fluid overload		http://www.guideline.gov/content.aspx?id=47080

KIDNEY DISEASE, CHRONIC

Disease Management	Organization	Date	Population	Recommendations	Comments	Source
Kidney Disease, Chronic	NICE	2008	Adults	1. Recommends the modification of diet in renal disease (MDRD) equation to estimate GFR. 　a. Advise patients not to eat any meat in the 12 h before a blood test for GFR estimation. 　b. Frequency of GFR testing by CKD stage: 　　i. Stages 1–2: annually 　　ii. Stage 3: every 6 months 　　iii. Stage 4: every 3 months 　　iv. Stage 5: every 6 weeks 2. Recommends urine albumin-to-creatinine ratio (ACR) to detect low levels of proteinuria. 　a. Levels ≥30 mg/mmol are significant 3. Recommends checking for urinary tract malignancy for persistent hematuria. 4. Recommends a renal ultrasound in CKD and if patient is/has: 　a. A GFR decline >5 mL/min/1.73 m² in 1 year or >10 mL/min/1.73 m² in 5 y 　b. Persistent hematuria 　c. Symptoms of urinary tract obstruction 　d. Age >20 y and has a family history of polycystic kidney disease 　e. Stages 4–5 CKD 　f. Being considered for a renal biopsy 5. Recommends nephrology referral for: 　a. Stages 4–5 CKD 　b. ACR ≥70 mg/mmol 　c. Proteinuria ≥1 g/24 h 　d. Poorly controlled HTN 　e. Suspected renal artery stenosis 　f. Rapidly progressive renal impairment 　g. Metabolic complications of CKD (anemia or hyperparathyroidism) 　h. Nephrolithiasis 6. Recommends a check of serum calcium, phosphate, intact parathyroid hormone (iPTH), 25-OH vitamin D, and hemoglobin levels for all stages 4–5 CKD.		http://www.nice.org.uk/nicemedia/live/12069/42117/42117.pdf
	Va/DoD	2014	Adults	1. Recommends dietary sodium restriction to reduce hypertension and proteinuria. 2. Protein restriction 0.6–0.8 g/kg/d for patients with Stage 3–4 CKD. 3. Recommend administration of vaccinations against influenza, Tdap, 13-valent pneumococcal conjugate vaccine, hepatitis B virus, Zoster, and MMR vaccines. 4. Recommend ACEI or ARB therapy for patients with diabetes, hypertension, or albuminuria. 5. Recommends bicarbonate supplementation in CKD with metabolic acidosis. 6. Recommends oral iron therapy for stage 3 or worse CKD. 7. Recommends erythropoietic-stimulating agents if hemoglobin <10 g/dL.		http://www.guideline.gov/content.aspx?id=48951

KIDNEY DISEASE, CHRONIC–MINERAL & BONE DISORDERS (CKD-MBDs)

Disease Management	Organization	Date	Population	Recommendations	Comments	Source
Kidney Disease, Chronic–Mineral and Bone Disorders (CKD-MBDs)	NKF	2009	Adults and children	1. Recommends monitoring serum calcium, phosphorus, immunoreactive parathyroid hormone (iPTH), and alkaline phosphatase levels for: a. Stage 3 CKD (adults) b. Stage 2 CKD (children) 2. Measure 25-OH vitamin D levels beginning in stage 3 CKD. 3. Recommends treating all vitamin D deficiency with vitamin D supplementat on. 4. In stages 3–5 CKD, consider a bone biopsy before bisphosphonate therapy if a dynamic bone disease is a possibility. 5. In stages 3–5 CKD, aim to normalize calcium and phosphorus levels. 6. In stage 5 CKD, maintain a parathyroid hormone (PTH) level of 130–600 pg/mL.	1. Options for oral phosphate binders: a. Calcium acetate b. Calcium carbonate c. Calcium citrate d. Sevelamer carbonate e. Lanthanum carbonate	http://kdigo.org/home/ mineral-bone-disorder/

KIDNEY STONES

Disease Management	Organization	Date	Population	Recommendations	Comments	Source

Kidney Stones	EAU
	AUA
		2010
		2014
			Adults and children with kidney stone disease	1. Recommended imaging study for patients with acute flank pain is a noncontrast CT urogram.
				2. Recommended evaluation for renal colic:
				  a. Urinalysis
				  b. Serum CBC, creatinine, uric acid, calcium, and albumin +/− intact parathyroid hormone
				  c. Stone analysis by x-ray crystallography or infrared spectroscopy
				3. Recommends 24-h urine analysis for complicated calcium stone disease: calcium; oxalate; citrate; creatinine; urate; magnesium; phosphate; sodium; and potassium.
				4. Recommends a thiazide diuretic for patients with hypercalciuria.
				5. Recommends treatment with an alkaline citrate for hypocitraturia, type 1 renal tubular acidosis (RTA), hypercalciuria, and hyperoxaluria.
				6. Recommends that adults with a history of urinary stones drink sufficient water to maintain a urine output >2.5 L/d.
				7. Consider use of an α-receptor blocker to facilitate spontaneous passage of ureteral stones <10 mm.
				8. Consider active ureteral stone removal for persistent obstruction, failure of spontaneous passage, or the presence of severe, unremitting colic.
				  a. Options include shockwave lithotripsy or ureteroscopy
				9. For calcium stones and hypercalciuria
				  a. Limit sodium intake and consume 1–2 g/d of dietary calcium
				  b. Thiazide diuretic
				10. For calcium oxalate stones
				  a. If high urinary oxalate, limit intake of oxalate-rich foods and maintain normal calcium consumption
				  b. If hyperuricosuria, treat with allopurinol
				11. For uric acid stones and high urinary uric acid, limit intake of non-dairy animal protein
				For struvite stones refractory to surgical management, consider acetohydroxamic acid therapy
				12. For uric acid or cystine stones, potassium citrate therapy to raise urinary pH to optimal level
					1. Patients at high risk for recurrent stone formation:
					  a. ≥3 stones in 3 y
					  b. Infection stones
					  c. Urate stones
					  d. Children and adolescents with stones
					  e. Cystinuria
					  f. Primary hyperoxaluria
					  g. Type 1 RTA
					  h. Cystic fibrosis
					  i. Hyperparathyroidism
					  j. Crohn disease
					  k. Malabsorption syndromes
					  l. Nephrocalcinosis
					  m. Family history of kidney stone disease
						http://www.uroweb.org/gls/pdf/18_Urolithiasis.pdf
						http://www.guideline.gov/content.aspx?id=48229

KIDNEY STONES					
Disease Management	**Organization**	**Date**	**Population**	**Recommendations**	**Comments**	**Source**

Kidney Stones (continued)	EAU	2013	Adults with kidney stone disease	• Recommended evaluation for renal colic:
				  ○ Sodium, potassium
				  ○ CRP
				  ○ PT, PTT (if intervention is likely)
				• Contrast-enhanced CT scan recommended if stone removal is planned and the renal anatomy needs to be assessed.
				• Hyperoxaluria
				  ○ Oxalate restriction
				  ○ Pyridoxine
				• Renal colic analgesia
				  ○ NSAIDs
				  ○ Opiates
				  ○ Alfa-blockers
				• Management of sepsis with obstructed kidney
				• Requires urgent decompression with a ureteral stent or percutaneous nephrostomy tubes
				  ○ Start antibiotics immediately
				• Indications for active kidney stone treatment:
				  ○ Stone growth
				  ○ Acute or chronic pain
				  ○ Kidney infection
				  ○ Kidney obstruction
						http://www.guideline.gov/content.aspx?id=45324

	EAU	2013	Adults with kidney stone disease	• Stop antiplatelets and anticoagulation before stone removal.
				• Goal is to drink water to maintain a urine output >2.5 L/d.
				• Struvite and infection stones:
				  ○ Surgical removal of stones
				  ○ Antibiotics
				  ○ Urinary acidification
				  ○ Urease inhibition
				• Cystine stones
				  ○ Potassium citrate
				  • Tiopronin		

			Children with kidney stone disease	• Recommend a complete metabolic workup based on stone analysis. • Ultrasound is the preferred imaging method in children. • Percutaneous nephrolithotripsy is recommended for treatment of renal pelvic or calyceal stones with a diameter >20 mm.		http://www.guideline.gov/content.aspx?id=45324

LARYNGITIS, ACUTE

Disease Management	Organization	Date	Population	Recommendations	Comments	Source
Laryngitis, Acute	Cochrane Database Systematic Reviews	2015	Adults	Insufficient evidence to support the use of antibiotics for acute laryngitis.	Many methodological flaws in studies evaluated.	http://www.cochrane.org/CD004783/ARI_antibiotics-to-treat-adults-with-acute-laryngitis

MENINGITIS, BACTERIAL

Disease Management	Organization	Date	Population	Recommendations	Comments	Source
Meningitis, Bacterial	Cochrane Database of Systematic Reviews	2013	Children and adults	Recommend corticosteroids prior to or when antibiotics are administered for presumed bacterial meningitis in high-income countries.	• Corticosteroids significantly reduced the incidence of hearing loss and neurological sequelae in bacterial meningitis. • Corticosteroids reduced mortality in meningitis from *Streptococcus pneumoniae*, but not with *Haemophilus influenzae* or *Neisseria meningitidis* infections. • No beneficial effect of corticosteroids in low-income countries.	http://onlinelibrary.wiley.com/doi/10.1002/14651858.CD004405.pub4/pdf/abstract

MENOPAUSE						
Disease Management	**Organization**	**Date**	**Population**	**Recommendations**	**Comments**	**Source**
Menopause	AACE	2011	Menopausal women	• Indications for menopausal hormone therapy: ◦ Severe menopausal symptoms ◦ Severe vulvovaginal atrophy ◦ Consider transdermal or topical estrogens which may reduce the risk of VTE ◦ Treatment of osteoporosis • Cautions with menopausal hormone therapy: ◦ Avoid unopposed estrogen use in women with an intact uterus ◦ Use hormonal therapy in the lowest effective dose for the shortest duration possible ◦ Custom compounded bioidentical hormone therapy is *not* recommended ◦ Not appropriate for prevention or treatment of dementia ◦ Avoid if at high risk for VTE ◦ Not recommended for prevention or treatment of cardiovascular disease • Contraindications of menopausal hormone therapy: ◦ History of breast CA ◦ Suspected estrogen-sensitive malignancy ◦ Undiagnosed vaginal bleeding ◦ Endometrial hyperplasia ◦ History of VTE ◦ Untreated hypertension ◦ Active liver disease ◦ Porphyria cutanea tarda	• Use of hormone therapy should always occur after a thorough discussion of the risks, benefits, and alternatives of this treatment with the patient.	https://www.aace.com/files/menopause.pdf

METABOLIC SYNDROME: IDENTIFICATION AND MANAGEMENT
Source: NCEP, ATP III, 2005

Clinical Identification

Risk Factor	Defining Level[a]
Abdominal obesity (waist circumference)[b]	
Men	>102 cm (>40 in)
Women	>88 cm (>35 in)
Triglycerides	≥150 mg/dL
HDL cholesterol	
Men	<40 mg/dL
Women	<50 mg/dL
Blood pressure	≥135 /≥85 mm Hg
Fasting glucose	≥100 mg/dL

Management

- First-line therapy: Lifestyle modification leading to weight reduction and increased physical activity
- Goal: ↓ Body weight by approximately 7%–10% over 6–12 mo
- At least 30 min of daily moderate-intensity physical activity
- Low intake of saturated fats, trans fats, and cholesterol
- Reduced consumption of simple sugars
- Increased intake of fruits, vegetables, and whole grains
- Avoid extremes in intake of either carbohydrates or fats
- Smoking cessation
- Drug therapy for HTN, elevated LDL cholesterol, and diabetes
- Consider combination therapy with fibrates or nicotinic acid plus a statin
- Low-dose ASA for patients at intermediate and high risk
- Bariatric surgery for BMI >35 mg/kg^2
- If one component is identified, a systematic search for the others is indicated, together with an active approach to managing all risk factors. (*Eur Heart J.* 2007;28:2375-2414)
- Metabolic syndrome is associated with the presence of subclinical ischemic brain lesions independent of other risk factors. (*Stroke.* 2008;39:1607-1609)
- In patients with atherosclerosis, the presence of metabolic syndrome is associated with an increased risk of cardiovascular event and all-cause mortality, independent of the presence of diabetes. (*Eur Heart J.* 2008;29:213-223)

ASA, aspirin; BMI, body mass index; HDL, high-density lipoprotein; HTN, hypertension; LDL, low-density lipoprotein.
[a]NCEP ATP III definition (*Circulation.* 2005;112:2735-2752) –Requires any three of the listed components.
[b]Waist circumference can identify persons at greater cardiometabolic risk than are identified by BMI alone. However, further studies are needed to establish waist circumference cutpoints that assess risk not adequately captured by BMI. (*Am J Clin Nutr.* 2007;85:1197-1202)
Note: The WHO and International Diabetes Federation (IDF, http://www.idf.org) define metabolic syndrome slightly differently. One study found a 5-fold difference in the prevalence of metabolic syndrome depending on which of seven diagnostic criteria were used (*Metabolism.* 2008;57:355-361). There is no official definition of metabolic syndrome in children, but a constellation of conditions confers significant increased risk of coronary heart disease. (*Circulation.* 2007;115:1948-1967)

TREATMENT OF METHICILLIN-RESISTANT *STAPHYLOCOCCUS AUREUS* INFECTIONS (MRSA) IN ADULTS AND CHILDREN

Source: IDSA 2011 Clinical Practice Guideline: *Clin Infect Dis.* 2011;52:1-38

Infection	Primary Therapy	Alternative Therapy	Comments

Abscess associated with extensive involvement; cellulitis; systemic illness; immunosuppression; extremes of age; involvement of face, hands, or genitalia; septic phlebitis; trauma; infected ulcer or burn; or poor response to incision and drainage	1. Incision and drainage
	2. Antibiotics
	 a. Outpatient
	  i. Clindamycin
	  ii. Trimethoprim-sulfamethoxazole (TMP-SMX)
	 b. Inpatient
	  i. Vancomycin
	  ii. Linezolid
	  iii. Daptomycin
		1. Outpatient antibiotics
		 a. Tetracycline
		 b. Linezolid
		2. Inpatient antibiotics
		 a. Telavancin
		 b. Clindamycin
			1. Tetracyclines should not be used in children age <8 y.
			2. Vancomycin is recommended for hospitalized children.
			3. Clindamycin and linezolid are alternative choices for children.

Recurrent skin and soft-tissue infections (SSTIs)	1. Cover draining wounds. 2. Maintain good hygiene. 3. Avoid reusing or sharing personal toiletries. 4. Use oral antibiotics only for active infections.	1. Decolonization only if recurrent SSTI despite good hygiene a. Mupirocin per nares bid × 5–10 d b. Chlorhexidine or dilute bleach baths twice weekly (BIW) × 1–2 wk	Screening cultures prior to decolonization or surveillance cultures after decolonization is not recommended.
Uncomplicated MRSA bacteremia[a]	Vancomycin × 2 wk	Daptomycin × 2 wk	Echocardiography is recommended for all MRSA bacteremia.
MRSA native valve endocarditis	Vancomycin × 6 wk	Daptomycin × 6 wk	1. Synergistic gentamicin or rifampin is not indicated for native valve endocarditis. 2. Vancomycin is the drug of choice for children.
MRSA prosthetic valve endocarditis	1. Vancomycin plus rifampin × 6 wk 2. Gentamicin 1 mg/kg IV q8h × 2 wk		Recommend early evaluation for valve replacement surgery.
MRSA pneumonia	1. Vancomycin 2. Linezolid	Clindamycin	1. Duration of therapy is 7–21 d. 2. Vancomycin for children.
MRSA osteomyelitis	1. Surgical débridement 2. Vancomycin 3. Daptomycin 4. Duration of therapy is at least 8 wk	1. Linezolid 2. TMP-SMX plus rifampin 3. Clindamycin	
MRSA septic arthritis	1. Drain or débride the joint space 2. Vancomycin	Daptomycin	Duration of therapy is 3–4 wk.
MRSA meningitis	1. Vancomycin × 2 wk	1. Linezolid 2. TMP-SMX	Consider adding rifampin.

[a]No endocarditis, no implanted prostheses, defervescence within 72 h, sterile blood cultures within 72 h, no evidence of metastatic sites of infection.

MULTIPLE SCLEROSIS

Disease Management	Organization	Date	Population	Recommendations	Comments	Source
Multiple Sclerosis (MS)	AAN	2014	Adults	1. Consider oral cannabis extract or Sativex oromucosal cannabinoid spray to patients with MS with spasticity and pain (central neuropathic pain). 2. May consider a trial of Gingko biloba or magnetic therapy for reducing fatigue. 3. Recommend against a low-fat diet with ω-3 fatty acid or lofepramine use or bee venom therapy to reduce relapses, depression or fatigue. 4. Reflexology may benefit paresthesias.		http://www.guideline.gov/content.aspx?id=47909

FEBRILE NEUTROPENIA (FN)

Disease Management	Organization	Population	Recommendations	Comments	Source

Febrile Neutropenia (FN)	Infectious Disease Society of America 2011	Patients with single temperature >100.9°F (38.3°C) or ≥100.4°F (38.0°C) for >1 h in the setting of neutropenia (absolute neutrophil count including granulocytes and bands <500/mm³)	• Two sets of blood cultures/urine C+S/chemistries. CXR/ancillary studies based on clinical evaluation. Begin antibiotics as rapidly as possible.
			• Stratify into **LOW RISK**[a] (absence of comorbidity, no cardiovascular compromise, expected duration of neutropenia <7 d, compliant) vs. **HIGH RISK**[a] (absolute neutrophil count [ANC] <100 comorbidity, cardiovascular compromise, unreliable, expected duration of neutropenia >7 d).
			• High-risk patients must be admitted to hospital with rapid initiation of single agent antibiotic (cefepime, imipenem, ceftazidime) or combination therapy (extended spectrum beta-lactam plus either aminoglycoside or fluoroquinolone) depending on clinical features. Add antifungal agent if continued fever and negative cultures after 4–7 d.
			• Selected low-risk patients can be treated with oral ciprofloxacin 500 mg bid and Augmentin 875 mg bid with <5% requiring hospitalization for worsening symptoms. Close communication with patient is essential.
			• Continue broad-spectrum antibiotics in both low- and high-risk groups until ANC >500. Adjust antibiotics based on positive cultures and switch to oral to complete a 10–14 d course of antibiotics.
				• Prophylactic granulocyte colony–stimulating factor (GCSF) should be used in patients on chemotherapy with an expected rate of FN of ≥20%. Secondary use of GCSF after FN shortens hospital stay by 1 d but no impact on survival.
				• Vancomycin should not be given empirically unless history of MRSA, catheter tunnel infection, presence of pneumonia, or soft-tissue infection.
				• Three other unique organisms requiring antibiotic adjustment:
				  ○ Vancomycin-resistant enterococci (VRE)—use linezolid or daptomycin
				  ○ Extended-spectrum beta-lactamase (ESBL) producing gram-negative bacteria—use carbapenem
				  ○ Carbapenemase-producing organism (*Klebsiella*)—use polymyxin-colistin or tigecycline
				• If central venous catheter (CVC) line infection suspected, draw blood cultures from CVC and peripheral vein. If CVC culture grows out >120 min before peripheral blood cultures, then CVC is source of infection.
				• CVC must be removed if infected with *Staphylococcus aureus*, *Pseudomonas* and other gram–negative bacteria, fungi, or mycobacteria, as well as tunnel or port pocket infection. If coagulation-negative *Staphylococcus*, retain CVC and treat with an antibiotic ×4–6 wk with 85% cure rate.
				• In afebrile patients with ANC <100 treat with oral fluoroquinolone to lower risk of severe infection. With ANC <100 risk of serious infection is 10% per day.
					Clin Infect Dis. 2011;52:e56–e93
					
					J Clin Oncol. 2013;31:794–810

[a]Multinational Association for Supportive Care in Cancer (MASCC)
• Symptoms → no or mild = 5, moderate = 3, severe = 0
• No hypotension—5
• No COPD—4
• No previous fungal infection—4
• No dehydration requiring parenteral fluids—3
• Outpatient status—3
• Age <60—2
• High risk = <21; Low risk = >21

ORAL DM2 AGENTS-CPG 2015

Category	Metformin	DDP-4I	GLP-1 RA	TZD	AGI	Colsevelam	BCR-QR	SU/MGN	Insulin	SGLT-2	Pramlintide
Hypoglycemia	Neutral	Neutral	Neutral	Neutral	Neutral	Neutral	Neutral	Moderate/severe/Mild	Moderate/severe/Mild	Neutral	Neutral
Weight	Slight loss	Neutral	Loss	Gain	Neutral	Neutral	Neutral	Gain	Gain	Loss	Loss
Renal/GU	CI if Crt>1.4 (W) Crt>1.5 (M) CrCl <50 mL/min	Dose adjust if CrCl <30 mL/min	CI if CrCl <30 mL/min	Fluid retention	Neutral	Neutral	Neutral	Renal impairment increases hypoglycemia	Renal impairment increases hypoglycemia	Infection; CI if CrCl <45 mL/min	Neutral
Gastrointestinal[a]	Moderate	Neutral	Moderate	CI in cirrhosis	Moderate	Mild	Moderate	Neutral	Neutral	Neutral	Moderate
CHF	Neutral	Neutral	Neutral	Moderate	Neutral	Neutral	Neutral	Neutral	Neutral	Neutral	Moderate
CVD	Benefit	Neutral	Neutral	Slight risk	Neutral	Neutral	Neutral	Unclear	Neutral	Orthostasis in elderly	Neutral
Bone loss	Neutral	Neutral	Neutral	Moderate	Neutral	Neutral	Neutral	Neutral	Neutral	Small	Neutral
Miscellaneous	B$_{12}$ deficiency	–	–	–	–	–	–	SIADH/headaches		–	Avoid with gastroparesis; headache

Side Effect Profile of the Different Antidiabetic Medications

DPP-4I = dipeptidyl peptidase-4 inhibitor; GLP-1 RA = glucagon-like peptide-1 receptor antagonist; TZD = thiazolidinediones; AGI = alphaglucosidase inhibitors; BCR-QR = bromocriptine quick release; SU = sulfonylurea; MGN = meglitinides; SGLT-2 = salt glucose contransporter 2; GU = genitourinary; CVD = cardiovascular disease; CI = contraindicated; SIADH = syndrome of inappropriate antidiuretic hormone

[a.]GI symptoms can include: nausea, vomiting, flatulence, diarrhea, anorexia, and pancreatitis (for GLP-1 RA)

Reference: *Endocrine Practice*, 2013; 19: 327.

MANAGEMENT OF OBESITY IN MATURE ADOLESCENTS AND ADULTS

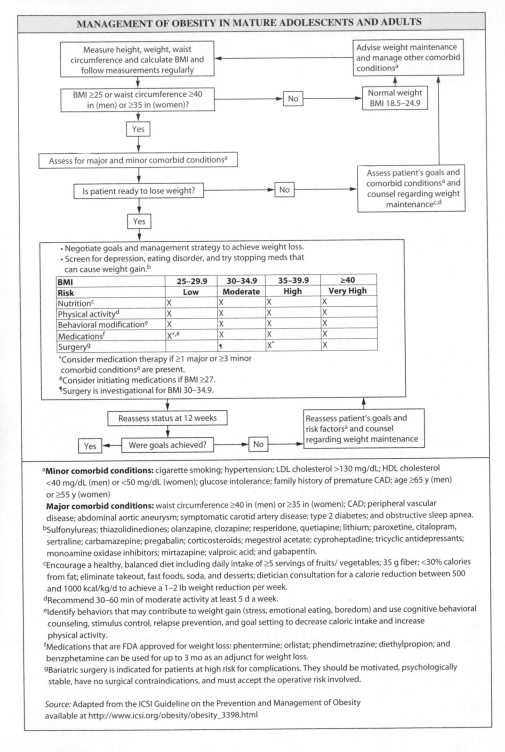

Measure height, weight, waist circumference and calculate BMI and follow measurements regularly

BMI ≥25 or waist circumference ≥40 in (men) or ≥35 in (women)? → No → Normal weight BMI 18.5–24.9 → Advise weight maintenance and manage other comorbid conditions[a]

Yes ↓

Assess for major and minor comorbid conditions[a]

Is patient ready to lose weight? → No → Assess patient's goals and comorbid conditions[a] and counsel regarding weight maintenance[c,d]

Yes ↓

- Negotiate goals and management strategy to achieve weight loss.
- Screen for depression, eating disorder, and try stopping meds that can cause weight gain.[b]

| BMI | 25–29.9 | 30–34.9 | 35–39.9 | ≥40 |
Risk	Low	Moderate	High	Very High
Nutrition[c]	X	X	X	X
Physical activity[d]	X	X	X	X
Behavioral modification[e]	X	X	X	X
Medications[f]	X*,#	X	X	X
Surgery[g]		¶	X*	X

*Consider medication therapy if ≥1 major or ≥3 minor comorbid conditions[a] are present.
#Consider initiating medications if BMI ≥27.
¶Surgery is investigational for BMI 30–34.9.

Reassess status at 12 weeks

Were goals achieved? → No → Reassess patient's goals and risk factors[a] and counsel regarding weight maintenance

Yes ←

[a]**Minor comorbid conditions:** cigarette smoking; hypertension; LDL cholesterol >130 mg/dL; HDL cholesterol <40 mg/dL (men) or <50 mg/dL (women); glucose intolerance; family history of premature CAD; age ≥65 y (men) or ≥55 y (women)
Major comorbid conditions: waist circumference ≥40 in (men) or ≥35 in (women); CAD; peripheral vascular disease; abdominal aortic aneurysm; symptomatic carotid artery disease; type 2 diabetes; and obstructive sleep apnea.
[b]Sulfonylureas; thiazolidinediones; olanzapine, clozapine; resperidone, quetiapine; lithium; paroxetine, citalopram, sertraline; carbamazepine; pregabalin; corticosteroids; megestrol acetate; cyproheptadine; tricyclic antidepressants; monoamine oxidase inhibitors; mirtazapine; valproic acid; and gabapentin.
[c]Encourage a healthy, balanced diet including daily intake of ≥5 servings of fruits/ vegetables; 35 g fiber; <30% calories from fat; eliminate takeout, fast foods, soda, and desserts; dietician consultation for a calorie reduction between 500 and 1000 kcal/kg/d to achieve a 1–2 lb weight reduction per week.
[d]Recommend 30–60 min of moderate activity at least 5 d a week.
[e]Identify behaviors that may contribute to weight gain (stress, emotional eating, boredom) and use cognitive behavioral counseling, stimulus control, relapse prevention, and goal setting to decrease caloric intake and increase physical activity.
[f]Medications that are FDA approved for weight loss: phentermine; orlistat; phendimetrazine; diethylpropion; and benzphetamine can be used for up to 3 mo as an adjunct for weight loss.
[g]Bariatric surgery is indicated for patients at high risk for complications. They should be motivated, psychologically stable, have no surgical contraindications, and must accept the operative risk involved.

Source: Adapted from the ICSI Guideline on the Prevention and Management of Obesity available at http://www.icsi.org/obesity/obesity_3398.html

OSTEOARTHRITIS (OA)

Disease Management	Organization	Date	Population	Recommendations	Comments	Source

Osteoarthritis (OA)	ACR	2012	Adults	• Nonpharmacologic recommendations for the management of hand OA
				  ○ Evaluate ability to perform activities of daily living (ADLs)
				  ○ Instruct in joint-protection technicues
				  ○ Provide assistive devices to help perform ADLs
				  ○ Instruct in use of thermal modalities
				  ○ Provide splints for trapeziometacarpal joint OA
				• Nonpharmacologic recommendations for the management of knee or hip OA
				  ○ Participate in aquatic exercise
				  ○ Lose weight
				  ○ Start aerobic exercise program
				  ○ Instruct in use of thermal modalities
				  ○ Consider for knee OA:
				    – Medially directed patellar taping
				    – Wedged insoles for either medial or lateral compartment OA
				• Pharmacologic options for OA
				  ○ Topical capsaicin
				  ○ Topical or PO NSAIDs
				  ○ Acetaminophen
				  ○ Tramadol
				  ○ Intraarticular steroids is an option for refractory knee or hip OA
					• The following should *not* be used for OA:
					  ○ Chondroitin sulfate
					  ○ Glucosamine
					  ○ Opiates (if possible)
						http://www.rheumatology.org/practice/clinical/guidelines/PDFs/ACR_OA_Guidelines_FINAL.pdf

OSTEOPOROSIS

Disease Management	Organization	Date	Population	Recommendations	Comments	Source

Osteoporosis	ICSI	2011	Adults at risk for osteoporosis or who have confirmed osteoporosis	• Evaluate all patients with a low-impact fracture for osteoporosis.
				• Advise smoking cessation and alcohol moderation (≤2 drinks per day).
				• Advise 1500-mg elemental calcium daily for established osteoporosis, glucocorticoid therapy, or age >65 y.
				• Assess for vitamin D deficiency with a 25-hydroxy vitamin D level
				  ○ Treat vitamin D deficiency if present.
				• Treatment of osteoporosis
				  ○ Bisphosphonate therapy
				  ○ Consider estrogen therapy in menopausal women <50 y of age
				  ○ Consider parathyroid hormone in women with very high risk for fracture
				• Fall prevention program
				  ○ Home safety evaluation
				  ○ Avoid medications that can cause sedation, orthostatic hypotension, or affect balance
				  ○ Assistive walking devices as necessary
					• All patients should have serial heights and observed for kyphosis.
					• Obtain a lateral vertebral assessment with DXA scan or x-ray if height loss exceeds 4 cm.
					• DXA bone mineral densitometry should be repeated no more than every 12–24 mo.
						https://www.icsi.org/_asset/vnw0c3/Osteo.pdf

	NAMS
	AACE
	ACOG
		2010
		2010
		2012
			Postmenopausal women	1. Recommend maintaining a healthy weight, eating a balanced diet, avoiding excessive alcohol intake, avoiding cigarette smoking, and utilizing measures to avoid falls.
				2. Recommend supplemental calcium 1200 mg/d and vitamin D_3 800–1000 international units (IU)/d.
				3. Recommend an annual check of height and weight, and assess for chronic back pain.
				4. DXA of the hip, femoral neck, and lumbar spine should be measured in women age ≥65 y or postmenopausal women with a risk factor for osteoporosis.[a]
				5. Recommend repeat DXA testing every 1–2 y for women taking therapy for osteoporosis and every 2–5 y for untreated postmenopausal women.
				6. Recommend against measurement of biochemical markers of bone turnover.
				7. Recommend drug therapy for osteoporosis for:
				  a. Osteoporotic vertebral or hip fracture
				  b. DXA with T score ≤ –2.5
				  c. DXA with T score ≤ –1 to –2.4 and a 10-y risk of major osteoporotic fracture ≥20% or hip fracture ≥3% based on FRAX calculator, available at http://www.shef.ac.uk/FRAX/
				8. Consider the use of hip protectors in women at high risk of falling.
					1. Options for osteoporosis drug therapy:
					  a. Bisphosphonates
					    i. First-line therapy
					    ii. Options include alendronate, ibandronate, risedronate, or zoledronic acid
					    iii. Potential risk for jaw osteonecrosis
					  b. Denosumab
					    i. Consider for women at high fracture risk
					  c. Raloxifene
					    i. Second-line agent in younger women with osteoporosis
					  d. Teriparatide is an option for high fracture risk when bisphosphonates have failed
					    i. Therapy should not exceed 24 months
					  e. Calcitonin
					    i. Third-line therapy for osteoporosis
					    ii. May be used for bone pain from acute vertebral compression fractures.
					2. Vitamin D therapy should maintain a 25-OH vitamin D level between 30 and 60 ng/mL.
						http://www.guidelines.gov/content.aspx?id=15500
						https://www.aace.com/files/osteo-guidelines-2010.pdf
						http://www.guidelines.gov/content.aspx?id=38413

[a]Previous fracture after menopause, weight <127 lb, BMI <21 kg/m², parent with a history of hip fracture, current smoker, rheumatoid arthritis, or excessive alcohol intake.

OSTEOPOROSIS, GLUCOCORTICOID-INDUCED

Disease Management	Organization	Date	Population	Recommendations	Comments	Source

Osteoporosis, Glucocorticoid-Induced	ACR	2010	Glucocorticoid-induced osteoporosis	1. All patients receiving glucocorticoid therapy should receive education and assess risk factors for osteoporosis.
				2. FRAX calculator should be used to place patients at low risk, medium risk, or high risk for major osteoporotic fracture.
				3. If glucocorticoid treatment is expected to last >3 mo, recommend:
				  a. Weight-bearing activities
				  b. Smoking cessation
				  c. Avoid >2 alcoholic drinks/day
				  d. Calcium 1200–1500 mg/day
				  e. Vitamin D 800–1000 IU/day
				  f. Fall risk assessment
				  g. Baseline DXA test and then every 2 y
				  h. Annual 25-OH vitamin D
				  i. Baseline and annual height measurement
				  j. Assessment of prevalent fragility fractures
				  k. X-rays of spine
				  l. Assessment of degree of osteoporosis medication compliance, if applicable
				4. For postmenopausal women or men age >50 y:
				  a. Low-risk group
				    i. Bisphosphonate if equivalent of prednisone ≥7.5 mg/d
				  b. Medium-risk group
				    i. Bisphosphonate if equivalent of prednisolone ≥5 mg/d
				  c. High-risk group
				    i. Bisphosphonate for any dose of glucocorticoid
				5. For premenopausal women or men age <50 y with a prevalent fragility (osteoporotic) fracture and glucocorticoid use ≥3 mo:
				  a. For prednisone ≥5 mg/d, use alendronate or risedronate
				  b. For prednisone ≥7.5 mg/d, use zoledronic acid
				  c. Consider teriparatide for bisphosphonate failures
					1. Clinical factors that may increase the risk of osteoporotic fracture estimated by FRAX calculator:
					  a. BMI <21 kg/m^2
					  b. Parental history of hip fracture
					  c. Current smoking
					  d. ≥3 alcoholic drinks/day
					  e. Higher glucocorticoid doses or cumulative dose
					  f. IV pulse glucocorticoid use
					  g. Declining central bone mineral density measurement
					2. Bisphosphonates recommended:
					  a. Low- to medium-risk patients
					    i. Alendronate
					    ii. Risedronate
					    iii. Zoledronic acid
					  b. High-risk patients
					    i. Same + teriparatide
						http://www.rheumatology.org/practice/clinical/guidelines/ACR_2010_GIOP_Recomm_Clinicians_Guide.pdf

OTITIS EXTERNA, ACUTE (AOE)

Disease Management	Organization	Date	Population	Recommendations	Comments	Source
Otitis Externa, Acute (AOE)	AAO-HNS	2014	Adults and children	1. Recommend topical antibiotics for uncomplicated AOE. 2. For a perforated tympanic membrane, prescribe a non-ototoxic topical formulation. 3. Recommend against systemic antibiotics for uncomplicated AOE.		http://www.guideline.gov/content.aspx?id=47795

OTITIS MEDIA, ACUTE (AOM)

Disease Management	Organization	Date	Population	Recommendations	Comments	Source

Otitis Media, Acute	AAP	2013	Children age 3 mo to 18 y	1. Diagnosis should be made with pneumatic otoscopy.
				2. Children at low risk should use a wait-and-see approach for 48–72 h with oral analgesics.
				3. Recommends symptomatic relief with acetaminophen or ibuprofen and warm compresses to the ear.
				4. Educate caregivers about prevention of otitis media: encourage breast-feeding, feed child upright if bottle fed, avoid passive smoke exposure, limit exposure to groups of children, careful handwashing prior to handling child, avoid pacifier use >10 mo, ensure immunizations are up to date.
				5. Amoxicillin is the first-line antibiotic for low-risk children.
				6. Alternative medication if failure to respond to initial treatment within 72 h; penicillin allergy; presence of a resistant organism found on culture.
				7. Recommends referral to an ear, nose, and throat (ENT) specialist for a complication of otitis media: mastoiditis, facial nerve palsy, lateral sinus thrombosis, meningitis, brain abscess, or labyrinthitis.
				8. Recommends against routine recheck at 10–14 d in children feeling well.
				9. Management of otitis media with effusion:
				  a. Educate that effusion will resolve on its own
				  b. Recommends against antihistamines or decongestants
				  c. Recommends a trial of antibiotics for 10–14 d prior to referral for tympanostomy tubes
					1. Amoxicillin is first-line therapy for low-risk children:
					  a. 40 mg/kg/d if no antibiotics used in last 3 mo
					  b. 80 mg/kg/d if child is not low risk
					2. Alternative antibiotics:
					  a. Amoxicillin- clavulanate
					  b. Cefuroxime axetil
					  c. Ceftriaxone
					  d. Cefprozil
					  e. Loracarbef
					  f. Cefdinir
					  g. Cefixime
					  h. Cefpodoxime
					  i. Clarithromycin
					  j. Azithromycin
					  k. Erythromycin
						Pediatrics. 2013;131: e964–e999.

	AAFP	2013		Do not prescribe antibiotics to children age 2–12 y with non-severe AOM when observation is an option.		http://www.choosingwisely.org/societies/american-academy-of-family-physicians/

	AAP	2013	Children 6 mo to 12 y	• Diagnosis of AOM
				  ○ Moderate-severe bulging of the tympanic membrane
				  ○ New-onset otorrhea not due to otitis externa
				  ○ Mild bulging of an intensely red tympanic membrane and new otalgia <48 h duration
				• Treatment of AOM
				  ○ Analgesics and antipyretics
				  ○ Indications for antibiotics
				   – Children <24 mo old with bilateral AOM
				   – Symptoms that are not improving or worsening during a 48- to 72-h observation period
				   – AOM associated with severe symptoms (extreme fussiness or severe otalgia)
				  ○ Observation for 48–72 h is recommended in the absence of severe symptoms and fever <102.2°F
				• Consider tympanostomy tubes for recurrent AOM (3 episodes in 6 mo or 4 episode in 1 y)
					• AOM is **not** present in the absence of a middle ear effusion based on pneumatic otoscopy or tympanometry.
					• Amoxicillin is the preferred antibiotics if the child has not received amoxicillin in the last 30 d.
					• Augmentin is the preferred antibiotic if the child has received amoxicillin in the last 30 d.
						http://www.guidelines.gov/content.aspx?id=43892

ªChildren older than age 2 y without severe disease (temperature >102°F [39°C] and moderate-severe otalgia), otherwise healthy, do not attend daycare, and have had no prior ear infections within the last month.

PAIN, NEUROPATHIC

Disease Management	Organization	Date	Population	Recommendations	Comments	Source

Pain, Neuropathic	NICE	2013	Adults with neuropathic pain	• Offer a choice of amitriptyline, duloxetine, gabapentin, or pregabalin as initial treatment for neuropathic pain (except trigeminal neuralgia).
				• Consider tramadol only if acute rescue therapy.
				• Consider capsaicin cream for localized neuropathic pain.
				• Recommend against the following agents:
				  ○ Cannabis sativa extract
				  ○ Capsaicin patch
				  ○ Lacosamide
				  ○ Lamotrigine
				  ○ Levetiracetam
				  ○ Morphine
				  ○ Oxcarbazepine
				  ○ Topiramate
				  ○ Tramadol (for long-term use)
				  ○ Venlafaxine
				• Recommend carbamazepine as initial therapy for trigeminal neuralgia.
						http://www.guideline.gov/content.aspx?id=47701

PALLIATIVE AND END-OF-LIFE CARE: PAIN MANAGEMENT

Principles of Analgesic Use

By the mouth	The oral route is the preferred route for analgesics, including morphine.
By the clock	Persistent pain requires around-the-clock treatment to prevent further pain. As-needed (PRN) dosing is irrational and inhumane; it requires patients to experience pain before becoming eligible for relief. Relief is accomplished with long-acting delayed-release preparations (fentanyl patch, slow-release morphine, or oxycodone).
By the WHO ladder	If a maximum dose of medication fails to adequately relieve pain, move up the ladder, not laterally to a different drug in the same efficiency group. Severe pain requires immediate use of an opioid recommended for controlling severe pain, without progressing sequentially through Steps 1 and 2. When using a long-acting opioid, the dose for breakthrough pain should be 10% of the 24-h opioid dose (ie, if a patient is on 100 mg/d of an extended-release morphine preparation, their breakthrough dose is 10 mg of morphine or equivalent every 1–2 h until pain relief is achieved).
Individualize treatment	The right dose of an analgesic is the dose that relieves pain with acceptable side effects for a specific patient.
Monitor	Monitoring is required to ensure the benefits of treatment are maximized while adverse effects are minimized.
Use adjuvant drugs	For example, a nonsteroidal antiinflammatory drug (NSAID) is often helpful in controlling bone pain. Nonopioid analgesics, such as NSAIDs or acetaminophen, can be used at any step of the ladder. Adjuvant medications also can be used at any step to enhance pain relief or counteract the adverse effects of medications. Neuropathic pain should be treated with gabapentin, duloxetine, nortriptyline, or pregabalin. Moderate-to-high-dose dexamethasone is effective as an adjunct to opioids in a pain crisis situation.

Source: Reprinted with permission from the American Academy of Hospice and Palliative Medicine. *Pocket Guide to Hospice/Palliative Medicine.*

PANCREATITIS, ACUTE (AP)

Disease Management	Organization	Date	Population	Recommendations	Comments	Source
Pancreatitis, Acute (AP)	ACG	2013	Individuals with acute pancreatitis	**The diagnosis of acute pancreatitis** usually includes the presence of two of the three following criteria: (i) abdominal pain consistent with the disease, (ii) serum amylase and/or lipase greater than three times the upper limit of normal, and/or (iii) characteristic findings from abdominal imaging. ○ Recommend a contrast-enhanced CT scan or MRI of the pancreas if the diagnosis is unclear or if symptoms are not improving within 72 h. ○ A gallbladder ultrasound should be performed in all patients with AP. ○ All patients without a history of alcohol abuse or gallstones should have a serum triglyceride level checked. ○ Consider ICU or intermediate-level monitoring for any organ dysfunction. **Initial management** ○ Aggressive isotonic fluids at 250–500 mL/h. ○ EERCP indicated for AP associated with choledocholithiasis. ○ In the absence of cholangitis or jaundice, recommend MRCP or endoscopic ultrasound to screen for choledocholithiasis. ○ Prophylactic antibiotics for severe necrotizing AP is not recommended. ○ In patients with infected necrosis, antibiotics known to penetrate pancreatic necrosis, such as carbapenems, quinolones, and metronidazole, may be useful in delaying or sometimes totally avoiding intervention, thus decreasing morbidity and mortality. ○ In mild AP, oral feedings with clear liquids or low-fat diet can be started immediately if there is no nausea and vomiting, and the abdominal pain has resolved. ○ In severe AP, enteral nutrition is recommended to prevent infectious complications. Parenteral nutrition should be avoided, unless the enteral route is not available, not tolerated, or not meeting caloric requirements. ○ Nasogastric delivery and nasojejunal delivery of enteral feeding appear comparable in efficacy and safety. ○ In patients with mild AP, found to have gallstones in the gallbladder, a cholecystectomy should be performed before discharge to prevent a recurrence of AP. ○ In a patient with necrotizing biliary AP, in order to prevent infection, cholecystectomy is to be deferred until active inflammation subsides and fluid collections resolve or stabilize. ○ In stable patients with infected necrosis, surgical, radiologic, and/or endoscopic drainage should be delayed preferably for more than 4 weeks to allow liquefaction of the contents and the development of a fibrous wall around the necrosis (walled-off necrosis).		http://www.guideline.gov/content.aspx?id=47155

ABNORMAL PAP SMEAR ALGORITHM

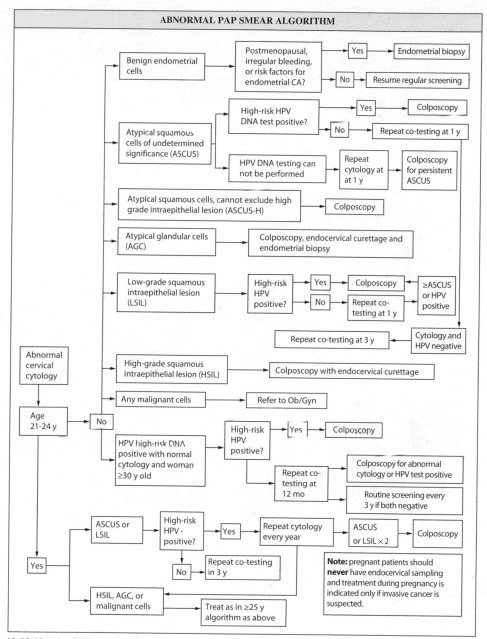

Modified from the ASCCP 2013 Updated Consensus Guidelines for Managing Abnormal Cervical Cancer Screening Tests and Cancer Precursors at http://www.asccp.org/ConsensusGuidelines/tabid/7436/Default.aspx.

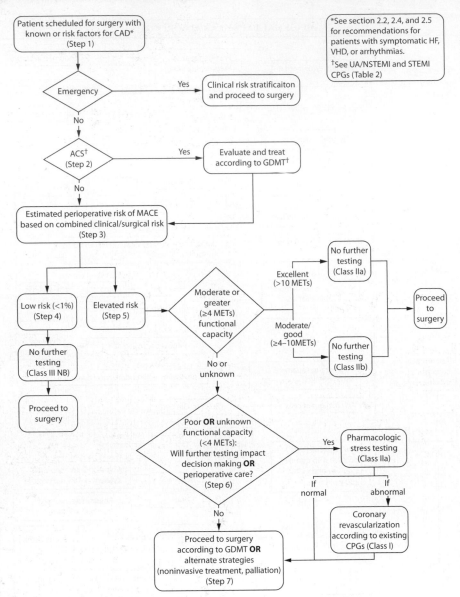

PERIOPERATIVE CARDIOVASCULAR EVALUATION AND MANAGEMENT OF PATIENTS UNDERGOING NONCARDIAC ACC/AHA/ESC 2014 GUIDELINES

Risk of surgical procedures:

– *Low risk:* when the combined surgical and patient characteristic predict a risk of a major adverse cardiac event (MACE) of death or MI of <1% (eg, cataract and plastic surgery)

– *Elevated risk:* when risk of MACE ≥1%

Calculation of risk to predict perioperative cardiac morbidity

- **RCRI** (Revised Cardiac Risk Index for perioperative risk) calculator (Lee index) assesses perioperative risk of major cardiac complications (MI, pulmonary edema, ventricular fibrillation or primary cardiac arrest, and complete heart block)
  - ○ It can be found at http://www.mdcalc.com/revised-cardiac-risk-index-for-pre-operative-risk/
  - ○ **For patients with a low risk of perioperative MACE, further testing is not recommended before the planned operation**
- The **NSQIP MICA** model (American College of Surgeons National Surgical Quality Improvement Program): http://www.surgicalriskcalculator.com/miorcardiacarrest

The NSQIP MICA model (American College of Surgeons National Surgical Quality Improvement Program) also known as myocardial infarction or cardiac arrest "GUPTA" risk calculator: http://www.surgicalriskcalculator.com/miorcardiacarrest

- ACS NSQIP Surgical Risk Calculator (American College of Surgeons) to calculate vascular surgery risk: http://riskcalculator.facs.org/PatientInfo/PatientInfo
- Revised Cardiac Risk Index for Pre-Operative Risk "LEE" calculator estimates risk of cardiac complications after surgery: http://www.mdcalc.com/revised-cardiac-risk-index-for-pre-operative-risk/

Perioperative β-blocker therapy ACC/AHA	Perioperative β-blocker therapy ESC
– β-blockers should be continued in patients undergoing surgery who have been on β-blockers chronically. – It is reasonable for the management of β-blockers after surgery to be guided by clinical circumstances (eg, hypotension, bradycardia, bleeding), independent of when the agent was started. – In patients with intermediate- or high-risk myocardial ischemia noted in preoperative risk stratification tests, it may be reasonable to begin perioperative β-blockers. Per ESC, for patients testing positive for preoperative stress, long-term β-blocker therapy should be used. – In patients with 3 or more RCRI risk factors (eg, diabetes mellitus, HF, CAD, renal insufficiency, cerebrovascular accident), it may be reasonable to begin β-blockers before surgery. – In patients with a compelling long-term indication for β-blocker therapy but no other RCRI risk factors, initiating β-blockers in the perioperative setting as an approach to reduce perioperative risk is of uncertain benefit. – In patients in whom β-blocker therapy is initiated, it may be reasonable to begin perioperative β-blockers long enough in advance to assess safety and tolerability, preferably more than 1 d before surgery. – **β-blocker therapy should not be started on the day of surgery!!!** – Abrupt withdrawal of long-term β-blockers is harmful.	– Perioperative continuation of β-blockers is recommended in patients currently receiving this medication. – Pre-operative initiation of β-blockers may be considered in patients scheduled for high-risk surgery and who have 2 clinical risk factors or ASA (American Society of Anesthesiologists) class III (patient has severe systemic disease that is not incapacitating). – Preoperative initiation of β-blockers may be considered in patients who have known IHD or myocardial ischemia – When oral β-blockade is initiated in patients who undergo noncardiac surgery, the use of atenolol or bisoprolol as a first choice may be considered. – β-blocker therapy should be initiated ideally >1 d (when possible at least 1 wk and up to 30 d) before surgery, starting with a low dose (atenolol or bisoprolol as first choice). – Initiation of perioperative high-dose β-blockers without titration **is not recommended**. – Preoperative initiation of β-blockers is not recommended in patients scheduled for low-risk surgery.
Perioperative statin therapy ACC/AHA	**Perioperative statin therapy ESC**
– Statins should be continued in patients currently taking statins and scheduled for noncardiac surgery. – Perioperative initiation of statin use is reasonable in patients undergoing vascular surgery. – Perioperative initiation of statins may be considered in patients with clinical indications according to GDMT who are undergoing elevated-risk procedures.	– Perioperative continuation of statins is recommended, favoring statins with a long half-life or extended-release formulation. (atorvastatin, lovastatin) – Preoperative initiation of statin therapy should be considered in patients undergoing vascular surgery, ideally at least 2 wk before surgery.
Perioperative antiplatelet therapy ACC/AHA	**Perioperative antiplatelet therapy ESC**
– In patients undergoing urgent noncardiac surgery during the first 4 to 6 wk after BMS or DES implantation, dual antiplatelet therapy (DAPT) should be continued unless the relative risk of bleeding outweighs the benefit of the prevention of stent thrombosis. – In patients who have received coronary stents and must undergo surgical procedures that mandate the discontinuation of $P2Y_{12}$ platelet receptor–inhibitor therapy, it is recommended that aspirin be continued if possible and the $P2Y_{12}$ platelet receptor–inhibitor be restarted as soon as possible after surgery. – Management of the perioperative antiplatelet therapy should be determined by a consensus of the surgeon, anesthesiologist, cardiologist, and patient, who should weigh the relative risk of bleeding versus prevention of stent thrombosis.	– It is recommended that aspirin be continued for 4 wk after BMS implantation and for 3–12 mo after DES implantation, unless the risk of life-threatening surgical bleeding on aspirin is unacceptably high. – Continuation of aspirin, in patients previously thus treated, may be considered in the perioperative period, and should be based on an individual decision that depends on the perioperative bleeding risk, weighed against the risk of thrombotic complications. – Discontinuation of aspirin therapy, in patients previously treated with it, should be considered in those in whom hemostasis is anticipated to be difficult to control during surgery.

PERIOPERATIVE CARDIOVASCULAR EVALUATION AND MANAGEMENT OF PATIENTS UNDERGOING NONCARDIAC ACC/AHA/ESC 2014 GUIDELINES (CONTINUED)	
– In patients undergoing nonemergency/nonurgent noncardiac surgery who have not had previous coronary stenting, it may be reasonable to continue aspirin when the risk of potential increased cardiac events outweighs the risk of increased bleeding. – Initiation or continuation of aspirin is not beneficial in patients undergoing elective noncardiac noncarotid surgery who have not had previous coronary stenting unless the risk of ischemic events outweighs the risk of surgical bleeding.	– Continuation of $P2Y_{12}$ inhibitor treatment should be considered for 4 wk after BMS implantation and for 3–12 mo after DES implantation, unless the risk of life-threatening surgical bleeding on this agent is unacceptably high. – In patients treated with $P2Y_{12}$ inhibitors, who need to undergo surgery, postponing surgery for at least 5 d after cessation of ticagrelor and clopidogrel—and for 7 d in the case of prasugrel—if clinically feasible, should be considered unless the patient is at high risk of an ischemic event.
Perioperative anticoagulation therapy ACC/AHA – The role of anticoagulants (warfarin, NOAC agents) other than platelet inhibitors in the secondary prevention of myocardial ischemia or MI has not been elucidated. – The risk of bleeding for any surgical procedure must be weighed against the benefit of remaining on anticoagulants on a case-by-case basis. – In minor procedures (cataract, minor dermatologic procedures) it may be reasonable to continue anticoagulation preoperatively. – NOAC agents do not appear to be acutely reversible, no reversible agent available at this time. – Patients with prosthetic valves taking vitamin K antagonists may require bridging therapy. – For patients with AF and normal renal function undergoing elective procedures during which hemostatic control is essential, such as major surgery, spine surgery, and epidural catheterization, discontinuation of anticoagulants for ≥48 h is suggested. Monitoring activated partial thromboplastin time for dabigatran and prothrombin time for apixaban and rivaroxaban may be helpful; a level consistent with control levels suggests a low serum concentration of the anticoagulant.	**Perioperative anticoagulation therapy ESC** – Patients at high risk of thrombo embolism treated with vitamin K antagonists (VKAs) such as AF with CHA_2DS_2-VASc score ≥4, or mechanical prosthetic heart valves, newly inserted biological prosthetic valves, mitral valvular repair (within the last 3 months) or recent venous thrombo embolism (within 3 months), or thrombophilia **WILL NEED BRIDGING** with unfractionated heparin (UFH) or therapeutic -dose LMWH. There is better evidence for the efficacy and safety of LMWH in comparison with UFH in bridging to surgery. – The overall recommendation is to stop NOACs for 2–3 times their respective biological half-lives prior to surgery in surgical interventions with "normal" bleeding risk, and 4–5 times the biological half-lives before surgery in surgical interventions with high bleeding risk. – Because of the fast "on" effect of NOACs (in comparison with VKAs), resumption of treatment after surgery should be delayed for 1–2 (in some cases 3–5) d, until postsurgical bleeding tendency is diminished.
Timing of elective noncardiac surgery in patients with previous PCI ACC/AHA – Elective noncardiac surgery should be delayed 14 d after balloon angioplasty and at least 30 days (ideally 3 mo) after BMS implantation. – Elective noncardiac surgery should optimally be delayed 365 d after drug-eluting stent (DES) implantation. – In patients in whom noncardiac surgery is required, a consensus decision among treating clinicians as to the relative risks of surgery and discontinuation or continuation of antiplatelet therapy can be useful. – Elective noncardiac surgery after DES implantation may be considered after 180 d if the risk of further delay is greater than the expected risks of ischemia and stent. – Elective noncardiac surgery should not be performed within 30 d after BMS implantation or within 12 mo after DES implantation in patients in whom dual antiplatelet therapy (DAPT) will need to be discontinued perioperatively. – Elective noncardiac surgery should not be performed within 14 d of balloon angioplasty in patients in whom aspirin will need to be discontinued perioperatively.	**Timing of elective noncardiac surgery in patients with previous PCI ESC** – It is recommended that, except for high-risk patients, asymptomatic patients who have undergone CABG in the past 6 y be sent for nonurgent, noncardiac surgery without angiographic evaluation. – Consideration should be given to performing non-urgent, non-cardiac surgery in patients with recent BMS implantation after a minimum of 4 wk and ideally 3 mo following the intervention. – Consideration should be given to performing non-urgent, non-cardiac surgery in patients who have had recent DES implantation no sooner than 12 mo following the intervention. This delay may be reduced to 6 mo for the new generation DES. – In patients who have had recent balloon angioplasty, surgeons should consider postponing non-cardiac surgery until at least 2 wk after the intervention.
Sources: Fleisher LA, Fleischmann KE, Auerbach AD, et al. 2014 ACC/AHA Guideline on perioperative cardiovascular evaluation and management of patients undergoing noncardiac surgery: executive summary. *J Am Coll Cardiol.* 2014. doi:10.1016/j.jacc.2014.07.945. 2014 ESC/ESA Guidelines on non-cardiac surgery: cardiovascular assessment and management. Kristensen SD, Knuuti J, Saraste A, et al. The Joint Task Force on non-cardiac surgery: cardiovascular assessment and management of the European Society of Cardiology (ESC) and the European Society of Anaesthesiology (ESA). *Eur Heart J.* 2014;35:2383-2431.doi:10.1093/eurheartj/ehu282.	

PREOPERATIVE CLEARANCE

Disease Management	Organization	Date	Population	Recommendations	Comments	Source
Preoperative Clearance	*Choosing Wisely* ACC	2014	Asymptomatic population without cardiac history	– Recommends against stress cardiac imaging or advanced noninvasive imaging as a preoperative assessment in patients scheduled to undergo low-risk noncardiac surgery.		http://www.choosingwisely.org/societies/american-college-of-cardiology/
	Choosing Wisely Society of Thoracic Surgeons	2013		– Recommends against preoperative stress testing prior to noncardiac thoracic surgery in patients who have no cardiac history and good functional status. – Recommends against routine evaluation of carotid artery disease prior to cardiac surgery in the absence of symptoms or other high-risk criteria.		http://www.choosingwisely.org/wp-content/uploads/2015/02/STS-Choosing-Wisely-List.pdf
	Choosing Wisely American College of Physicians	2013		– Recommends against preoperative chest radiography in the absence of a clinical suspicion for intrathoracic pathology.		http://www.choosingwisely.org/societies/american-college-of-physicians/
	Choosing Wisely American Society of Echocardiography	2013		– Recommends avoiding echocardiograms for preoperative/perioperative assessment of patients with no history of symptoms of heart disease.		http://www.choosingwisely.org/societies/american-society-of-echocardiography/

APPROACH TO ACUTE PHARYNGITIS
Source: IDSA 2012 GUIDELINES ON GROUP A
STREPTOCOCCUS (GAS) PHARYNGITIS

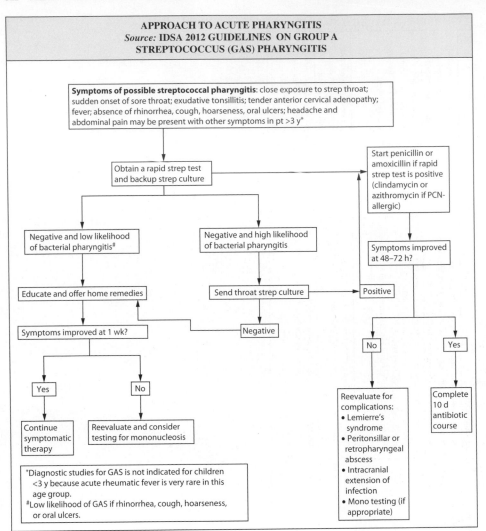

Symptoms of possible streptococcal pharyngitis: close exposure to strep throat; sudden onset of sore throat; exudative tonsillitis; tender anterior cervical adenopathy; fever; absence of rhinorrhea, cough, hoarseness, oral ulcers; headache and abdominal pain may be present with other symptoms in pt >3 y*

Obtain a rapid strep test and backup strep culture

Start penicillin or amoxicillin if rapid strep test is positive (clindamycin or azithromycin if PCN-allergic)

Symptoms improved at 48–72 h?

Negative and low likelihood of bacterial pharyngitis#

Negative and high likelihood of bacterial pharyngitis

Educate and offer home remedies

Send throat strep culture

Positive

Symptoms improved at 1 wk?

Negative

No

Yes

Yes

No

Continue symptomatic therapy

Reevaluate and consider testing for mononucleosis

Reevaluate for complications:
• Lemierre's syndrome
• Peritonsillar or retropharyngeal abscess
• Intracranial extension of infection
• Mono testing (if appropriate)

Complete 10 d antibiotic course

*Diagnostic studies for GAS is not indicated for children <3 y because acute rheumatic fever is very rare in this age group.
#Low likelihood of GAS if rhinorrhea, cough, hoarseness, or oral ulcers.

PLATELET TRANSFUSION

Disease Management	Organization	Date	Population	Recommendations	Comments	Source
Platelet Transfusion	American Association of Blood Banks (AABB)	2014	Adults and children	1. Transfusion with a single apheresis unit or a pool of 4 to 6 whole blood derived platelet concentrates is indicated for patients with therapy-induced platelet counts of <10,000 (<20,000 if infection). 2. Prophylactic platelet transfusions are indicated for patients having elective central venous catheter (CVC) placement with platelet count <20,000 and for those having elective diagnostic lumbar puncture or major non-neurological surgery with <50,000 platelets. 3. Platelet transfusions are not recommended for non-thrombocytopenic patients having cardicpulmonary bypass surgery unless they have perioperative bleeding with thrombocytopenia or evidence of platelet dysfunction.	1. These guidelines do not pertain to ITP, TTP, or heparin-induced thrombocytopenia. Platelet transfusion may worsen these immune-mediated diseases and should not be given unless there is major life-threatening bleeding. (*Blood.* 2015; 125:1470) 2. No strong evidence was found for platelet transfusion with intracranial bleed in patients taking anti-platelet drugs or in patients undergoing neurosurgery with platelets <100,000 although platelets >100,000 is current clinical practice. 3. Guidelines emphasize that clinical judgment and not a specific platelet count should be paramount in decision making. 4. Beware that risk of bacterial infection with platelet transfusion is 1 in 3000 (5 times more common than RBC transfusions). (*Transfusion.* 2013; 55:1603)	*Ann Intern Med.* 2015; 162:205-213 *Blood.* 2014;123: 1146-1151

PNEUMONIA, COMMUNITY-ACQUIRED: EVALUATION
Source: IDSA, ATS, 2007

Diagnostic Testing

- CXR or other chest imaging required for diagnosis
- Sputum Gram stain and culture
  - Outpatients: optional
  - Inpatients: if unusual or antibiotic resistance suspected

Admission Decision

- Severity of illness (eg, CURB-65) and prognostic indices (eg, PSI) support decision
- One must still recognize social and individual factors

CURB-65
(*Thorax.* 2003;58:337-382)

Clinical Factor	Points
Confusion	1
BUN >19 mg/dL	1
Respiratory rate ≥30 breaths/min	1
Systolic BP <90 mm Hg or Diastolic BP ≤60 mm Hg	1
Age >65 y	1
Total points	

- CURB-65 ≥2 suggest need for hospitalization

Score	In-hospital mortality
0	0.7%
1	3.2%
2	3.0%
3	17%
4	42%
5	57%

Pneumonia Severity Index
(*N Engl J Med.* 1997;336:243-250)

Demographic Factor	Points
Demographic factor	
Men age	Age in years
Women age	Age in years −10
Nursing home resident	+10
Coexisting illnesses	
Neoplastic disease	+30
Liver disease	+20
Congestive heart failure	+10
Cerebrovascular disease	+10
Renal disease	+10
Physical exam findings	
Altered mental status	+20
Respiratory rate 30 breaths/min	+20
Systolic BP <90 mm Hg	+20
Temperature <95°F (35°C)	+15
Temperature >104°F (40°C)	+15
Pulse >125 beats/min	+10
Laboratory and radiographic findings	
Arterial blood pH <7.35	+30
BUN >30 mg/dL	+20
Sodium level <130 mmol/L	+20
Glucose level >250 mg/dL	+10
Hematocrit <30%	+10
PaO_2 <60 mm Hg or O_2 saturation <90%	+10
Pleural effusion	+10

Add up total points to estimate mortality risk

Class	Points	Overall Mortality
I	<51	0.1%
II	51–70	0.6%
III	71–90	0.9%
IV	91–130	9.5%
V	>130	26.7%

BP, blood pressure; BUN, blood urea nitrogen; CURB-65, confusion, urea nitrogen, respiratory rate, blood pressure, 65 years of age and older; CXR, chest x-ray; PSI, pneumonia severity index.

Sources: Mandell LA, Wunderink RG, Anzueto A, et al; Infectious Diseases Society of America; American Thoracic Society. Infectious Diseases Society of America/American Thoracic Society consensus guidelines on the management of community-acquired pneumonia in adults. *Clin Infect Dis.* 2007;44 Suppl 2:S27-S72. Fine MJ, Auble TE, Yealy DM, et al. A prediction rule to identify low-risk patients with community-acquired pneumonia. *N Engl J Med.* 1997;336:243-250.

PNEUMONIA, COMMUNITY-ACQUIRED: SUSPECTED PATHOGENS
Source: IDSA, ATS, 2007

Condition and Risk Factors	Commonly Encountered Pathogens
Alcoholism	*Streptococcus pneumoniae*, oral anaerobes, *Klebsiella pneumoniae*, *Acinetobacter* species, *Mycobacterium tuberculosis*
COPD and/or smoking	*Haemophilus influenzae, Pseudomonas aeruginosa, Legionella* species, *S. pneumoniae, Moraxella catarrhalis, Chlamydia pneumoniae*
Aspiration	Gram-negative enteric pathogens, oral anaerobes
Lung abscess	CA-MRSA, oral anaerobes, endemic fungal pneumonia, *M. tuberculosis,* and atypical mycobacteria
Exposure to bat or bird droppings	Histoplasma capsulatum
Exposure to birds	*Chlamydophila psittaci* (if poultry: avian influenza)
Exposure to rabbits	*Francisella tularensis*
Exposure to farm animals or parturient cats	*Coxiella burnetii* (Q fever)
HIV infection (early)	*S. pneumoniae, H. influenzae,* and *M. tuberculosis*
HIV infection (late)	The pathogens listed for early infection plus *Pneumocystis jiroveci, Cryptococcus, Histoplasma, Aspergillus,* atypical mycobacteria (especially *Mycobacterium kansasii), P. aeruginosa, H. influenzae*
Hotel or cruise ship stay in previous 2 wk	*Legionella* species
Travel to or residence in southwestern United States	*Coccidioides* species, *hantavirus*
Travel to or residence in Southeast and East Asia	*Burkholderia pseudomallei,* avian influenza, SARS
Influenza active in community	Influenza, *S. pneumoniae, Staphylococcus aureus, H. influenzae*
Cough ≥2 wk with whoop or posttussive vomiting	*Bordetella pertussis*
Structural lung disease (eg, bronchiectasis)	*P. aeruginosa, Burkholderia cepacia,* and *S. aureus*
Injection drug use	*S. aureus,* anaerobes, *M. tuberculosis,* and *S. pneumoniae*
Endobronchial obstruction	Anaerobes, *S. pneumoniae, H. influenzae, S. aureus*
In context of bioterrorism	*Bacillus anthracis* (anthrax), *Yersinia pestis* (plague), *F. tularensis* (tularemia)

CA-MRSA, community-acquired methicillin-resistant *S. aureus*; COPD, chronic obstructive pulmonary disease; SARS, severe acute respiratory syndrome.

POLYCYSTIC OVARY SYNDROME

Disease Management	Organization	Date	Population	Recommendations	Comments	Sources

Polycystic ovary Syndrome	Endocrine Society	2013	Adolescent and adult women	1. Diagnosis if 2 of 3 criteria are met:
				  a. Androgen excess
				  b. Ovulatory dysfunction
				  c. Polycystic ovaries
				2. Treatment
				  a. Hormonal contraceptives for menstrual irregularities, acne, and hirsutism
				  b. Exercise and diet for weight management
				  c. Clomiphene citrate recommended for infertility
				  d. Recommends against the use of metformin, inositols, or thiaolidinediones
						http://www.guideline.gov/content.aspx?id=47899

POSTPARTUM HEMORRHAGE (PPH)					
Disease Management	**Organization**	**Date**	**Population**	**Recommendations**	**Comments**	**Source**

Postpartum Hemorrhage (PPH)	WHO	2012	Pregnant women	• Uterotonics for the treatment of PPH
				  ○ Intravenous oxytocin is the recommended agent
				  ○ Alternative uterotonics:
				    – Misoprostol 800 μg sublingual
				    – Methylergonovine 0.2 mg IM
				    – Carboprost 0.25 mg IM
				• Additional interventions for PPH
				  ○ Isotonic crystalloid resuscitation
				  ○ Bimanual uterine massage
				• Therapeutic options for persistent PPH
				  ○ Tranexamic acid is recommended for persistent PPH refractory to oxytocin
				  ○ Uterine artery embolization
				  ○ Balloon tamponade
				• Therapeutic options for a retained placenta
				  ○ Controlled cord traction with oxytocin 10 IU IM/IV
				  ○ Manual removal of placenta
				    – Give single dose of first-generation antibiotic for prophylaxis against endometritis
				  ○ Recommend against methylergonovine, misoprostol, or carboprost (Hemabate) for retained placenta
					• Misoprostol 800–1000 μg can also be administered as a rectal suppository for PPH related to uterine atony.	http://www.guidelines.gov/content.aspx?id=39383

ROUTINE PRENATAL CARE

Preconception Visit

1. Measure height, weight, blood pressure, and total and HDL cholesterol.
2. Determine rubella, rubeola, and varicella immunity status.
3. Assess all patients for pregnancy risk: substance abuse, domestic violence, sexual abuse, psychiatric disorders, risk factors for reterm labor, exposure to chemicals or infectious agents, hereditary disorders, gestational diabetes, or chronic medical problems.
4. Educate patients about proper nutrition; offer weight reduction strategies for obese patients.
5. Immunize if not current on the following: Tdap (combined tetanus, diphtheria, and pertussis vaccine), MMR (measles, mumps, rubella), varicella, or hepatitis B vaccine.
6. Initiate folic acid 400–800 µg/d; 4 mg/d for a history of a child affected by a neural tube defect.

Initial Prenatal Visit

1. Medical, surgical, social, family, and obstetrical history and do complete examination.
2. Pap smear, urine NAAT for gonorrhea and *Chlamydia*, and assess for history of genital herpes.
3. Consider a varicella antibody test if the patient unsure about prior varicella infection.
4. Urinalysis for proteinuria and glucosuria, and urine culture for asymptomatic bacteriuria.
5. Order prenatal labs to include a complete blood count, blood type, antibody screen, rubella titer, VDRL, hepatitis B surface antigen, and an HIV test.
6. Order an obstetrical ultrasound for dating if any of the following: beyond 16-wk gestational age, unsure last menstrual period, size/dates discrepancy on examination, or for inability to hear fetal heart tones by 12 gestational weeks.
7. Discuss fetal aneuploidy screening and counseling regardless of maternal age.
8. Prenatal testing offered for: sickle cell anemia (African descent), thalassemia (African, Mediterranean, Middle Eastern, Southeast Asians), Canavan disease and Tay-Sachs (Jewish patients), cystic fibrosis (whites and Ashkenazi Jews), and fragile X syndrome (family history of nonspecified mental retardation).
9. Place a tuberculosis skin test for all medium-to-high-risk patients.[a]
10. Consider a 1-h 50-g glucose tolerance test for certain high-risk groups.[b]
11. Obtain an operative report in all women who have had a prior cesarean section.
12. Psychosocial risk assessment for mood disorders, substance abuse, or domestic violence.

Frequency of Visits for Uncomplicated Pregnancies

1. Every 4 wk until 28 gestational wk; q 2 wk from 28 to 36 wk; weekly >36 wk.

Routine Checks at Follow-up Prenatal Visits

1. Assess weight, blood pressure, and urine for glucose and protein.
2. Exam: edema, fundal height, and fetal heart tones at all visits; fetal presentation starting at 36 wk.
3. Ask about regular uterine contractions, leakage of fluid, vaginal bleeding, or decreased fetal movement.
4. Discuss labor precautions.

Antepartum Lab Testing

1. All women should be offered either first trimester, second trimester, or combined testing to screen for fetal aneuploidy; invasive diagnostic testing for fetal aneuploidy should be available to all women regardless of maternal age.
   a. First trimester
   b. Second trimester screening options: amniocentesis at 14 wk; a Quad Marker Screen at 16–18 wk; and/or a screening ultrasound with nuchal translucency assessment
2. Consider serial transvaginal sonography of the cervix every 2–3 wk to assess cervical length for patients at high risk for preterm delivery starting at 16 wk.
3. No role for routine bacterial vaginosis screening.
4. 1-h 50-g glucose tolerance test in all women between 24 and 28 wk.
5. Rectovaginal swab for group B streptococcal (GBS) testing between 35 and 37 wk.
6. Recommend weekly amniotic fluid assessments and twice weekly nonstress testing starting at 41 wk.

Prenatal Counseling

1. Cessation of smoking, drinking alcohol, or use of any illicit drugs.
2. Avoid cat litter boxes, hot tubs, certain foods (ie, raw fish or unpasteurized cheese)
3. Proper nutrition and expected weight gain: National Academy of Sciences advises weight gain 28–40 lb (prepregnancy BMI <20), 25–35 lb (BMI 20–26), 15–25 lb (BMI 26–29), and 15–20 lb (BMI ≥30).
4. Inquire about domestic violence and depression at initial visit, at 28 wk, and at postpartum visit.
5. Recommend regular mild-to-moderate exercise 3 or more times a week.
6. Avoid high-altitude activities, scuba diving, and contact sports during pregnancy.
7. Benefits of breastfeeding vs bottle feeding.
8. Discuss postpartum contraceptive options (including tubal sterilization) during third trimester.
9. Discuss analgesia and anesthesia options and offer prenatal classes at 24 wk.
10. Discuss repeat C-section vs vaginal birth after cesarean (if applicable).
11. Discuss the option of circumcision if a boy is delivered.
12. Avoid air travel and long train or car trips beyond 36 wk.

ROUTINE PRENATAL CARE (CONTINUED)

Prenatal Interventions

1. Suppressive antiviral medications starting at 36 wk for women with a history of genital herpes.
2. Cesarean delivery is indicated for women who are HIV-positive or have active genital herpes and are in labor.
3. For patients who report a history of abuse, offer interventions and resources to increase their safety during and after pregnancy.
4. For patients with severe depression, consider treatment with an SSRI (avoid paroxetine if possible).
5. Rh immune globulin 300 μg IM for all Rh-negative women with negative antibody screens between 26 and 28 wk.
6. Refer for nutrition counseling at 10–12 wk for BMI <20 kg/m^2 or at any time during pregnancy for inadequate weight gain.
7. Start prenatal vitamins with iron and folic acid 400–800 μg/d and 1200 mg elemental calcium/day starting at 4 wk preconception (or as early as possible during pregnancy) and continued until 6 wk postpartum.
8. Give inactivated influenza vaccine IM to all pregnant women during influenza season.
9. Consider progesterone therapy IM weekly or intravaginally daily to women at high risk for preterm birth.
10. Recommend an external cephalic version at 37 wk for all noncephalic presentations.
11. Offer labor induction to women at 41 wk by good dates.
12. Treat all women with confirmed syphilis with penicillin G during pregnancy.
13. Treat all women with gonorrhea with ceftriaxone; follow treatment with a test of cure.
14. Treat all women with *Chlamydia* with azithromycin; follow treatment with a test of cure.
15. Treat all GBS-positive women with penicillin G when in labor or with spontaneous rupture of membranes.

Postpartum Interventions

1. Treat all infants born to HBV-positive women with hepatitis B immunoglobulin (HBIG) and initiate HBV vaccine series within 12 h of life.
2. All women with a positive tuberculosis skin test and no evidence of active disease should receive a postpartum chest x-ray; treat with isoniazid 300 mg PO daily for 9 mo if chest x-ray is negative.
3. Administer a Tdap booster if tetanus status is unknown or the last Td (tetanus-diphtheria) vaccine was >10 y ago.
4. Administer an MMR vaccine to all rubella nonimmune women.
5. Offer HPV vaccine to all women ≤26 wk who have not been immunized.
6. Initiate contraception.
7. Repeat Pap smear at 6-wk postpartum check.

[a] Postgastrectomy, gastric bypass, immunosuppressed (HIV-positive, diabetes, renal failure, chronic steroid/immunosuppressive therapy, head/neck or hematologic malignancies), silicosis, organ transplant recipients, malabsorptive syndromes, alcoholics, intravenous drug users, close contacts of persons with active pulmonary tuberculosis, medically underserved, low socioeconomic class, residents/employees of long-term care facilities and jails, health care workers, and immigrants from endemic areas.

[b] Overweight (BMI ≥25 kg/m^2 and an additional risk factor: physical inactivity; first-degree relative with DM; high-risk ethnicity (eg, African American, Latino, Native American, Asian American, Pacific Islander); history of gestational diabetes mellitus (GDM); prior baby with birthweight >9 lb; unexplained stillbirth or malformed infant; HTN on therapy or with BP ≥140/90 mm Hg; HDL cholesterol level <35 mg/dL (0.90 mmol/L) and/or a triglyceride level >250 mg/dL (2.82 mmol/L); polycystic ovary syndrome; history of impaired glucose tolerance or HgbA1c ≥5.7%; acanthosis nigricans; cardiovascular disease; or >2+ glucosuria.

Adapted from ACOG ICSI Guideline on Routine Prenatal Care, July 2010. http://www.icsi.org/prenatal_care_4/prenatal_care_routine_full_version_2.html.

RED BLOOD CELL (RBC) TRANSFUSION

Disease Management	Organization/ Population	Recommendation	Comments	Source
Red Blood Cell (RBC) Transfusion	American Association of Blood Banks (AABB)	A. Hospitalized, hemodynamically stable patients—restrictive transfusion strategy preferred (See Table I). 1. For non-surgical patients transfusion considered at hemoglobin of 7 g/dL or less. 2. In post-op surgical patients transfusion considered at hemoglobin of 8 g/dL or less. 3. Patients with heart disease should be treated with restrictive transfusion strategy (trigger hemoglobin 7–8 g/dL). Erythrocyte stimulating agents should not be used because of increased thrombotic risk. 4. In symptomatic patients (chest pain, tachycardia, hypotension, or heart failure) or with continued hemorrhage clinical judgment should supervene. 5. In patients meeting criteria for transfusion, give only as much as necessary to raise hemoglobin to recommended levels (1 unit of red blood cells will raise hemoglobin by 1 g/dL). 6. Leukocyte reduction (either at the time of collection or filtration at the time of transfusion) is necessary to decrease febrile, nonhemolytic transfusion reactions, decrease risk of cytomegalovirus (CMV) transmission, and decrease risk of HLA-allo immunization but does not prevent transfusion associated graft vs. host disease (TA-GVHD).	1. 15 million units of red blood cells are transfused annually in the US and 85 million transfused annually worldwide. 2. Transfusion carries significant risk of infection, immunosupression, hemolytic transfusion reaction, transfusion related acute lung injury (TRALI) (see Table II). 3. Nineteen trials were evaluated by AABB assessing noninferiority of restrictive vs liberal transfusion policy. There was no statistically significant difference although a trend for lower mortality in the patients treated by the restrictive transfusion policy was noted. 4. Patients with pharmacologically treatable anemia such as iron deficiency or B_{12} or folate deficiency should not be transfused unless they are significantly symptomatic. 5. Transfusion of red cells should be given slowly over first 15 min and completed within 4 h.	*Ann Intern Med.* 2012;157:49-58. *Blood.* 2012;119:1757-1767. *N Engl J Med.* 2011;365:2433-2462. *Crit Care Med.* 2008;36:2667-2674.
	AABB	B. Prevention of TA-GVHD—High risk 1. High-risk situation include product donated by family member or HLA selected donor. 2. Acute leukemia and Hodgkin and non-Hodgkin lymphoma patients on therapy. 3. Allogenic or autologous hemopoietic progenitor cell transplant recipient. 4. Aplastic anemia patients on anti-thymocyte globulin and/or cyclosporine. 5. Purine analogues and other drugs affecting T-cell count and function—fludarabine, clofarabine, bendamustine, nelarabine, alemtuzumab, and temozolomide. 6. Recommended preventive strategy is 2500 cGy of radiation to product to be transfused. This dose will destroy T cells. Shelf life of irradiated product is 28 d. C. Infection complications of transfusion now very very rare (see Table III).	1. Must be aware of circumstances that increase risk of TA-GVHD in order to initiate protective strategy. If TA-GVHD does occur mortality approaches 100%. 2. In immunosuppressed patients and in family members with shared genes, targeting T cells from the donor may not be eliminated through immunologic attack. These surviving T cells then interact with host cellular antigens damaging skin, liver, GI tract, and lung with high mortality. 3. With polymerase chain reaction (PCR) and antibody screening transfusion related infection complications are rare. Bacterial infection and sepsis occurs 50 fold more commonly with platelet transfusion vs red blood cell transfusion. 4. Immune compromised patients needing transfusion should have CMV serology checked and if antibodies not present CMV negative blood should be given (60%–80% are antibody positive).	

Table I

RED BLOOD CELL—TRANSFUSION GUIDELINES FOR HEMODYNAMICALLY STABLE PATIENTS		
Patient Situation	**Transfusion Threshold**	**Strength of Evidence**
ICU[a]	Hgb ≤7 g/dL	High
Post-op	Hgb ≤8 g or symptoms[b]	High
Cardiovascular disease	Hgb ≤8 or symptoms[b]	Moderate

[a]Guidelines for non-ICU hospitalized patients have not been determined.
[b]Includes chest pain, hypoxia, hypotension and tachycardia, CHF, ischemic bowel.

Table II

NONINFECTIOUS COMPLICATIONS OF BLOOD TRANSFUSION			
Complication	**Incidence**	**Diagnosis**	**Rx and Outcome**
Acute hemolytic transfusion reaction (AHTR)	1:40,000	Serum free hemoglobin, Coombs	Fluids to keep urine output >1 mL/kg/h, pressors, treat DIC, fatal in 1:1.8 × 10⁶ RBC exposures
Delayed transfusion reaction (HTR)	1:3000–5000	Timing (10—14 d after tx)−(+) Coombs, ↑-LDH, indirect bili, retic ct.—Ab often to Kidd or Rh	Identify responsible antigen, transfuse compatible blood if necessary
Febrile non-HTR	0.1%–1%	Exclude AHTR —↓- risk with leucocyte depletion—starts within 2 h of transfusion	Acetaminophen po, support and reassurance
Allergic (urticarial)	1%–3%	Urticaria, pruritus, no fever caused by antibody to donor-plasma proteins	Hold tx—give antihistamines and complete tx. when symptoms resolve
Anaphylactic	1:20–50,000	Hypotension, bronchospasm, urticaria, anxiety, rule out hemolysis	Epinephrine 1:1000 –0.2–0.5 mL. SQ, steroids, antihistamine
Transfusion-related acute lung injury (TRALI)	1:10,000	HLA or neutrophil antibodies in donor blood-hypoxia, bilat lung infiltrates, and fever within 6 h of transfusion	Supportive care—steroids ineffective mortality—10%–20%

Table III

INFECTIOUS COMPLICATIONS OF TRANSFUSION	
Transfusion Transmitted Organism	**Risk per Unit of Blood Transfused**
HIV Hepatitis C Hepatitis B West Nile virus Cytomegalovirus (CMV)	1 in 1,467,000 1 in 1,149,000 1 in 282,000 Rare 60%–80% of donors are carriers, leukodepletion ↓-risk but in situation of significant immunosuppression give CMV negative blood
Bacterial infection	1 in 3000—5-fold more common in platelet vs RBC transfusion
Parasitic infection (Babesiosis, malaria, Chagas disease)	Rare

				PARACENTESIS		
Disease Management	**Organization**	**Date**	**Population**	**Recommendations**	**Comments**	**Source**
Paracentesis	AASLD	2014		Do not routinely administer fresh frozen plasma prior to a paracentesis.		http://www.choosingwisely. org/societies/ american-association-for-the-study-of-liver-diseases/

PERINATAL & POSTNATAL GUIDELINES *Source:* AAP, AAFP	
Breast-feeding	Strongly recommends education and counseling to promote breast-feeding.
Hemoglobinopathies	Strongly recommends ordering screening tests for hemoglobinopathies in neonates.
Hyperbilirubinemia	Perform ongoing systematic assessments during the neonatal period for the risk of an infant developing severe hyperbilirubinemia.
Phenylketonuria	Strongly recommends ordering screening tests for phenylketonuria in neonates.
Thyroid function abnormalities	Strongly recommends ordering screening tests for thyroid function abnormalities in neonates.
Source: Pediatrics. 2004;114:297-316. *Pediatrics.* 2005;115:496-506.	

PREGNANCY, PREMATURE RUPTURE OF MEMBRANES

Disease Management	Organization	Date	Population	Recommendations	Comments	Source
Pregnancy, Premature Rupture of Membranes	ACOG	2013	Pregnant women	• Women with preterm premature rupture of membranes before 32 gestational weeks at risk for imminent delivery should be considered for intravenous magnesium sulfate treatment for its fetal neuroprotective effect. • For women with premature rupture of membranes at 37 gestational weeks or more, labor should be induced if spontaneous labor does not occur near the time of presentation. • At 34 gestational weeks or greater, delivery is recommended for all women with ruptured membranes. • In the setting of ruptured membranes, therapeutic tocolysis is not recommended. • Outpatient management of preterm premature rupture of membranes is not recommended.		http://www.guideline.gov/content.aspx?id=47106
	Cochrane Database of Systematic Reviews	2013		Routine antibiotics should be prescribed for women with preterm rupture of membranes prior to 37 gestational weeks.	22 studies involving over 6800 pregnant women with PROM prior to 37 gestational weeks were analyzed. Routine antibiotics decreased the incidence of chorioamnionitis (RR 0.66), prolonged pregnancy by at least 7 d (RR 0.79), and decreased neonatal infection (RR 0.67), but had no effect on perinatal mortality compared with placebo.	http://www.cochrane.org/CD001058/PREG_antibiotics-for-preterm-rupture-of-membranes

PREGNANCY, PRETERM LABOR

Disease Management	Organization	Date	Population	Recommendations	Comments	Source

Pregnancy, Preterm labor	ACOG	2012	Pregnant women	• Single dose of corticosteroids for pregnant women between 24 and 34 gestational weeks who may deliver within 7 d.
				• Magnesium sulfate for possible preterm delivery prior to 32 wk for neuroprotection.
				• Tocolytic options for up to 48 h
				  ○ β-agonists
				  ○ Nifedipine
				  ○ Indomethacin
				• No role for antibiotics in preterm labor and intact membranes.
				• Bedrest and hydration have not been shown to prevent preterm birth and should not be routinely recommended.
					• Magnesium sulfate administered prior to 32 wk reduces the severity and risk of cerebral palsy.
					• Cochrane analysis found no difference in the incidence of preterm delivery comparing hydration and bedrest with bedrest alone.
						http://www.guidelines.gov/content.aspx?id=38621

	Cochrane Database of Systematic Reviews	2013				http://www.cochrane.org/CD003096/PREG_hydration-for-treatment-of-preterm-labour

PREGNANCY, PRETERM LABOR, TOCOLYSIS

Disease Management	Organization	Date	Population	Recommendations	Comments	Source
Pregnancy, Preterm labor, Tocolysis	RCOG	2011	Pregnant women in preterm labor	• There is no clear evidence that tocolysis improves perinatal outcomes and therefore it is reasonable not to use them. • Nifedipine and atosiban have comparable effectiveness in delaying birth up to 7 d. • Avoid the use of multiple tocolytic drugs simultaneously. • Maintenance tocolytic therapy following threatened preterm labor is not recommended.	• Tocolysis may be considered for women with suspected preterm labor who require in utero transfer or to complete a course of corticosteroids.	http://www.rcog.org.uk/files/rcog-corp/GTG1b26072011.pdf

PRESSURE ULCERS

Disease Management	Organization	Date	Population	Recommendations	Comments	Sources
Pressure Ulcers	NICE	2014	Adults at risk for pressure ulcers	1. Regular documentation of ulcer size. 2. Debride any necrotic tissue if present with sharp debridement or autolytic debridement. 3. Nutritional supplementation for patients who are malnourished. 4. Recommend a pressure-redistributing foam mattresses. 5. Negative pressure wound therapy, electrotherapy, or hyperbaric oxygen therapy is not routinely recommended. 6. Antibiotics are only indicated for superimposed cellulitis or underlying osteomyelitis.		http://www.guideline.gov/content.aspx?id=48026

	PROCEDURAL SEDATION				
Disease Management	Organization	Date	Population	Recommendations	Comments	Sources
Procedural sedation	ACEP	2014	Adults or children	1. No preprocedural fasting needed prior to procedural sedation. 2. Recommend continuous capnometry and oximetry to detect hypoventilation. 3. During procedural sedation, a nurse or other qualified individual must be present for continuous monitoring in addition to the procedural operator. 4. Safe options for procedural sedation in children and adults include ketamine, propofol, and etomidate.	The combination of ketamine and propofol is also deemed to be safe for procedural sedation in children and adults. Alfentanil can be safely administered to adults for procedural sedation.	http://www.guideline.gov/content.aspx?id=47772

PSORIASIS, PLAQUE-TYPE

Disease Management	Organization	Date	Population	Recommendations	Comments	Sources
Psoriasis, Plaque-Type	AAD	2009	Adults	**Topical Therapies** 1. Topical therapies are most effective for mild-to-moderate disease. 2. Topical corticosteroids daily—bid: 　a. Cornerstone of therapy 　b. Limit class 1 topical steroids to 4 weeks maximum 3. Topical agents that have proven efficacy when combined with topical corticosteroids: 　a. Topical vitamin D analogues 　b. Topical tazarotene 　c. Topical salicylic acid 4. Emollients applied 1–3 times daily are a helpful adjunct.	1. Approximately, 2% of population has psoriasis. 2. 80% of patients with psoriasis have mild-to-moderate disease. 3. Topical steroid toxicity: 　a. Local: skin atrophy, telangiectasia, striae, purpura, or contact dermatitis 　b. Hypothalamic–pituitary—adrenal axis may be suppressed with prolonged use of medium-to-high potency steroids	http://www.aad.org/File%20 Library/Global%20 navigation/Education%20 and%20quality%20care/ Guidelines-psoriasis-sec-3.pdf
	AAD	2009	Adults	**Systemic Therapies** 1. Indicated for severe, recalcitrant, or disabling psoriasis. 2. Methotrexate (MTX): 　a. Dose: 7.5–30 mg PO weekly 　b. Monitor CBC and liver panel monthly 3. Cyclosporine: 　a. Initial dose: 2.5–3 mg/kg divided bid 　b. Monitor for nephrotoxicity, HTN, and hypertrichosis 4. Acitretin: 　a. Dose: 10–50 mg PO daily 　b. Monitor: liver panel	1. MTX contraindications: pregnancy; breastfeeding; alcoholism; chronic liver disease; immunodeficiency syndromes; cytopenias; hypersensitivity reaction. 2. Cyclosporine contraindications: CA; renal impairment; uncontrolled HTN. 3. Acitretin contraindications: pregnancy, chronic liver, or renal disease.	http://www.aad.org/File%20 Library/Global%20 navigation/Education%20 and%20quality%20care/ Guidelines-psoriasis-sec-4.pdf

PSORIASIS AND PSORIATIC ARTHRITIS

Disease Management	Organization	Date	Population	Recommendations	Comments	Source

Psoriasis and Psoriatic Arthritis	AAD	2010	Adults	• Treatment options for patients with limited plaque-type psoriasis
				  ○ First-line therapy
				    – Topical corticosteroids
				    – Topical calcipotriene/calcitriol
				    – Topical calcipotriene/steroid
				    – Topical tazarotene
				    – Topical calcineurin inhibitors (flexural surfaces and face)
				    – Targeted phototherapy
				  ○ Second-line therapy
				    – Systemic agents
				• Treatment of extensive plaque-type psoriasis
				  ○ First-line therapy
				    – UVB phototherapy ± acitretin
				    – Topical PUVA
				  ○ Second-line therapy
				    – Acitretin + biologic
				    – Cyclosporine + biologic
				    – Cyclosporine + methotrexate
				    – Methotrexate + biologic
				    – UVB + biologic
				• Treatment of palmoplantar psoriasis
				  ○ First-line therapy
				• Topical corticosteroids
				• Topical calcipotriene/calcitriol
				• Topical calcipotriene/steroid
				• Topical tazarotene
				  ○ Second-line therapy
				    – Acitretin
				    – Targeted UVB
				    – Topical PUVA
				  ○ Third-line therapy
				    – Adalimumab
				    – Alefacept
				    – Cyclosporine
				    – Etanercept
				    – Infliximab
				    – Methotrexate
				    – Ustekinumab
					• Use of potent topical corticosteroids should be limited to 4 wk duration.	http://www.guideline.gov/content.aspx?id=15650
						http://www.aad.org/File%20Library/Global%20navigation/Education%20and%20quality%20care/Guidelines-psoriasis-sec-2.pdf

PSORIASIS AND PSORIATIC ARTHRITIS

Disease Management	Organization	Date	Population	Recommendations	Comments	Source

Psoriasis and Psoriatic Arthritis (continued)				• Treatment of erythrodermic psoriasis
				  ○ Acitretin
				  ○ Adalimumab
				  ○ Cyclosporine
				  ○ Infliximab
				  ○ Methotrexate
				  ○ Ustekinumab
				• Treatment of psoriatic arthritis
				  ○ First-line therapy
				    – Adalimumab
				    – Etanercept
				    – Golimumab
				    – Infliximab
				    – Methotrexate
				    – Tumor necrosis factor (TNF) blocker + methotrexate
				  ○ Second-line therapy
				    – Ustekinumab and methotrexate		

RESPIRATORY TRACT INFECTIONS

Disease Management	Organization	Date	Population	Recommendations	Comments	Source

Lower Respiratory Tract Infections	ESCMID	2011	Adults	• For *Streptococcus* pneumonia:
				  ○ Erythromycin MIC >0.5 mg/L predicts clinical failure
				  ○ Penicillin MIC ≤8 mg/L predicts IV penicillin susceptibility
				• The role of community-acquired MRSA in community-acquired pneumonia (CAP) is poorly defined in Europe.
				• A C-reactive protein (CRP) <2 mg/dL at presentation with symptoms >24 h makes pneumonia highly unlikely; a CRP >10 mg/dL makes pneumonia likely.
				• Indications for antibiotics in lower respiratory tract infections (LRTIs):
				  ○ Suspected pneumonia
				  ○ Acute exacerbation of COPD with increased dyspnea, sputum volume, and sputum purulence
				• Evaluation of patients admitted for CAP
				  ○ Two sets of blood cultures
				  ○ Pleural fluid analysis is indicated when a significant parapneumonic effusion exists
				  ○ Sputum Gram stain and culture should be obtained if a purulent sputum sample can be obtained
				  ○ Consider testing for urine pneumococcal antigen
				  ○ Antibiotic duration for CAP should not exceed 8 d
					• Consider aspiration pneumonia in patients with a pneumonia and dysphagia.
					• Empiric antibiotics of choice for LRTI in outpatient setting are amoxicillin or tetracycline.
						http://www.escmid.org/fileadmin/src/media/PDFs/4ESCMID_Library/2Medical_Guidelines/ESCMID_Guidelines/Woodhead_et_al_CMI Sep_2011_LRTI_GL_fulltext.pdf

Upper Respiratory Tract Infections	IDSA	2015		Do not prescribe antibiotics for upper respiratory tract infections.		http://www.choosingwisely.org/societies/infectious-diseases-society-of-america/

Acute Bacterial Sinusitis	AAP	2013	Children aged 1–18 y	• Presumptive diagnosis of acute bacterial sinusitis when a child with a URI presents with:
				  ○ Persistent symptoms without improvement for over 10 d
				  ○ Worsening course
				  ○ Severe onset (T >102.2°F and purulent rhinorrhea for at least 3 d)
				• Recommend against imaging studies to differentiate viral URI from bacterial sinusitis
				• Recommend a CT or MRI with contrast of the paranasal sinuses if globe or CNS complications from sinusitis are suspected
				• Amoxicillin or amoxicillin-clavulanate is recommended for severe symptoms, worsening symptoms, or persistent symptoms beyond 13 d.
					• Improvement of symptoms should occur within 72 h of antibiotic initiation.	http://www.guideline.gov/content.aspx?id=46939

Sinusitis	ACEP	2013		Avoid prescribing antibiotics in the ER for patients presenting with uncomplicated acute sinusitis.		http://www.choosingwisely.org/societies/american-college-of-emergency-physicians/

RESTLESS LEGS SYNDROME & PERIODIC LIMB MOVEMENT DISORDERS

Disease Management	Organization	Date	Population	Recommendations	Comments	Source

Restless Legs Syndrome and Periodic Limb Movement Disorders	American Academy of Sleep Medicine	2012	Adults	• Recommended treatments for restless legs syndrome (RLS):
				  ○ Dopaminergic medication
				    – Pramipexole
				    – Ropinirole
				  ○ Second-line agents
				    – Carbidopa/levodopa
				    – Opioids
				  ○ Third-line agents
				    – Gabapentin
				    – Pregabalin
				    – Carbamazepine
				    – Clonidine
				  ○ Consider iron supplementation for RLS with low ferritin levels
					• Potential for heart valve damage with Pergolide and Cabergoline.
					• Insufficient evidence to support any pharmacological treatment for periodic limb movement disorder.
						www.guidelines.gov/content.aspx?id=38320

Disease Management	**Organization**	**Date**	**Population**	**Recommendations**	**Comments**	**Source**

Rheumatoid Arthritis (RA), Biologic Disease-Modifying Antirheumatic Drugs (DMARDs)	ACR	2008	Adults	1. Anti–TNF-α agents
				  a. A tuberculosis (TB) skin test or IGRA must be checked before initiating these medications
				  b. Any patient with latent TB needs at least 1 mo treatment prior to the initiation of a TNF-α or biologic agent.
				  c. Recommended for all patients with high disease activity and presence of poor prognostic features of any duration of disease
				2. Recommended for patients with disease ≥6 mo who have failed nonbiologic DMARD therapy and have moderate-high disease activity, especially if poor prognostic features are present.
				3. Abatacept has same indications as anti–TNF-α agents.
				4. Rituximab has same indications as a ti–TNF-α agents.
				5. Recommends withholding all biologic DMARDs 1 wk before or after surgery.
					1. Anti–TNF-α agents, abatacept, and rituximab all contraindicated in:
					  a. Serious bacterial, fungal, and viral infections, or with latent TB
					  b. Acute viral hepatitis or Child's B or Child's C cirrhosis
					  c. Instances of a lymphoproliferative disorder treated ≤5 y ago; decompensated congestive heart failure (CHF); or any demyelinating disorder
						http://www.rheumatology.org/practice/clinical/guidelines/Singh_ACR_RA_GL_May_2012_AC-R.pdf

	ACR	2012	Adults	1. Target low disease activity or remission.
				2. MTX or leflunomide monotherapy may be used for patients with any disease severity or duration
				3. Hydroxychloroquine or minocycline monotherapy recommended if low disease activity and duration ≤24 mo.
				4. Sulfasalazine recommended for all d sease durations and without poor prognostic features.[a]
				5. MTX plus either hydroxychloroquine or leflunomide recommended for moderate-tc–high disease activity regardless of disease duration.
				6. MTX plus sulfasalazine recommended for high disease activity and poor prognostic features.
					1. Contraindications to DMARD therapy:
					  a. Serious bacterial, fungal, or viral infections
					  b. Only DMARDs safe with latent TB are hydroxychloroquine, minocycline, and sulfasalazine
					  c. Avoid MTX for interstitial pneumonitis and for creatinine clearance <30 mL/min
					  d. Avoid MTX and leflunomide for cytopenias, hepatitis, pregnancy, and breastfeeding (also minocycline)
					  e. Avoid all DMARDs in Child's B or Child's C cirrhosis
						http://www.rheumatology.org/practice/clinical/guidelines/Singh_ACR_RA_GL_May_2012_AC-R.pdf

[a]Functional limitation, presence of rheumatoid nodules, secondary Sjögren syndrome, RA vasculitis, Felty syndrome, and RA lung disease.

RHEUMATOID ARTHRITIS (RA), BIOLOGIC DISEASE-MODIFYING ANTIRHEUMATIC DRUGS (DMARDs)

MANAGEMENT OF NONINFECTIOUS RHINITIS
Sources: ICSI, JANUARY 2011 AND AAO-HNS 2015

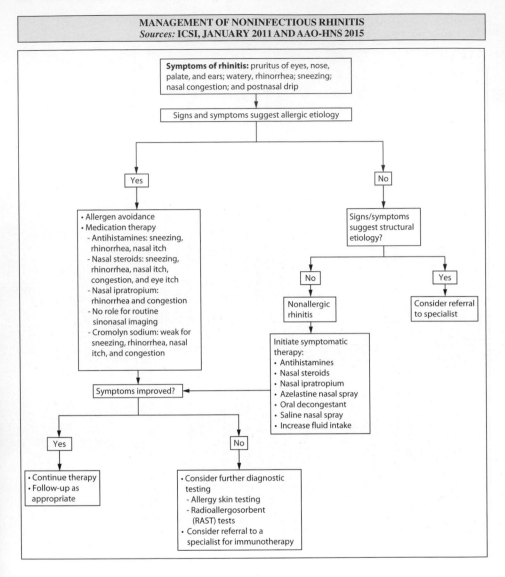

Symptoms of rhinitis: pruritus of eyes, nose, palate, and ears; watery, rhinorrhea; sneezing; nasal congestion; and postnasal drip

Signs and symptoms suggest allergic etiology

Yes

- Allergen avoidance
- Medication therapy
  - Antihistamines: sneezing, rhinorrhea, nasal itch
  - Nasal steroids: sneezing, rhinorrhea, nasal itch, congestion, and eye itch
  - Nasal ipratropium: rhinorrhea and congestion
  - No role for routine sinonasal imaging
  - Cromolyn sodium: weak for sneezing, rhinorrhea, nasal itch, and congestion

No

Signs/symptoms suggest structural etiology?

No

Nonallergic rhinitis

Yes

Consider referral to specialist

Initiate symptomatic therapy:
- Antihistamines
- Nasal steroids
- Nasal ipratropium
- Azelastine nasal spray
- Oral decongestant
- Saline nasal spray
- Increase fluid intake

Symptoms improved?

Yes

- Continue therapy
- Follow-up as appropriate

No

- Consider further diagnostic testing
  - Allergy skin testing
  - Radioallergosorbent (RAST) tests
- Consider referral to a specialist for immunotherapy

SEIZURES

Disease Management	Organization	Date	Population	Recommendations	Comments	Source

Seizures, Febrile	AAP	2011	Children 6 mo to 5 y old	• A lumbar puncture should be performed in any child who presents with a fever and seizure and has meningeal signs or whose history is concerning for meningitis.
				• Lumbar puncture is an option in children 6–12 mo of age who present with a fever and seizure and are not up to date with their *Haemophilus influenzae* or *Streptococcus pneumoniae* vaccinations.
				• Lumbar puncture is an option in a child presenting with a fever and a seizure who has been pretreated with antibiotics.
				• Studies that should not be performed for a simple febrile seizure:
				  ○ An EEG
				  ○ Routine labs including a basic metabolic panel, calcium, phosphorus, magnesium, glucose, or CBC
				  ○ Neuroimaging
					• A febrile seizure is a seizure accompanied by fever (T ≥100.4°F [38°C]) without CNS infection in a child age 6 mo to 5 y.	http://pediatrics.aappublications.org/content/127/2/389.full.pdf+html

Seizures	ACEP	2014	Adults	1. For first generalized convulsive seizure, ED physicians need not initiate chronic antiepileptic therapy.
				  a. A precipitating medical condition should be sought.
				  b. Need not admit patients who have returned to their clinical baseline.
				2. If known seizure disorder, antiepileptic therapy in ED can be administered orally or by IV.
				3. For status epilepticus:
				  a. First-line therapy is benzodiazepines
				  b. Options for second line therapy: phenytoin, fosphenytoin, valproic acid, levetiracetam
					For refractory status epilepticus, consider intubation and use of a propofol infusion.	http://www.guideline.gov/content.aspx?id=47921

SEXUALLY TRANSMITTED DISEASES TREATMENT GUIDELINES
ADAPTED FROM CDC GUIDELINES, *MMWR Recomm Rep.* 2010;59(RR-12):1-116

Infection	Recommended Treatment	Alternative Treatment
Chancroid	• Azithromycin 1 g PO × 1 • Ceftriaxone 250 mg IM × 1	• Ciprofloxacin 500 mg PO bid for 3 d • Erythromycin base 500 mg PO tid for 7 d
First episode of genital HSV	• Acyclovir 400 mg PO tid × 7–10 d[a] • Famciclovir 250 mg PO tid × 7–10 d[a] • Valacyclovir 1 g PO bid × 7–10 d[a]	• Acyclovir 200 mg PO 5 times a day for 7–10 d[a]
Suppressive therapy for genital HSV	• Acyclovir 400 mg PO bid • Famciclovir 250 mg PO bid	• Valacyclovir 1 g PO daily
Episodic therapy for recurrent genital HSV	• Acyclovir 400 mg PO tid × 5 d • Famciclovir 125 mg PO bid × 5 d • Valacyclovir 500 mg PO bid × 3 d	• Acyclovir 800 mg PO bid × 5 d • Acyclovir 800 mg PO tid × 2 d • Famciclovir 1000 mg PO bid × 1 d • Famciclovir 500 mg PO × 1 then 250 mg bid × 2 d • Valacyclovir 1 g PO daily × 5 d
Suppressive therapy for HIV-positive patients	• Acyclovir 400–800 mg PO bid-tid • Famciclovir 500 mg PO bid • Valacyclovir 500 mg PO bid	
Episodic therapy for recurrent genital HSV in HIV-positive patients	• Acyclovir 400 mg PO tid × 5–10 d • Famciclovir 500 mg PO bid × 5–10 d • Valacyclovir 1 g PO bid × 5–10 d	
Granuloma inguinale (Donovanosis)	• Doxycycline 100 mg PO bid × ≥3 wk and until all lesions have completely healed	• Azithromycin 1 g PO weekly × ≥3 wk • Ciprofloxacin 750 mg PO bid × ≥3 wk • Erythromycin base 500 mg PO QID × ≥3 wk • TMP-SMX 1 double-strength (160/800 mg) tablet PO bid × ≥3 wk • Continue all of these treatments until all lesions have completely healed
Lymphogranuloma venereum	• Doxycycline 100 mg PO bid for × 21 d	• Erythromycin base 500 mg PO qid × 21 d
Syphilis in adults	• Benzathine penicillin G 2.4 million units IM × 1	
Syphilis in infants and children	• Benzathine penicillin G 50,000 units/kg IM, up to the adult dose of 2.4 million units × 1	
Early latent syphilis in adults	• Benzathine penicillin G 2.4 million units IM × 1	
Early latent syphilis in children	• Benzathine penicillin G 50,000 units/kg IM, up to the adult dose of 2.4 million units × 1	
Late latent syphilis or latent syphilis of unknown duration in adults	• Benzathine penicillin G 2.4 million units IM weekly × 3 doses	
Late latent syphilis or latent syphilis of unknown duration in children	• Benzathine penicillin G 50,000 units/kg, up to the adult dose of 2.4 million units, IM weekly × 3 doses	
Tertiary syphilis	• Benzathine penicillin G 2.4 million units IM weekly × 3 doses	
Neurosyphilis	• Aqueous crystalline penicillin G 3–4 million units IV q4h × 10–14 d	• Procaine penicillin 2.4 million units IM daily × 10–14 d **PLUS** • Probenecid 500 mg PO QID × 10–14 d
Syphilis, pregnant women	• Pregnant women should be treated with the penicillin regimen appropriate for their stage of infection	
Congenital syphilis	• Aqueous crystalline penicillin G 50,000 units/kg/dose IV q12h × 7 d; then q8h × 3 more days	• Procaine penicillin G 50,000 units/kg/dose IM daily × 10 d • Benzathine penicillin G 50,000 units/kg/dose IM × 1
Older children with syphilis	• Aqueous crystalline penicillin G 50,000 units/kg IV q4–6h × 10 days	
Nongonococcal urethritis	• Azithromycin 1 g PO × 1 • Doxycycline 100 mg PO bid × 7 d	• Erythromycin base 500 mg PO QID × 7 d • Erythromycin ethylsuccinate 800 mg PO QID × 7 d • Levofloxacin 500 mg PO daily × 7 d • Ofloxacin 300 mg PO bid × 7 d
Recurrent or persistent urethritis	• Metronidazole 2 g PO × 1 • Tinidazole 2 g PO × 1 • Azithromycin 1 g PO × 1	

	SEXUALLY TRANSMITTED DISEASES TREATMENT GUIDELINES (CONTINUED) ADAPTED FROM CDC GUIDELINES, *MMWR Recomm Rep.* 2010;59(RR-12):1-116	
Infection	**Recommended Treatment**	**Alternative Treatment**
Cervicitis[b]	• Azithromycin 1 g PO × 1 • Doxycycline 100 mg PO bid × 7 d	
Chlamydia infections in adolescents, adults[b]	• Azithromycin 1 g PO × 1 • Doxycycline 100 mg PO bid × 7 d	• Erythromycin base 500 mg PO QID × 7 d • Erythromycin ethylsuccinate 800 mg PO QID × 7 d • Levofloxacin 500 mg PO daily × 7 d • Ofloxacin 300 mg PO BID × 7 d
Chlamydia infections in pregnancy[b]	• Azithromycin 1 g PO × 1 • Amoxicillin 500 mg PO tid × 7 d	• Erythromycin base 500 mg PO QID × 7 d • Erythromycin ethylsuccinate 800 mg PO QID × 7 d
Ophthalmia neonatorum from *Chlamydia*	• Erythromycin base or ethylsuccinate 50 mg/kg/day PO QID × 14 d	
Chlamydia trachomatis pneumonia in infants	• Erythromycin base or ethylsuccinate 50 mg/kg/day PO QID × 14 d	
Chlamydia infections in children <45 kg	• Erythromycin base or ethylsuccinate 50 mg/kg/day PO QID × 14 d	
Chlamydia infections in children ≥45 kg and age <8 y	• Azithromycin 1 g PO × 1	
Chlamydia infections in children age ≥8 y	• Azithromycin 1 g PO × 1 • Doxycycline 100 mg PO bid × 7 d	
Uncomplicated gonococcal infections of the cervix, urethra, pharynx, or rectum in adults or children >45 kg	• Ceftriaxone 250 mg IM × 1 **PLUS** • Azithromycin 1 g PO × 1 **OR** • Doxycycline 100 mg daily × 7 d	
Gonococcal conjunctivitis in adults or children >45 kg	• Ceftriaxone 1 g IM × 1	
Gonococcal meningitis or endocarditis in adults or children >45 kg	• Ceftriaxone 1 g IV q12h	
Disseminated gonococcal infection in adults or children >45 kg	• Ceftriaxone 1 g IV/IM daily	• Cefotaxime 1 g IV q8h • Ceftizoxime 1 g IV q8h
Ophthalmia neonatorum caused by gonococcus	• Ceftriaxone 25–50 mg/kg, not to exceed 125 mg, IV/IM × 1	
Prophylactic treatment of infants born to mothers with gonococcal infection	• Ceftriaxone 25–50 mg/kg, not to exceed 125 mg, IV/IM × 1	
Uncomplicated gonococcal infections of the cervix, urethra, pharynx, or rectum in children ≤45 kg	• Ceftriaxone 125 mg IM × 1	
Gonococcal infections with bacteremia or arthritis in children or adults	• Ceftriaxone 50 mg/kg (maximum dose 1 g) IM/IV daily × 7 d	
Ophthalmia neonatorum prophylaxis	• Erythromycin (0.5%) ophthalmic ointment in each eye × 1	
Bacterial vaginosis	• Metronidazole 500 mg PO bid × 7 d[c] • Metronidazole gel 0.75%, 1 applicator (5 g) IVag daily × 5 d • Clindamycin cream 2%, 1 applicator (5 g) IVag qhs × 7 d[d]	• Tinidazole 2 g PO daily × 3 d • Clindamycin 300 mg PO bid × 7 d • Clindamycin ovules 100 mg IVag qhs × 3 d
Bacterial vaginosis in pregnancy	• Metronidazole 500 mg PO bid × 7 d • Metronidazole 250 mg PO tid × 7 d • Clindamycin 300 mg PO bid × 7 d	

SEXUALLY TRANSMITTED DISEASES TREATMENT GUIDELINES (CONTINUED)
ADAPTED FROM CDC GUIDELINES, *MMWR Recomm Rep.* **2010;59(RR-12):1-116**

Infection	Recommended Treatment	Alternative Treatment
Trichomoniasis	• Metronidazole 2 g PO × 1[c] • Tinidazole 2 g PO × 1	• Metronidazole 500 mg PO bid × 7 d[c]
Candidal vaginitis	• Butoconazole 2% cream 5 g IVag × 3 d • Clotrimazole 1% cream 5 g IVag × 7–14 d • Clotrimazole 2% cream 5 g IVag × 3 d • Nystatin 100,000-unit vaginal tablet, 1 tablet IVag × 14 d • Miconazole 2% cream 5 g IVag × 7 d • Miconazole 4% cream 5 g IVag × 3 d • Miconazole 100-mg vaginal suppository, one suppository IVag × 7 d • Miconazole 200-mg vaginal suppository, one suppository IVag × 3 d • Miconazole 1200-mg vaginal suppository, one suppository IVag × 1 • Tioconazole 6.5% ointment 5 g IVag × 1 • Terconazole 0.4% cream 5 g IVag × 7 d • Terconazole 0.8% cream 5 g IVag × 3 d • Terconazole 80-mg vaginal suppository, 1 suppository IVag × 3 d	• Fluconazole 150-mg oral tablet, 1 tablet in single dose
Severe pelvic inflammatory disease	• Cefotetan 2 g IV q12h **OR** • Cefoxitin 2 g IV q6h **PLUS** • Doxycycline 100 mg PO/IV bid	• Clindamycin 900 mg IV q8h **PLUS** • Gentamicin loading dose IV or IM (2 mg/kg of body weight), followed by a maintenance dose (1.5 mg/kg) q8h. Single daily dosing (3–5 mg/kg) can be substituted. **OR** • Ampicillin/sulbactam 3 g IV q6h **PLUS** • Doxycycline 100 mg PO/IV bid
Mild-moderate pelvic inflammatory disease	• Ceftriaxone 250 mg IM × 1 OR • Cefoxitin 2 g IM × 1 and probenecid 1 g PO × 1 **PLUS** • Doxycycline 100 mg PO bid × 14 d ± metronidazole 500 mg PO bid × 14 d[c]	
Epididymitis	• Ceftriaxone 250 mg IM × 1 **PLUS** • Doxycycline 100 mg PO bid × 10 d	• Levofloxacin 500 mg PO daily × 10 d • Ofloxacin 300 mg PO BID × 10 d
External genital warts	**Provider-Administered:** • Cryotherapy every 1–2 wk • Podophyllin resin 10%–25% in a compound tincture of benzoin • TCA or BCA 80%–90% • Surgical removal either by tangential scissor excision, tangential shave excision, curettage, or electrosurgery	**Patient-Applied:** • Podofilox 0.5% solution or gel • Imiquimod 5% cream • Sinecatechins 15% ointment
Cervical warts	• Biopsy to exclude high-grade SIL must be performed before treatment is initiated	
Vaginal warts	• TCA or BCA 80%–90% applied only to warts, repeated weekly	
Urethral meatal warts	• Cryotherapy every 1–2 wk • TCA or BCA 80%–90% applied only to warts, repeated weekly	
Anal warts	• Cryotherapy every 1–2 wk • TCA or BCA 80%–90% applied only to warts, repeated weekly	• Surgical removal either by tangential scissor excision, tangential shave excision, curettage, or electrosurgery
Proctitis	• Ceftriaxone 250 mg IM × 1 **PLUS** • Doxycycline 100 mg PO bid × 7 d	

SEXUALLY TRANSMITTED DISEASES TREATMENT GUIDELINES (CONTINUED) ADAPTED FROM CDC GUIDELINES, *MMWR Recomm Rep.* 2010;59(RR-12):1-116		
Infection	**Recommended Treatment**	**Alternative Treatment**
Pediculosis pubis	• Permethrin 1% cream rinse applied to affected areas and washed off after 10 min • Pyrethrins with piperonyl butoxide applied to the affected area and washed off after 10 min	• Malathion 0.5% lotion applied for 8–12 h and then washed off • Ivermectin 250 µg/kg PO, repeated in 2 wk
Scabies	• Permethrin cream (5%) applied to all areas of the body from the neck down and washed off after 8–14 h • Ivermectin 200 µg/kg PO, repeat in 2 wk	• Lindane (1%) 1 oz of lotion (or 30 g of cream) applied in a thin layer to all areas of the body from the neck down and thoroughly washed off after 8 h

BCA, bichloracetic acid; bid, twice a day; h, hour(s); HIV, human immunodeficiency virus; HSV, herpes simplex virus; IM, intramuscular; IV, intravenous; IVag, intravaginally; PO, by mouth; q, every; qhs, at bedtime; QID, four 4 times a day; SIL, squamous intraepithelial lesion; TCA, trichloroacetic acid; tid, three 3 times a day; TMP-SMX, trimethoprim-sulfamethoxazole.
[a]Treatment can be extended if healing is incomplete after 10 d of therapy.
[b]Consider concomitant treatment of gonorrhea.
[c]Avoid alcohol during treatment and for 24 h after treatment is completed.
[d]Clindamycin cream may weaken latex condoms and diaphragms during treatment and for 5 d thereafter.

SINUSITIS, ACUTE BACTERIAL

Secondary Prevention	Organization	Date	Population	Recommendations	Comments	Source

Sinusitis, Acute Bacterial	AAP	2013	Children aged 1–18 y	• Presumptive diagnosis of acute bacterial sinusitis when a child with a URI presents with:
				  ○ Persistent symptoms without improvement for over 10 d
				  ○ Worsening course
				  ○ Severe onset (T >102.2°F and purulent rhinorrhea for at least 3 d)
				• Recommend against imaging studies to differentiate viral URI from bacterial sinusitis.
				• Recommend a CT or MRI with contrast of the paranasal sinuses if globe or CNS complications from sinusitis are suspected.
				• Amoxicillin or amoxicillin-clavulanate is recommended for severe symptoms, worsening symptoms, or persistent symptoms beyond 13 d.
					• Improvement of symptoms should occur within 72 h of antibiotic initiation.	http://www.guideline.gov/content.aspx?id=46939

2014 AHA/ASA GUIDELINES FOR SECONDARY PREVENTION OF STROKE IN PATIENTS WITH STROKE AND TIA

Secondary Prevention	Organization	Date	Population	Recommendations	Comments	Source
Stroke Recurrence	AHA/ASA	2014	Atrial fibrillation	1. For most patients with a stroke or TIA in the setting of AF, it is reasonable to initiate oral anticoagulation within 14 d after the onset of neurological symptoms. In the presence of high risk for hemorrhagic conversion (ie, large infarct, hemorrhagic transformation on initial imaging, uncontrolled hypertension, or hemorrhage tendency), it is reasonable to delay initiation of oral anticoagulation beyond 14 d. 2. VKA therapy (Class I; Level of Evidence A), apixaban (Class I; Level of Evidence A), and dabigatran (Class I; Level of Evidence B) are all indicated for the prevention of recurrent stroke in patients with nonvalvular AF, whether paroxysmal or permanent. Rivaroxaban is reasonable for the prevention of recurrent stroke in patients with nonvalvular AF. 3. For patients with ischemic stroke or TIA and AF who are unable to take oral anticoagulants, aspirin alone is recommended. The addition of clopidogrel to aspirin therapy might be reasonable. 4. The usefulness of closure of the left atrial appendage with the WATCHMAN device in patients with ischemic stroke or TIA and AF is uncertain.		Guidelines for the Prevention of Stroke in Patients With Stroke and Transient Ischemic Attack. A Guideline for Healthcare Professionals From the American Heart Association/American Stroke Association. *Stroke*. 2014:45. http://stroke.ahajournals.org
			Hypertension	• Initiation of BP therapy is indicated for previously untreated patients with ischemic stroke or TIA who after the first several days have an established SBP ≥140 mm Hg or DBP ≥90 mm Hg. In patients previously treated for HTN, resumption of BP therapy is indicated beyond the first several days for both prevention of recurrent stroke and other vascular events. Goals: <140/90 mm Hg; for recent lacunar stroke reasonable SBP target <130 mm Hg.		
			Dyslipidemia	• Intensive lipid-lowering effects are recommended in patients with ischemic stroke or TIA presumed to be of atherosclerotic origin, an LDL-C ≥100 mg/dL and with/without evidence of other clinical ASCVD.		
			Glucose disorders	• All patients should be screened for DM (HgbA1c).		
			Obesity	• Calculate BMI for all patients and start weight-loss management when necessary.		
			Sleep apnea	• A sleep study might be considered for patients with history of CVA or TIA on the basis of very high prevalence in this population.		
			MI and thrombus	• VKA therapy (INR: 2–3) for 3 mo may be considered in patients with ischemic stroke or TIA in the setting of acute anterior STEMI.		

2014 AHA/ASA GUIDELINES FOR SECONDARY PREVENTION OF STROKE IN PATIENTS WITH STROKE AND TIA (CONTINUED)

Secondary Prevention	Organization	Date	Population	Recommendations	Comments	Source
Stroke Recurrence (continued)			Cardiomyopathy	• In patients with ischemic stroke or TIA in sinus rhythm who have left atrial or left ventricular thrombus demonstrated by echocardiography or other imaging modality, anticoagulant therapy with a VKA is recommended for ≥3 mo.		
			Valvular heart disease	• For patients with ischemic stroke or TIA who have rheumatic mitral valve disease and AF, long-term VKA therapy with an INR target of 2.5 (range, 2.0–3.0) is recommended. • For patients with ischemic stroke or TIA and native aortic or nonrheumatic mitral valve disease who do not have AF or another indication for anticoagulation, antiplatelet therapy is recommended.		
			Prosthetic heart valve	• For patients with a mechanical aortic valve and a history of ischemic stroke or TIA before its insertion, VKA therapy is recommended with an INR target of 2.5 (range, 2.0–3.0). • For patients with a mechanical mitral valve and a history of ischemic stroke or TIA before its insertion, VKA therapy is recommended with an INR target of 3.0 (range, 2.5–3.5). • For patients with a mechanical mitral or aortic valve who have a history of ischemic stroke or TIA before its insertion and who are at low risk for bleeding, the addition of aspirin 75 to 100 mg/d to VKA therapy is recommended. • For patients with a bioprosthetic aortic or mitral valve, a history of ischemic stroke or TIA before its insertion, and no other indication for anticoagulation therapy beyond 3 to 6 mo from the valve placement, long-term therapy with aspirin 75 to 100 mg/d is recommended in preference to long-term anticoagulation.		
			Aortic arch atheroma	• For patients with an ischemic stroke or TIA and evidence of aortic arch atheroma, antiplatelet therapy is recommended.		
			PFO	• For patients with an ischemic stroke or TIA and a PFO who are not undergoing anticoagulation therapy, antiplatelet therapy is recommended. • For patients with an ischemic stroke or TIA and both a PFO and a venous source of embolism, anticoagulation is indicated, depending on stroke characteristics. When anticoagulation is contraindicated, an inferior vena cava filter is reasonable. • For patients with a cryptogenic ischemic stroke or TIA and a PFO without evidence for DVT, available data do not support a benefit for PFO closure. • In the setting of PFO and DVT, PFO closure by a transcatheter device might be considered, depending on the risk of recurrent DVT.		
			Homocysteinemia	• Routine screening for hyperhomocysteinemia among patients with a recent ischemic stroke or TIA is not indicated.		
			Hypercoagulation	• The usefulness of screening for thrombophilic states in patients with ischemic stroke or TIA is unknown. • Antiplatelet therapy is recommended in patients who are found to have abnormal findings on coagulation testing after an initial ischemic stroke or TIA if anticoagulation therapy is not administered.		

2014 AHA/ASA GUIDELINES FOR SECONDARY PREVENTION OF STROKE IN PATIENTS WITH STROKE AND TIA (CONTINUED)

Secondary Prevention	Organization	Date	Population	Recommendations	Comments	Source
Stroke Recurrence (continued)			**Sickle cell disease**	• For patients with sickle cell disease ad prior ischemic stroke or TIA, chronic blood transfusions to reduce hemoglobin S to <30% of total hemoglobin are recommended.		

			Pregnancy	• In the presence of a high-risk condition that would require anticoagulation outside of pregnancy, the following options are reasonable:
				  a. LMWH twice daily throughout pregnancy, with dose adjusted to achieve the LMWH manufacturer's recommended peak anti-Xa level 4 h after injection, or
				  b. Adjusted-dose UFH throughout pregnancy, administered subcutaneously every 12 h in doses adjusted to keep the midinterval aPTT at least twice control or to maintain an anti-Xa heparin level of 0.35 to 0.70 U/mL, or
				  c. UFH or LMWH (as above) until the 13th week, followed by substitution of a VKA until close to delivery, when UFH or LMWH is resumed
				• For pregnant women receiving adjusted-dose LMWH therapy for a high-risk condition that would require anticoagulation outside of pregnancy, and when delivery is planned, it is reasonable to discontinue LMWH ≥24 h before induction of labor or cesarean section.
				• In the presence of a low-risk situation in which antiplatelet therapy would be the treatment recommendation outside of pregnancy, UFH or LMWH, or no treatment may be considered during the first trimester of pregnancy depending on the clinical situation.		

			Breastfeeding	• In the presence of a high-risk condition that would require anticoagulation outside of pregnancy, it is reasonable to use warfarin, UFH, or LMWH. • In the presence of a low-risk situation in which antiplatelet therapy would be the treatment recommendation outside of pregnancy, low-dose aspirin use may be considered.		

AHA/ASA ISCHEMIC STROKE GUIDELINES 2013

- Physicians should use *stroke assessment tools* like the Cincinnati Prehospital Stroke Scale or the Los Angles Prehospital Stroke Screen to aid in prompt assessment.
- The role of *9-1-1 emergency systems* should be recommended to ensure prompt transport of patients to the appropriate emergency system.
- Physicians should encourage their local hospitals to become *Primary Care Centers* or *Comprehensive Care Centers*.
- *Neurology imaging* is essential. If not available, teleradiology systems should be encouraged to allow for prompt diagnosis.
- A multidisciplinary *stroke team* should be established including physicians, nurses and laboratory and radiology personnel.
- An emergency department *stroke protocol* should exist to allow prompt evaluation and initiation of fibrinolytic treatment within 60 min. This should include a stroke severity scale such as NIHSS.
- Noncontrast CT of the head is the first imaging test suggested to exclude intracerebral hemorrhage. A noncontrast CT or MRI is recommended before fibrinolysis is started. These tests should be interpreted within 45 min of patient's arrival.
- Consideration of intravenous recombinant tissue-type plasminogen activator (rtPA) should be considered in all ischemic stroke patients who meet the indications and have no exclusion criteria.
- Imaging with noncontrast CT or MRI imaging is indicated in all patients presenting with transient neurologic symptoms (TIA). The MRI is the test of choice. The test should be performed within 24 h of presentation.
- Sources of hyperthermia should be investigated and treatment should be started.
- Hypertension for hypertension during a stroke should be withheld until BP 220/120 mm Hg. If the BP exceeds that level, it should be lowered by 15% during the first 24 h. BP goals are lower if the patient is to receive rtPA.
- Treat persistent hyperglycemia at ranges of 140–180 mg/dL.
- Intravenous rtPA should be administered to all eligible patients even if intraarterial treatments are being considered. Intraarterial fibrinolysis should be considered with major strokes of <6 h duration involving the middle cerebral artery. This procedure should be performed only in stroke centers.
- Urgent anticoagulation to prevent recurrent stroke or improve symptoms is not recommended.
- Aspirin within 24–48 h after stroke is recommended. ASA administration within 24 h postfibrinolysis is not recommended.
- Stroke Units, which give comprehensive specialized stroke care, are recommended.

Source: Jauch EC, Saver JL, Adams HP, et al. Guidelines for the early management of patients with acute ischemic stroke. Guideline for healthcare professionals from the American Heart Association/American Stroke Association. *Stroke.* 2013;44:870-947.

INTRACRANIAL STROKEAHA/ASA GUIDELINES 2014

- For patients with recent (<30 d) stroke or TIA attributable to severe stenosis (70%–99%) of a major intracranial artery, the addition of Clopidogrel 75 mg daily in addition to ASA for 90 days might be reasonable.
- The combination of aspirin and clopidogrel might be considered for initiation within 24 h of a minor ischemic stroke or TIA and for continuation for 90 d.
- For patients with a stroke or TIA attributable to 50%–99% stenosis of a major intracranial artery, maintenance of SBP <140 mm Hg, and high-intensity statin therapy are recommended.
- For patients with a stroke or TIA attributable to moderate stenosis (50%–69%) of a major intracranial artery, angioplasty or stenting is not recommended given the low rate of stroke on medical management and the inherent periprocedural risk of endovascular treatment.
- For patients with stroke or TIA attributable to severe stenosis (70%–99%) of a major intracranial artery, stenting with the Wingspan stent system is not recommended as an initial treatment, even for patients who were taking an antithrombotic agent at the time of the stroke or TIA.
- For patients with stroke or TIA attributable to severe stenosis (70%–99%) of a major intracranial artery, the usefulness of angioplasty alone or placement of stents other than the Wingspan stent is unknown and is considered investigational.
- For patients with severe stenosis (70%–99%) of a major intracranial artery and recurrent TIA or stroke after institution of aspirin and clopidogrel therapy, achievement of systolic BP <140 mm Hg, and high-intensity statin therapy, the usefulness of angioplasty alone or placement of a Wingspan stent or other stents is unknown and is considered investigational.

Source: Bushnell C, McCullough LD, Awad IA, et al. Guidelines for the prevention of stroke in women a Statement for healthcare professionals from the American Heart Association/American Stroke Association. *Stroke.* 2014;45. doi: 10.1161/01.str.0000442009.06663.48.

SYPHILIS

Disease Management	Organization	Date	Population	Recommendations	Comments	Source

Syphilis	IDSA	2011	Adults	• Penicillin G 2.4 million units is drug of choice for early syphilis.
				• Cerebrospinal fluid (CSF) analysis is indicated if:
				  ○ Early syphilis infection and neurologic symptoms
				  ○ Late latent syphilis
				• HIV-infected patients with rapid plasma reagent (RPR) titer ≥1:32 or CD4 <350 cells/mm³.
				• Patients with early syphilis do not achieve a ≥4-fold decline in RPR titers within 12 mo.
				• Doxycycline is second-line therapy for early syphilis in penicillin-allergic patients.
				• Ceftriaxone is second-line therapy for neurosyphilis in penicillin-allergic patients.
					• Avoid doxycycline in pregnancy.	http://cid.oxfordjournals.org/content/53/suppl_3/S110.abstract

IMMUNE THROMBOCYTOPENIA PURPURA (ITP)

Disease Management	Organization	Population	Recommendations	Comments	Source
Immune Thrombocytopenia Purpura (ITP)	American Society of Hematology (ASH) 2011—evidence-based practice guidelines for ITP	Adults	• **Diagnosis**—diagnosis of exclusion—no reliable diagnostic test (including antiplatelet antibody studies). Bone marrow examination not necessary irrespective of age in patients with typical ITP (healthy with isolated thrombocytopenia with large normal-appearing platelets on peripheral blood smear). Testing patients for underlying hepatitis C and HIV is recommended. Testing for another underlying illness (rheumatologic disorders, lymphoproliferative disease, *Helicobacter pylori* infection, antiphospholipid syndrome) is based on history and physical exam. • **Treatment of newly diagnosed ITP** Treat if platelet count <30,000 with or without bleeding. Longer courses of corticosteroids (prednisone 0.5–2 mg/kg daily with taper) is preferred over shorter courses of high-dose corticosteroids or intravenous immune globulin (IVIG). IVIG should be used with corticosteroids when a more rapid rise in platelet count is required. Either IVIG or anti-D immune globulin (in patients that are Rh(+) and spleen in place) can be used as first-line therapy if corticosteroids are contraindicated. Dose of IVIG should be 1 g/kg as a one-time dose that may be repeated if necessary (see Table I). • **Treatment of patients who are unresponsive or relapse after initial therapy** Splenectomy either laparoscopic or open at least 2–4 wk after vaccination with pneumococcal, meningococcal, and *Haemophilus influenzae* b vaccine. Thrombopoietin receptor agonists (romiplostim or eltrombopag) are recommended for patients at risk for bleeding who relapse after splenectomy or who have contraindication to splenectomy and who have failed one other therapy. (*Lancet*. 2008;371:537)	• Be aware of autosomal dominant hereditary macrothrombocytopenia. Platelets are large, hypogranular, and misshapen with counts between 30 and 60,000. Bleeding is modest but is often confused with ITP. The treatment is with platelet transfusion for significant bleeding. Treatment for ITP is ineffective. • TTP (thrombotic thrombocytopenic purpura) should always be excluded. These patients will be ill with low-grade fever, muscle aches, chest pain, and altered mental status. They will have thrombocytopenia and a hemolytic anemia with red cell fragmentation, elevated reticulocyte count, and significant elevation of lactate dehydrogenase. This is a medical emergency and should be treated urgently with plasma exchange. • In the elderly, myelodysplastic syndrome is common, but isolated thrombocytopenia occurs in <10%. ITP is by far the most common cause of isolated thrombocytopenia, even in elderly patients. • Treating patients for active *H. pylori* infection with new-onset ITP will result in a durable complete remission in up to 50% of patients. • Be alert to pseudothrombocytopenia caused by platelet clumping in response to ethylenediaminetetraacetic acid (EDTA). Review the peripheral smear or repeat the platelet count in a citrated tube to make the diagnosis. • Platelet transfusion should be considered along with standard therapy when there is life-threatening hemorrhage (usually brain or GI tract). The platelet count usually will not rise significantly, but bleeding can be slowed. Do not give prophylactic platelets based on platelet counts <5000 or for minor bleeding. • Anti-D immune globulin therapy is associated with disseminated intravascular coagulation (DIC) and resultant death. Close monitoring of patients is required.	*Blood.* 2011;117:4190-4207 *Blood.* 2010;115:168-186

Blood. 2013;121:537 (within Recommendations)

	IMMUNE THROMBOCYTOPENIA PURPURA (ITP)			
Disease Management	Organization	Population	Recommendations	Comments	Source

Immune Thrombocytopenia Purpura (ITP)

Recommendations

- Thrombopoietin receptor agonists can be used in patients at risk for bleeding who have failed one line of therapy but have not had a splenectomy. Response rate is 80%–90%. Rituximab may be considered in patients at risk of bleeding who have failed one line of therapy, including splenectomy. (*N Engl J Med.* 2011;366:734. *Blood.* 2014;124:3228;

- **Treatment of ITP after splenectomy** No further treatment in asymptomatic patients with platelet count >30,000. If platelets <30,000 second-line therapy (Rituxan, thrombopoietin receptor agonists, and immunosuppression) should be used (see Table II).

- **Treatment of ITP in pregnancy** In pregnant patients requiring therapy corticosteroids or IVIG should be used. For refractory patients splenectomy should be performed during second trimester. For pregnant women with ITP, mode of delivery is based upon obstetrical indications.

- **Treatment of specific forms of secondary ITP** (see Table III).

1. **HCV-associated**—antiviral therapy should be considered in absence of contraindications. Initial therapy in this setting should be IVIG.

2. **HIV-associated**—HIV treatment should be considered first unless patient has significant bleeding complications. If ITP therapy is required use corticosteroids, IVIG, anti-D immune globulin, and romiplostim or eltrombopag. Refractory patients should have a splenectomy.

3. **H. pylori-associated**—eradication therapy if active *H. pylori* infection found (stool Ag, urea breath test, endoscopic biopsy).

Comments

- Splenectomy is the most effective of all treatments for chronic ITP. 75%–80% of patients will achieve a remission with 60%–65% demonstrating durable response. Postsplenectomy sepsis is life-threatening—patients need to be educated and receive appropriate vaccinations (pneumococcal, meningococcal and *Haemophilus influenzae*). It is common practice for these patients to have a supply of antibiotics (eg. Levaquin, Augmentin) which can be started at the first sign of chills and fever as they begin their trip to the emergency department. (*Ann Intern Med.* 2009;151:546)

- More than half of patients with ITP have a reduction in platelet production, as well as enhanced peripheral destruction. Thrombopoietin agonists are small molecules that interact with the MPL receptor on bone marrow megakaryocytes causing maturation and proliferation of new platelet production. (*Blood.* 2013;121:537)

- In clinical trials, 80%–90% of patients who have failed initial primary therapy respond with platelet counts rising to more than 50,000. Thus far, toxicity has been minimal, with mild marrow fibrosis with romiplostim and liver enzyme elevation with eltrombopag. These 2 drugs have significantly altered our approach to treatment of ITP.

- Significant thrombocytopenia in infants of ITP mothers is infrequent (<10%) and intracranial bleeding is very rare. Platelets can drop precipitously in a newborn of an ITP mother in the first 5 d of life as the spleen rapidly matures. Infant platelet counts should be monitored.

- Drug-induced ITP is impossible to separate from idiopathic ITP except by history. The precipitating drug usually has been started within 2–3 wk of onset of ITP. Most common precipitating drugs include trimethoprim-sulfa, quinine, carbamazepine, and rifampin. Recovery of platelet count usually occurs within 1 wk, but patients with platelet counts <10,000 are usually treated with corticosteroids and IVIG although evidence for benefit is weak.

IMMUNE THROMBOCYTOPENIA PURPURA (ITP)

Disease Management	Organization	Population	Recommendations	Comments	Source
Immune Thrombocytopenia Purpura (ITP) (continued)	ASH	Pediatric	• Diagnosis. Bone marrow (BM) examination unnecessary in children and adolescents with typical features of ITP (isolated thrombocytopenia, large, morphologically normal platelets, asymptomatic except for bleeding). BM also not necessary in patients failing intravenous, IVIG therapy or before splenectomy. • Initial management. Children with no or mild bleeding (bruising, petechiae) can be managed with observation alone *regardless of platelet count*. For patients requiring therapy, a single dose of IVIG (0.8–1 g/kg) or short course corticosteroid should be used as first-line therapy. Anti-D immune globulin (WinRho) can be used as first-line therapy in Rh positive, nonsplenectomized children needing treatment. • Second-line treatment for pediatric. ITP—Rituximab can be considered if ongoing bleeding despite IVIG, anti-D immune globulin, and steroids. Rituximab can be considered an alternative to splenectomy or in patients not responding to splenectomy. High-dose dexamethasone (0.6/kg/d × 4 d q 4 wk) may be considered for patients with bleeding and persistent thrombocytopenia despite appropriate therapy. • Splenectomy—consider for children and adolescents with chronic ITP who have significant or persistent bleeding and lack of responsiveness or intolerance to other standard therapies. It is recommended not to do splenectomy for at least 12 mo after start of ITP treatment unless severe disease with significant serious bleeding risks. (*Blood.* 2013;121:4457-4462. *Blood.* 2010;115:168-186. *Pediatr Blood Cancer.* 2009;53:652-654 *Blood.* 2014;124:3295)	1. Measurement of immunoglobulin to exclude common variable immune deficiency (CVID) is common practice as ITP can be the presenting feature of CVID. 2. Study of 332 children with typical ITP with bone marrow—no leukemia—only 1 with BM aplasia. 3. Recommendation for treatment focuses on severity of bleeding not platelet cell count. In a study of 505 children with platelets <20,000 and skin bleeding only 3 patients developed severe bleeding but none had intracranial hemorrhage. 4. The older the child or adolescent, the more likely they are to have chronic ITP (defined as platelet count <150,000 at 6-mo follow-up). Rate for children age 3 mo–12 mo = 23%; children >12 mo and <10 y = 28%; and children >10 y = 47%. 5. Anti-D immune globulin therapy more effective at 75 vs 50 μg/kg, but increased toxicity including small percentage with DIC. Drop in hemoglobin averages 1.6 g/dL. 6. Response rate to splenectomy is 70%–80%, but unless child has severe unresponsive disease delay the splenectomy for at least 12 mo since 20%–30% will have spontaneous remission. Patients undergoing splenectomy should be immunized at least 2 weeks before surgery with pneumococcal, meningococcal, and *H. influenzae* type b vaccine. 7. Effectiveness of Rituximab varies from 20% to 50% in different trials. Serious side effects include serum sickness, severe hepatitis in hepatitis B carriers, and rare cases of multifocal leukoencephalopathy. 8. MMR (measles, mumps, rubella) vaccination-induced ITP occurs in 2.6 per 100,000 vaccine doses. ITP following natural measles or rubella infection ranges from 600 to 1200 per 100,000 cases, justifying the overall clinical benefit of the vaccine. 9. Thrombopoietin receptor agonists (romiplostim and eltrombopag) are active agents for ITP in adults but have not been adequately studied in children.	

THROMBOTIC THROMBOCYTOPENIA PURPURA (TTP)					
Disease Management	**Organization**	**Population**	**Recommendations**	**Comments**	**Source**
Thrombotic Thrombocytopenia Purpura (TTP)	2012 British Committee For Standards in Haematology (*Br J Haematol.* 2012; 150:323)	• Acquired TTP in adults and children	• Diagnosis of TTP should be made on clinical history, laboratory tests, and review of peripheral blood smear. Diagnosis suspected if evidence of Coombs-negative microangiopathic hemolytic anemia (MAHA), elevated lactate dehydrogenase (LDH), and thrombocytopenia. TTP should be treated as a medical emergency. ADAMTS-13 (von Willebrand factor [vWF] cleaving enzyme) is low in >90% of patients with TTP, but treatment should be started as rapidly as possible and not wait for test results to return. • Three units of fresh-frozen plasma should be given while a large-bore catheter is placed for plasma exchange, which should begin within 6 h of presentation. Serologic testing for HIV, hepatitis B and hepatitis C viruses, and autoantibodies should be done. Young women should have a pregnancy test. Plasma exchange (PEX) should be started with 1.5 plasma volume (PV) exchanges. The volume of exchange can be reduced to 1.0 PV as clinical conditions and lab studies improve. Intensification in frequency of PEX to twice a day should be considered if platelet count is not rising and LDH remains high. (*Transfusion.* 2008;48:349) Daily PEX should continue for a minimum of 2 days after platelet count >150,000 and then stopped. Steroids (usually 1 mg/kg of prednisone equivalent) is often given, although benefits uncertain. In patients with neurologic and/or cardiac pathology (associated with increased mortality), rituximab should be used at a dose of 375 mg/m² weekly for 4 doses. (*Blood.* 2011;118:1746. *N Engl J Med.* 2014;370:847) Cyclosporin or tacrolimus should be considered in patients with acute and chronic relapsing TTP. The benefit of aspirin in TTP is uncertain, but it is safe at a dose of 81 mg/d with a platelet count >50,000. In patients who relapse (~20% with majority in first 30 d)	1. Classic pentad of MAHA, thrombocytopenia, fever, CNS symptoms, hematuria—now most commonly MAHA and thrombocytopenia only at diagnosis. Time is critical to outcome. Expedited treatment associated with better survival. 2. Autoimmune disease with IgG antibody to ADAMTS-13 which prevents cleavage of large high-molecular-weight vWF. vWF binds to platelet receptor GPIB and the resulting complex obstructs the microvasculature leading to red cell fragmentation, thrombocytopenia, and organ ischemia. Plasma exchange is not a curative therapy, but protects the patient until antibody level declines either spontaneously or with use of corticosteroids and rituximab. 3. Mortality prior to intervention of plasma exchange in the early 1980s was 85%–90%; today the mortality is 10%–15%. 4. Prognosis can be predicted using the Wyllie index of adverse features including age >40 y, hemoglobin <9.0, and fever >100.5°F (38°C) at time of diagnosis. Predictions based on 0, 1, 2, or 3 of these features resulted in mortality at 6 months of 12.5%, 14.0%, 31.3%, and 61%, respectively. (*Br J Haematol.* 2005;132:204). 5. Precipitating factors associated with the onset of acquired TTP include drugs (quinine, ticlopidine, clopidogrel, simvastatin, trimethoprim, and interferon), HIV infection, and pregnancy (usually in the second trimester). Removal of the fetus has not shown to affect the course of TTP in pregnancy.	*Sem Throm Haemat.* 2006;32:81 *N Engl J Med.* 354:1927 *Br J Haematol.* 2008;142:819 *Transfusion.* 2010;50:868 *Br J Haematol.* 2011;153:277

THROMBOTIC THROMBOCYTOPENIA PURPURA (TTP)

Disease Management	Organization	Population	Recommendations	Comments	Source
Thrombotic Thrombocytopenia Purpura (TTP) (continued)			PEX should be restarted if platelets <50,000 with the addition of rituximab. If ADAMTS-13 level drops to <5% without a drop in platelets, rituximab alone should be considered. (*Blood.* 2010;116:4060) • Supportive Therapy 1. Red cell transfusion as clinically indicated. 2. Folate supplementation during active hemolysis. 3. Platelet transfusions are CONTRAINDICATED in TTP unless life-threatening hemorrhage. 4. Thromboprophylaxis with LMWH once platelet count >50,000.	6. Congenital TTP is rare, with <200 patients described worldwide. Onset usually is in later infancy or childhood. Patients may present as adults, with pregnancy a common precipitant. Diagnosis is made by ADAMTS-13 activity <5%, with absence of antibody and confirmation of mutations in ADAMTS-13 gene. Treatment is with fresh-frozen plasma administration prophylactically every 10–20 days. 7. Responding patients with acquired TTP will relapse at a rate of 20%–40%, most commonly in the first month following successful therapy. Studies show monitoring ADAMTS-13 levels and instituting rituximab proactively can decrease the rate of disease relapse. (*Br J Haematol* 2007; 136–145. *Blood.* 2011;118:1746) 8. Hemolytic uremic syndrome (HUS) clinically resembles TTP, but has a different pathophysiology, and PEX is of minimal benefit. This illness is commonly caused by bacterial toxins (*Shiga*-like toxin from *Escherichia coli*) or drugs (quinine, gemcitabine, mitomycin C). It is also associated with malignancy and autoimmune disease. In HUS, there is disruption of the endothelium and release of high-molecular-weight vWF that overwhelms the cleaving capacity of ADAMTS-13. An antibody to ADAMTS-13 is not involved. Renal failure dominates the clinical picture and 15%–20% succumb to the disease. (*Br J Haematol.* 2010;148:37) (*N Engl J Med.* 2014;371:654)	*Blood.* 2012;120:243

			HEPARIN-INDUCED THROMBOCYTOPENIA (HIT)	
Disease Management	Organization	Population	Recommendations	Comments
Heparin-Induced Thrombocytopenia (HIT)	ACCP 2012 ASH 2009	Adults	• Diagnosis—Maintain high suspicion. If no prior heparin in last 90 days, monitor platelet count every 2 d from days 4 to 14. If previous exposure to heparin within 90 days, monitor from day 1. If platelets drop 30%–50%, suspect HIT and use 4Ts scoring model (see Table IV) to assess likelihood of HIT. If intermediate-to-high probability, treat for HIT and send immunologic (enzyme-linked immunosorbent assay [ELISA] assay) and functional testing (platelet serotonin release assay). • Treatment—Stop all sources of heparin and give vitamin K if on warfarin to restore protein C and S. Begin a direct thrombin inhibitor (argatroban, or danaparoid). Fondaparinux is also a safe and effective alternative. (*N Engl J Med.* 2013;368:737-744) Avoid platelet transfusion unless life-threatening bleeding. DO NOT start warfarin until platelet count is >150,000 and overlap with argatroban for at least 5 days with the INR therapeutic for the last 2 d. Patients who have not had clot should be anticoagulated for 6–8 wk. In patients with clot, systemic anticoagulation should be continued for a minimum of 3 mo. Patients with renal insufficiency should be treated with argatroban, and in patients with liver dysfunction, fondaparinux and danaparoid are preferred. In patients with acute HIT and those who are antibody-positive should be treated with bivalirudin if urgent cardiac surgery is needed, but it is preferable to delay surgery if possible. Patients with a past history of HIT with acute thrombosis with negative heparin antibodies should be treated with fondaparinux at full therapeutic dose until transition to warfarin. (*Blood.* 2012;119:2209-2218. *Annu Rev Med.* 2010;61:77-90)	1. Highest risk for HIT is in postsurgical patients treated with UFH. 2. UFH is 8–10x more likely to cause HIT compared to LMWH. 3. Fondaparinux (Arixtra®)—Synthetic pentasaccharide inhibits factor X activity through antithrombin and is safe to be used in HIT, although direct thrombin inhibitors are preferred. 4. Platelet counts can mildly decrease in the first 4 days after starting heparin but this is not immunologically mediated and is not associated with thrombosis. 5. HIT is an immune-mediated disorder triggered by the formation of antibodies to a heparin/platelet factor 4 antigen complex. The complex binds to platelet FC receptors, causing activation of the platelet microparticle release and increased risk of clotting. 6. Both VTE and arterial clotting occur in the HIT syndrome in a ratio of 3:1. Adrenal infarction with shock from arterial thrombosis has been reported. 7. HIT occurs very rarely in patients <40 y old. HIT is increased in females 2.4-fold compared to males. 8. The median platelet count in HIT is 60,000 and seldom falls below 20,000. HIT-associated thrombosis shows a propensity to occur in areas of vessel injury (sites of central venous catheter, arterial line insertion, or other vascular interventions). 9. The development of HIT is not related to the degree of exposure to heparin. A single flush of an IV line or 1 dose of prophylactic heparin can trigger the HIT syndrome. If HIT is not recognized, further administration of heparin will lead to significant increased risk of clot, morbidity, and mortality. (*N Engl J Med.* 2006;355:809-817. *JAMA.* 2004;164:361-369) 10. The 4T scoring system is most accurate in the low-risk subset, with a negative predictive value of 0.998. (*Blood.* 2012;120: 4160-4167) (See Table IV.)

TABLE I

FIRST-LINE THERAPY FOR ITP		
CORTICOSTEROIDS	**RR**	**% WITH SUSTAINED RESPONSE**
Prednisone 0.5–2 mg/kg/d for 2 wk followed by taper	70–80%	10 year disease free—13%–15%
Dexamethasone 40 mg daily for 4 d every 2–4 wk for 1–4 cycles	90%	As high as 50% (2–5-y follow-up)
IV anti-D immune globulin 50–75 μg/kg—warning regarding brisk hemolysis and rare DIC	80%	Usually lasts 3–4 wk, but may persist for months in some patients
IVIG 0.4 g/kg/d × 5 d or 1 g/kg/d for 1–2 d	80%	Transient benefit lasting 2–4 wk

TABLE II

SELECTED SECOND-LINE THERAPY OPTIONS IN ADULT ITP	
TPO RECEPTOR AGONIST	**RR**
Eltrombopag 25–75 mg orally daily	70%–80%
Romiplostim 1–10 μg/kg SQ weekly	80%–90%
IMMUNOSUPPRESSION	
Azathioprine 1–2 mg/kg	40%
Cyclosporine 5 mg/kg/d for 6 d then 2.5–3 m/kg/d to titrate blood levels of 100–200 mg/mL	50%–60%
Cytoxan 1–2 mg/kg orally or IV (0.3–1 g/m²) for 1–3 doses every 2–4 wk	30%–60%
Rituximab 375 mg/m² weekly × 4	50%–60% respond—sustained >3–5 y in 10%–15%
UNCERTAIN MECHANISM IV	
Danazol 200 mg 2–4× daily	~50%
Vinca alkaloid 1–2 mg IV weekly to max of 6 mg	~30% variable

TABLE III

UNDERLYING CAUSES ASSOCIATED WITH ITP
• Drug induced (trimethoprim-sulfa, rifampin, carbamazepine, vancomycin, quinine derivatives, and many more)
• Systemic Lupus/Sjögren syndrome, and other rheumatologic diseases
• Infections—hepatitis C, HIV, cytomegalovirus (CMV), *Helicobacter pylori*, Epstein-Barr virus (EBV), varicella, and autoimmune
• Indolent lymphomas breast and colon cancer
• Vaccinations—mostly in children
• Common variable immunodeficiency—almost exclusively in children

TABLE IV

4Ts	2 POINTS	1 POINT	0 POINT
Thrombocytopenia	• Fall in platelet count >50% and nadir of ≥20,000 and • No surgery in preceding 3 d	• >50% fall in platelets but with surgery in preceding 3 d • 30%–50% platelet fall with nadir 10–19,000	• <30% fall in platelets • Any platelet fall with nadir <10,000
Timing of platelet fall	• 5–10 d after start of heparin • Platelet fall <5 d with heparin exposure within past 30 d	• Platelet fall after day 10 • Platelet fall <5 d with heparin exposure in past 100 d	• Platelet fall ≤ day 4 without exposure to heparin in last 100 days
Thrombosis or other sequelae	• Confirmed new venous or arterial thrombosis • Skin necrosis at heparin injection sites • Anaphylactoid reaction to IV heparin	• Progressive or recurrent thrombosis while on heparin • Erythematous skin reaction at heparin injection sites	Thrombosis suspected
Other causes of thrombocytopenia	• No alternative cause of or platelet drop evident	• At least one other possible cause of drop in platelet count	Definite or highly likely cause present • Sepsis • Chemotherapy within 20 d • DIC • Drug-induced ITP • Posttransfusion purposes
High probability: 6–8 points; intermediate probability: 4–5 points; low probability: ≤3 points			

MANAGEMENT OF THYROID NODULES
SOURCES: AACE, JUNE 2010 AND ATA, NOVEMBER 2009

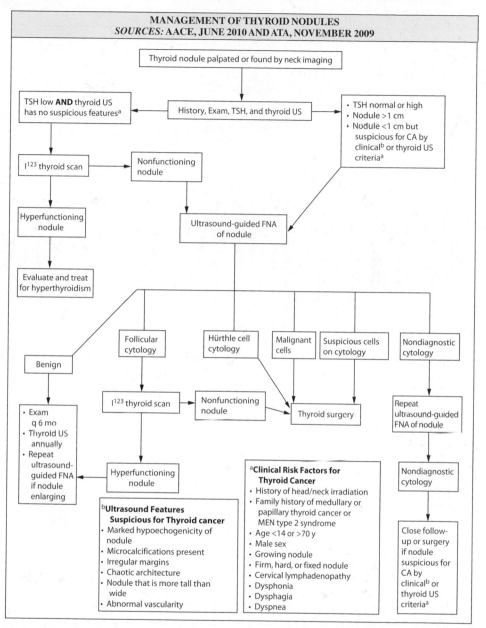

FNA, fine-needle aspiration; MEN, multiple endocrine neoplasia; TSH, thyroid-stimulating hormone; US, ultrasound

THYROID DISEASE, HYPERTHYROIDISM

Disease Management	Organization	Date	Population	Recommendations	Comments	Source

Thyroid Disease, Hyperthyroidism	AACE	2011	Adults	• Radioactive iodine uptake scan should be performed when the etiology of thyrotoxicosis is unclear.
				• β-blockade should be prescribed to elderly patients and considered for all patients with symptomatic thyrotoxicosis.
				• Graves disease
				  ○ Options for Graves disease treatment:
				    – ^{131}I therapy
				    – Antithyroid medications
				    – Thyroidectomy
				• Patients with Graves disease and increased risk of complications should be pretreated with methimazole and beta-blockers prior to ^{131}I therapy.
				  ○ Advise smoking cessation
				  ○ Graves' ophthalmopathy should have steroids and ^{131}I therapy
				• 131 I therapy
				  ○ A pregnancy test should be checked within 48 h of administering ^{131}I therapy
				  ○ Assess patients 1–2 mo after ^{131}I therapy with a free T_4 and total triiodothyronine (T_3) level
				  ○ Consider retreatment with ^{131}I therapy if hyperthyroidism persists 6 mo after ^{131}I treatment
				• Antithyroid drug therapy
				  ○ Methimazole is the preferred antithyroid drug except during the first trimester of pregnancy
				  ○ A CBC with differential should be obtained whenever a patient taking antithyroid drugs develops a febrile illness or pharyngitis
				  ○ Recommend measurement of TSH receptor antibody level prior to stopping antithyroid drug therapy
				• Thyroidectomy
				  ○ Indicated for toxic multinodular goiter or toxic adenoma
				  ○ Wean beta-blockers postoperative
				  ○ Follow serial calcium or intact PTH levels postoperative
				  ○ Start levothyroxine 1.6 µg/kg/d immediately postoperative
				  ○ Check a serum TSH level 6–8 wk postoperative
				• Thyroid storm should be treated with β-blockers, antithyroid drugs, inorganic iodide, corticosteroid therapy, volume resuscitation, and acetaminophen.
						https://www.aace.com/files/hyper-guidelines-2011.pdf

	AACE	2012	Adults	• Replacement dosing of levothyroxine is 1.6 µg/kg/d.
				• Recommend checking anti-thyroid peroxidase antibodies (TPOAb) in patients with subclinical hypothyroidism or recurrent miscarriages.
				• Recommend treating hypothyroid patients with levothyroxine if:
				  ○ TSH >10 mIU/L
				  ○ Symptomatic
				  ○ Positive TPOAb
						https://www.aace.com/files/hypothyroidism_guidelines.pdf

THYROID DISEASE, PREGNANCY & POSTPARTUM

Disease Management	Organization	Date	Population	Recommendations	Comments	Source
Thyroid Disease, Pregnancy and Postpartum	ATA	2011	Women during and immediately after pregnancy	• Hypothyroidism in pregnancy is defined as: 　○ An elevated TSH (>2.5 mIU/L) and a suppressed free thyroxine (FT_4) 　○ TSH ≥10 mIU/L (irrespective of FT_4) 　○ Subclinical hypothyroidism is defined as a TSH 2.5–9.9 mIU/L) and a normal FT_4 • Insufficient evidence to support treatment of subclinical hypothyroidism in pregnancy. • Goal therapy is to normalize TSH levels. • PTU is the preferred antithyroid drug in pregnancy. • Monitor TSH levels every 4 wk when treating thyroid disease in pregnancy. • Measure a TSH receptor antibody level at 20–24 wk for any history of Graves disease. • All pregnant and lactating women should ingest at least 250 µg iodine daily. • All pregnant women with thyroid nodules should undergo thyroid ultrasound and TSH testing. • Patients found to have thyroid cancer during pregnancy would ideally undergo surgery during second trimester.	• Surgery for well-differentiated thyroid carcinoma can often be deferred until postpartum period.	http://thyroidguidelines.net/sites/thyroidguidelines.net/files/file/thy.2011.0087.pdf

TINNITUS

Disease Management	Organization	Date	Population	Recommendations	Comments	Source
Tinnitus	AAO-HNS	2014	Adults and children	1. Recommend a thorough history and exam on patients with tinnitus. 2. Recommend a comprehensive audiologic examination for unilateral or persistent tinnitus or any associated hearing impairment. 3. Recommend imaging studies only for unilateral tinnitus, pulsatile tinnitus, asymmetric hearing loss, or focal neurological abnormalities. 4. Recommend a hearing aid for tinnitus with hearing loss. 5. Consider cognitive behavioral training or sound therapy for persistent, bothersome tinnitus. 6. Recommend against medical or herbal therapy or transcranial magnetic stimulation for tinnitus.		http://www.guideline.gov/content.aspx?id=48751

TOBACCO CESSATION TREATMENT ALGORITHM
Source: US PUBLIC HEALTH SERVICE

Five As

1. Ask about tobacco use.

2. Advise to quit through clear, personalized messages.

3. Assess willingness to quit.

4. Assist to quit,[a] including referral to Quit Lines (eg, 1-800-NO-BUTTS).

5. Arrange follow-up and support.

[a]Physicians can assist patients to quit by devising a quit plan, providing problem-solving counseling, providing intratreatment social support, helping patients obtain social support from their environment/friends, and recommending pharmacotherapy for appropriate patients. Use caution in recommending pharmacotherapy in patients with medical contraindications, those smoking <10 cigarettes per day, pregnant/breast-feeding women, and adolescent smokers. As of March 2005, Medicare covers costs for smoking cessation counseling for those who (1) have a smoking-related illness; (2) have an illness complicated by smoking; or (3) take a medication that is made less effective by smoking. (http://www.cms.hhs.gov/mcd/viewdecisionmemo.asp?id=130)

Source: Fiore MC, Jaén CR, Baker TB, et al. *Treating Tobacco Use and Dependence. Quick Reference Guide for Clinicians.* Rockville, MD: U.S. Department of Health and Human Services. Public Health Service; 2008. http://www.ahrq.gov/legacy/clinic/tobacco/tobaqrg.pdf.

MOTIVATING TOBACCO USERS TO QUIT

Five R's

1. Relevance: personal

2. Risks: acute, long term, environmental

3. Rewards: have patient identify (eg, save money, better food taste)

4. Road blocks: help problem solve

5. Repetition: at every office visit

TOBACCO CESSATION TREATMENT OPTIONS[a]

Pharmacotherapy	Precautions/ Contraindications	Side Effects	Dosage	Duration	Availability
First-Line Pharmacotherapies (approved for use for smoking cessation by the FDA)					
Bupropion SR	History of seizure, History of eating disorder	Insomnia, Dry mouth	150 mg every morning for 3 d, then 150 mg bid. (Begin treatment 1–2 wk prequit.)	7–12 wk maintenance up to 6 mo	Zyban (prescription only)
Nicotine gum	—	Mouth soreness Dyspepsia	1–24 cigarettes/day: 2-mg gum (up to 24 pieces/d) 25+ cigarettes/day: 4-mg gum (up to 24 pieces/d)	Up to 12 wk	Nicorette, Nicorette Mint (OTC only)
Nicotine inhaler	—	Local irritation of mouth and throat	6–16 cartridges/d	Up to 6 mo	Nicotrol Inhaler (prescription only)
Nicotine nasal spray	—	Nasal irritation	8–40 doses/d	3–6 mo	Nicotrol NS (prescription only)
Nicotine patch	—	Local skin reaction, Insomnia	21 mg/24 h, 14 mg/24 h, 7 mg/24 h, 15 mg/16 h	4 wk, Then 2 wk, Then 2 wk, 8 wk	NicoDerm CQ (OTC only), generic patches (prescription and OTC), Nicotrol (OTC only)
Varenicline	Renal impairment	Nausea, Abnormal dreams	0.5 mg qd for 3 d, then 0.5 mg bid for 4 d, then 1.0 mg PO bid	12 wk or 24 wk	Chantix (prescription only)
Second-Line Pharmacotherapies (not approved for use for smoking cessation by the FDA)					
Clonidine	Rebound hypertension	Dry mouth, Drowsiness, Dizziness, Sedation	0.15–0.75 mg/d	3–10 wk	Oral clonidine–generic, Catapres (prescription only), transdermal Catapres (prescription only)
Nortriptyline	Risk of arrhythmias	Sedation, Dry mouth	75–100 mg/d	12 wk	Nortriptyline HCL–generic (prescription only)

BID, twice daily; FDA, Food and Drug Administration; OTC, over-the-counter; PO, by mouth; qd, every day.
[a]The information contained within this table is not comprehensive. Please see package inserts for additional information.
Source: U.S. Public Health Service.

TONSILLECTOMY

Disease Management	Organization	Date	Population	Recommendations	Comments	Source

Tonsillectomy	AAO-HNS	2011	Children	• Recommends against routine perioperative antibiotics for tonsillectomy.
				• Tonsillectomy indicated for:
				  ○ Tonsillar hypertrophy with sleep disordered breathing
				  ○ Recurrent throat infections for ≥7 episodes of recurrent throat infection in last year; ≥5 episodes of recurrent throat infection per year in last 2 y; or ≥3 episodes of recurrent throat infection per year in last 3 y
				• Recommend posttonsillectomy pain control.
						http://www.entnet.org/HealthInformation/upload/CPG-TonsillectomyInChildren.pdf

TRAUMATIC BRAIN INJURY

Disease Management	Organization	Date	Population	Recommendations	Comments	Source
Traumatic Brain Injury	ACEP	2013		Avoid CT scan of head for minor head trauma in patients who are low risk based on validated decision rules.		http://www.choosingwisely.org/ societies/american-college-of-emergency-physicians/

TREMOR, ESSENTIAL

Disease Management	Organization	Date	Population	Recommendations	Comments	Source
Tremor, Essential	AAN	2011	Adults	• Recommends treatment with propranolol or primidone. • Alternative treatment options include alprazolam, atenolol, gabapentin, sotalol, or topiramate. • Recommend against treatment with levetiracetam, pindolol, trazodone, acetazolamide, or 3,4–diaminopyridine.	• Unilateral thalamotomy may be effective for severe refractory essential tremors.	http://www.neurology.org/content/77/19/1752.full.pdf+html

TUBERCULOSIS, MULTIDRUG-RESISTANT (MDR-TB)

Disease Management	Organization	Date	Population	Recommendations	Comments	Source
Tuberculosis, Multidrug-Resistant (MDR-TB)	WHO	2011	Patients with suspected or proven drug-resistant tuberculosis	• Rapid drug susceptibility testing of isoniazid and rifampicin is recommended at the time of TB diagnosis. • Recommend sputum smear microscopy and culture to monitor patients with MDR-TB. • Recommend addition of a later-generation fluoroquinolone, ethionamide, pyrazinamide, and a parenteral agent ± cycloserine for ≥8 mo. • Recommend total treatment duration of 20 mo.		http://whqlibdoc.who.int/publications/2011/9789241501583_eng.pdf

TYMPANOSTOMY TUBES

Disease Management	Organization	Date	Population	Recommendations	Comments	Source

Tympanostomy Tubes	AAO	2013	Children 6 mo to 12 y	• Clinicians should not perform tympanostomy tube insertion for children with:
				  ○ A single episode of otitis media with effusion (OME) of <3 mo duration
				  ○ Recurrent acute otitis media without effusion
				• Clinicians should obtain a hearing test if OME persists for at least 3 mo or if tympanostomy tube insertion is being considered.
				• Clinicians should offer bilateral tympanostomy tube insertion to children with:
				  ○ Bilateral OME for at least 3 mo **AND** documented hearing impairment.
				  ○ Recurrent acute otitis media with effusions
				  ○ Tympanostomy tube insertion is an option for chronic symptomatic OME associated with balance problems, poor school performance, behavioral problems, or ear discomfort **thought to be due to OME**.
					• No need for prophylactic water precautions (avoidance of swimming or water sports or use of earplugs) for children with tympanostomy tubes.	http://www.guideline.gov/content.aspx?id=46909

URINARY CATHETERS

Disease Management	Organization	Date	Population	Recommendations	Comments	Source
Indwelling Urinary Catheters or Intermittent Catheterization	AUA	2015		Recommend against empiric antibiotics unless the patient has symptoms of a urinary tract infection.		http://www.choosingwisely.org/clinician-lists/american-urological-association-antimicrobials-indwelling-or-intermittent-bladder-catheterization/

ULCERS, STRESS

Disease Management	Organization	Date	Population	Recommendations	Comments	Source
Stress Ulcers	SHM	2013		Do not prescribe medications for stress ulcer prophylaxis to medical inpatients unless they are at high risk for GI complications.		http://www.choosingwisely.org/societies/society-of-hospital-medicine-adult/

URINARY INCONTINENCE, OVERACTIVE BLADDER

Disease Management	Organization	Date	Population	Recommendations	Comments	Source

Urinary Incontinence, Overactive Bladder	American Urologic Association	2014	Adults	• Rule out a urinary tract infection.
				• Recommend checking a post-void residual to rule out overflow incontinence.
				• First-line treatments
				   ○ Bladder training
				   ○ Bladder control strategies
				   ○ Pelvic floor muscle training
				• Second-line treatments
				   ○ Antimuscarinic meds
				     – Darifenacin, fesoterodine, oxybutynin, solifenacin, tolterodine, or trospium
				     – Contraindicated with narrow-angle glaucoma or gastroparesis
				• Third-line treatments
				   ○ Sacral neuromodulation
				   ○ Peripheral tibial nerve stimulation
				   ○ Intradetrusor botulinum toxin A
				• Recommend against indwelling urinary catheters.
						http://www.guideline.gov/content.aspx?id=4826

URINARY INCONTINENCE, STRESS

Disease Management	Organization	Date	Population	Recommendations	Comments	Source
Urinary Incontinence, Stress	AUA	2009	Adult women	1. Recommends an exam: to assess the degree of urethral mobility, pelvic floor relaxation, pelvic organ prolapse, and assess whether any urethral abnormalities exist. 2. Recommends a urinalysis. 3. Assess the postvoid residual volume. 4. Surgical options for refractory stress urinary incontinence include periurethral injections, laparoscopic bladder suspensions, midurethral slings, pubovaginal slings, and retropubic suspensions.		http://www.auanet.org/content/media/stress2009-chapter1.pdf
	ACP	2014		Recommends pelvic floor muscle training and bladder training for urinary incontinence in women		http://www.guideline.gov/content.aspx?id=48543

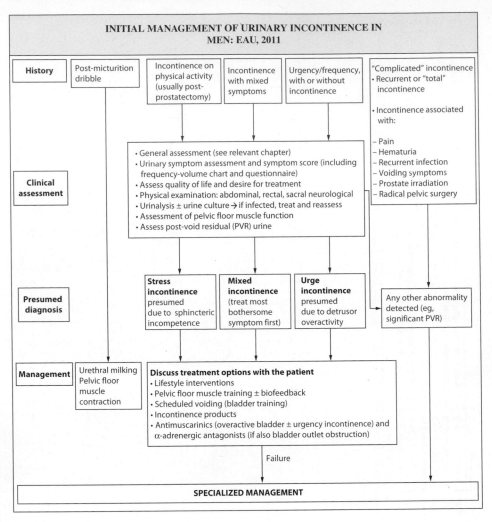

INITIAL MANAGEMENT OF URINARY INCONTINENCE IN MEN: EAU, 2011

History

- Post-micturition dribble
- Incontinence on physical activity (usually post-prostatectomy)
- Incontinence with mixed symptoms
- Urgency/frequency, with or without incontinence
- "Complicated" incontinence
  - Recurrent or "total" incontinence
  - Incontinence associated with:
    - Pain
    - Hematuria
    - Recurrent infection
    - Voiding symptoms
    - Prostate irradiation
    - Radical pelvic surgery

Clinical assessment

- General assessment (see relevant chapter)
- Urinary symptom assessment and symptom score (including frequency-volume chart and questionnaire)
- Assess quality of life and desire for treatment
- Physical examination: abdominal, rectal, sacral neurological
- Urinalysis ± urine culture → if infected, treat and reassess
- Assessment of pelvic floor muscle function
- Assess post-void residual (PVR) urine

Presumed diagnosis

- **Stress incontinence** presumed due to sphincteric incompetence
- **Mixed incontinence** (treat most bothersome symptom first)
- **Urge incontinence** presumed due to detrusor overactivity
- Any other abnormality detected (eg, significant PVR)

Management

- Urethral milking
- Pelvic floor muscle contraction

Discuss treatment options with the patient
- Lifestyle interventions
- Pelvic floor muscle training ± biofeedback
- Scheduled voiding (bladder training)
- Incontinence products
- Antimuscarinics (overactive bladder ± urgency incontinence) and α-adrenergic antagonists (if also bladder outlet obstruction)

Failure

SPECIALIZED MANAGEMENT

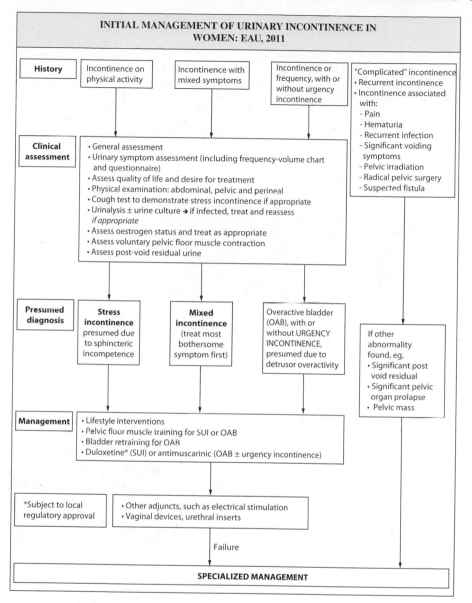

INITIAL MANAGEMENT OF URINARY INCONTINENCE IN WOMEN: EAU, 2011

History

Incontinence on physical activity

Incontinence with mixed symptoms

Incontinence or frequency, with or without urgency incontinence

"Complicated" incontinence
- Recurrent incontinence
- Incontinence associated with:
  - Pain
  - Hematuria
  - Recurrent infection
  - Significant voiding symptoms
  - Pelvic irradiation
  - Radical pelvic surgery
  - Suspected fistula

Clinical assessment
- General assessment
- Urinary symptom assessment (including frequency-volume chart and questionnaire)
- Assess quality of life and desire for treatment
- Physical examination: abdominal, pelvic and perineal
- Cough test to demonstrate stress incontinence if appropriate
- Urinalysis ± urine culture → if infected, treat and reassess *if appropriate*
- Assess oestrogen status and treat as appropriate
- Assess voluntary pelvic floor muscle contraction
- Assess post-void residual urine

Presumed diagnosis

Stress incontinence presumed due to sphincteric incompetence

Mixed incontinence (treat most bothersome symptom first)

Overactive bladder (OAB), with or without URGENCY INCONTINENCE, presumed due to detrusor overactivity

If other abnormality found, eg,
- Significant post void residual
- Significant pelvic organ prolapse
- Pelvic mass

Management
- Lifestyle interventions
- Pelvic floor muscle training for SUI or OAB
- Bladder retraining for OAB
- Duloxetine* (SUI) or antimuscarinic (OAB ± urgency incontinence)

*Subject to local regulatory approval

- Other adjuncts, such as electrical stimulation
- Vaginal devices, urethral inserts

Failure

SPECIALIZED MANAGEMENT

URINARY TRACT INFECTIONS (UTIs)

Disease Management	Organization	Date	Population	Recommendations	Comments	Source
Asymptomatic bacteriuria	IDSA	2015	Nonpregnant women	Do not treat asymptomatic bacteriuria with antibiotics.		http://www.choosingwisely.org/societies/infectious-diseases-society-of-america/

Urinary Tract Infections (UTIs)	ACOG
	EAU
	IDSA
	ACOG
	IDSA
		2008
		2010
		2011
		2008
		2011
			Adult women	1. Screening for and treatment of asymptomatic bacteriuria is not recommended.
				2. Recommend duration of antibiotics:
				  a. Uncomplicated cystitis: 3 d
				    i. Nitrofurantoin requires 5–7 d of therapy
				  b. Uncomplicated pyelonephritis: 7–10 d
				  c. Complicated pyelonephritis or UTI: 3–5 d after control/elimination of complicating factors and defervescence
				3. Recommended empiric antibiotics for uncomplicated cystitis[a]:
				  a. TMP-SMX
				  b. Fluoroquinolones
				  c. Nitrofurantoin macrocrystals
				  d. Beta-lactam antibiotics are alternative agents[b]
				4. Recommended empiric antibiotics for complicated UTI or uncomplicated pyelonephritis:
				  a. Fluoroquinolones
				  b. Ceftriaxone
				  c. Aminoglycosides
				5. Recommended empiric antibiotics for complicated pyelonephritis:
				  a. Fluoroquinolones
				  b. Piperacillin-tazobactam
				  c. Carbapenem
				  d. Aminoglycosides
				• Recommend a urinalysis or dipstick testing for symptoms of a UTI: dysuria, urinary frequency, suprapubic pain, or hematuria.
				• Empiric antibiotics for UTI
				  ○ Trimethoprim-sulfamethoxazole × 3 d (not recommended if local resistance rate >20%)
				  ○ Nitrofurantoin monohydrate × 5 d
				  ○ Fosfomycin 3 g PO × 1
				• Consider a fluoroquinolone for symptoms of pyelonephritis or for refractory UTI.
					1. EAU recommends 7 d of antibiotics for men with uncomplicated cystitis.
					2. EAU suggests the following options for antimicrobial prophylaxis of recurrent uncomplicated UTIs in nonpregnant women:
					  a. Nitrofurantoin 50 mg PO daily
					  b. TMP-SMX 40/200 mg/d
					3. EAU suggests the following options for antimicrobial prophylaxis of recurrent uncomplicated UTIs in pregnant women:
					  a. Cephalexin 125 mg PO daily
					4. Once urine culture and sensitivity results are known, antibiotics can be adjusted to the narrowest spectrum antibiotic.
						http://www.guidelines.gov/content.aspx?id=12628
						http://www.uroweb.org/gls/pdf/Urological%20Infections%202010.pdf
						http://www.guidelines.gov/content.aspx?id=25652
						http://guidelines.gov/content.aspx?id=12628
						http://cid.oxfordjournals.org/content/52/5/e103.full.pdf+html

Disease Management	Organization	Date	Population	Recommendations	Comments	Source
Urinary Tract Infections (UTIs) (continued)	AAP	2011	Febrile children 2–24 mo	• Diagnosis of a UTI f: ○ Pyuria ≥50,000 colonies/mL single uropathogenic organism • Recommend a renal and bladder ultrasound in all infants 2–24 mo with a febrile UTI • Treat febrile UTIs with 7–14 d of antibiotics. • Antibiotic prophylaxis is not indicated for a history of febrile UTI. • A voiding cystourethrogram (VCUG) is indicated if ultrasound reveals hydronephrosis, renal scarring, or other findings of high-grade vesicoureteral reflux, and for recurrent febrile UTIs.	• Urine obtained through catheterization has a 95% sensitivity and 99% specificity for UTI. • Bag urine cultures have a specificity of approximately 63% with an unacceptably high false-positive rate. **Only useful if the cultures are negative.**	http://pediatrics.aappublications.org/content/128/3/595.full.pdf+html?sid=c1de42b3-c89b-4fd2-9592-35908782317

ᵃTMP-SMX only if regional *Escherichia coli* resistance is <20%; fluoroquinolones include ciprofloxacin, ofloxacin, or levofloxacin.
ᵇAmoxicillin-clavulanate, cefdinir, cefaclor, or cefpodoxime-proxetil. Cephalexin may be appropriate in certain settings.

URINARY TRACT SYMPTOMS, LOWER

Disease Management	Organization	Date	Population	Recommendations	Comments	Source
Urinary Tract Symptoms, Lower	NICE EAU	2010 2011	Adult men	1. All men with LUTS should have a thorough history and exam, including a prostate examination, and a review of current medications. 2. Recommends supervised bladder training exercises and consider anticholinergic medications for symptoms suggestive of an overactive bladder. 3. Recommends an α-blocker for men with moderate-to-severe LUTS.[a] 4. Consider a 5-α-reductase inhibitor for men with LUTS with prostate size larger than 30 g. 5. For men with refractory obstructive urinary symptoms despite medical therapy, offer 1 of 3 surgeries: transurethral resection, transurethral vaporization, or laser enucleation of the prostate.		http://www.nice.org.uk/nicemedia/live/12984/48557/48557.pdf http://www.uroweb.org/gls/pdf/12_Male_LUTS.pdf

[a]Alfuzosin, doxazosin, tamsulosin, or terazosin.

Figure I

DIAGNOSIS AND TREATMENT OF VENOUS THROMBOEMBOLISM (VTE) WELLS CRITERIA

Source: Goldhaber SZ, Bounameaux H. Pulmonary embolism and deep vein thrombosis. *Lancet.* 2012;379:1835.

Pretest probability (PTP) of VTE guides clinical evaluation–Wells criteria for PTP of DVT and PE

DVT		PE	
VARIABLE	SCORE	VARIABLE	SCORE
Active cancer	1	Clinical evidence of DVT	3.0
Paralysis/immobilization	1	Other dx less likely than PE	3.0
Bedridden for >3 d or major surgery within 4 wk	1	Heart rate >100	1.5
Entire leg swollen	1	Immobile >3 d or major surgery within 4 wk	1.5
Tenderness along deep vein	1	Previous DVT/PE	1.5
Calf swelling >3 cm	1	Hemoptysis	1.0
Pitting edema (unilateral)	1	Malignancy	1.0
Collateral superficial veins	1		
Alternative dx more likely than DVT	–2		
Score and Probability-DVT		**Score and Probability-PE**	
High—3 or greater (75% risk of DVT) Moderate—1 or 2 (20% risk of DVT) Low—0 (3% risk of DVT)		High—6 or greater (>70% risk of PE) Moderate—2–6 (20–30% risk of PE) Low—less than 2 (2–3% risk of PE)	

DEEP VEIN THROMBOSIS (DVT)

Disease Management	Organization	Date	Population	Recommendations	Comments	Source
Deep Vein Thrombosis (DVT)	ACCP ACP	2012 2011	Patients with DVT (lower and upper extremity)	For diagnostic workup of DVT/PE see **Figures I, II,** and **III.** • Initial heparin based regimen with unfractionated heparin (UFH) 80 units/kg bolus, then 18 units/kg per hour titrated to partial thromboplastin time (PTT), enoxaparin 1 mg/kg SQ q12h or 1.5 mg/kg SQ daily • Fondaparinux 5 mg (<50 kg), 7.5 mg (50–100 kg) or 10 mg (>100 kg) SQ daily • Start warfarin (≤10 mg) on day 1 and overlap with heparin for at least 5 d with therapeutic INR for last 2 d. Rivaroxaban now approved by FDA to treat acute DVT and PE. Apixaban and dabigatran are also approved to treat venous thromboembolism. Extended treatment has shown protection from further clot with minimal bleeding risk. Rivaroxaban is not approved in acute coronary syndrome (*N Engl J Med.* 2010;363:2499–2510. *N Engl J Med.* 2012;366:1287-1297) See Table I	1. Clinical findings alone are poor predictors of DVT. 2. Early ambulation on heparin is safe. 3. With iliofemoral thrombosis and significant swelling thrombolysis or surgical thrombectomy not recommended unless significant symptoms. 4. Inferior vena cava (IVC) filter indicated if pulmonary embolus while on therapeutic anticoagulation or significant uncontrolled bleeding precluding anticoagulation. 5. With provoked clot, anticoagulate for 3 mo if precipitating problem solved.[a] 6. Continue anticoagulation indefinitely if provoking problem continues. 7. In cancer-related clots, continue low-molecular-weight heparin (LMWH), do not transition to warfarin if cancer still active. (*Blood.* 2014;123:3972) 8. In unprovoked clot, anticoagulate for 3 mo then weigh risk of bleeding to benefit of prolonged anticoagulation to prevent clot; consider thrombophilia evaluation, including hereditary factors and antiphospholipid antibody syndrome.	*Chest.* 2012;141: e419s–e494s
				Women have 50% increased risk of recurrent clot compared to men. (*Am J Med.* 2014;127:530).		
				• Outpatient management of VTE with rivaroxaban, apixaban, or dabigatran is acceptable if the patient does not have any of the following: >80 y/o, hx of cancer, hx of COPD, CHF, pulse >110, BP <100, O₂ sat <90. • Knee high GCS (graduated compression stockings) with 30–40 mm Hg pressure at ankles for 2 y will reduce postthrombotic syndrome by 50%)	9. Rivaroxaban should not be used in pregnancy or in patients with liver disease. 10. Risk factors for warfarin bleeding—age >65 y, history of stroke, history of GI bleed, and recent comorbidity (MI, Hct <30, creatinine >1.5, diabetes). If all 4 factors present, 40% risk of significant bleed in 12 mo; 0.4% of patients on warfarin die of bleeding yearly. (*Chest.* 2006;130;1296. *Am J Med.* 2011;124:111). 11. Patients with mild symptoms and good support system can be treated as outpatient either with rivaroxaban (direct factor Xa inhibitor) or with lovenox and warfarin. 12. Calf and iliofemoral thrombosis have increased incidence of false negative compression ultrasound–recommend CT or MR venogram or venography for suspected iliofemoral thrombosis–for calf thrombosis follow-up compression ultrasound (CUS) in 5–7 d is acceptable.	

DEEP VEIN THROMBOSIS (DVT)

Disease management	Organization	Date	Population	Recommendations	Comments	Source
Deep Vein Thrombosis (DVT) (continued)					13. Normal d-dimer with abnormal CUS in leg with previous DVT makes new clot unlikely. (*J Thromb Haemost.* 2007;5:1076) 14. Consider high thrombophilic risk in patients with recurrent VTE or patients with first unprovoked VTE who: • Are <50 y old • Family history of VTE • Unusual site of thrombosis • Massive venous thrombosis 15. In unprovoked VTE 3% of patients are found to have associated malignancy with another 10% diagnosed with cancer over next 2 y. (*N Engl J Med.* 1998;338:1169. *Ann Intern Med.* 2008;149:323)	

[a]Surgery, cancer, hormones, pregnancy, travel, inflammatory bowel disease, hemolytic anemia, immobilization, trauma, CHF, myeloproliferative disorders, stroke, central venous catheter, rheumatologic disorders.

Figure II

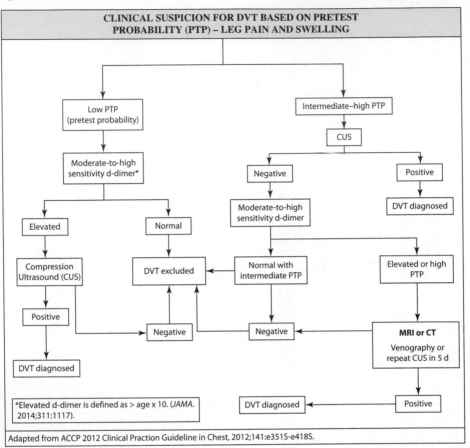

Disease Management	Organization	Date	Population	Recommendations	Comments	Source
Pulmonary Embolus (PE)	ACCP ACP	2012 2011	Diagnosed Pulmonary embolism	• Approach to initial anticoagulation is the same as DVT. • If patient hypotensive without high bleeding risk, and tachycardiac systemically administered thrombolytic therapy is recommended. • In a patient with acute PE associated with hypotension with contraindications to or failed thrombolysis or in shock that is likely to lead to rapid death, catheter assisted thrombus removal is indicated if appropriate expertise and resources are available. • In patients whose first episode of VTE is an unprovoked PE, extended anticoagulation beyond 3 mo is preferred unless high risk of bleeding.	• Patients whose first VTE is a PE, will have a 3-fold increase risk of a second clot being a PE compared to patients with DVT only. (*N Engl J Med.* 2010;363:266) • In patients with unprovoked PE or DVT elevated d-dimer at the time of discontinuation of warfarin or 2–3 wk after stopping anticoagulants predicts for a 3- to 5-fold increase in risk of clot over the next 12 mo. (*Blood.* 2010;115:481) • The presence of a permanent IVC filter does not mandate continuous anticoagulation unless documented recurrent clot problems • Unprovoked clot has risk of recurrent clot in first 12 mo of 8–12% vs 3% for patients with provoked clot. (*JAMA.* 2011;305:1336) • Patients with intermediate or high PTP of PE should be treated with heparin before diagnostic workup is complete. • Asymptomatic PE (found incidentally on chest CT) should be treated with same protocol as symptomatic PE. • Emerging data suggest the use of aspirin (100 mg PO daily) may reduce the risk of recurrent clot in patients with unprovoked VTE after 6–12 mo of warfarin therapy. (*N Engl J Med.* 2012;366:1959).	*Chest.* 2012;141: e152s–e184s *Chest.* 2012;141: e24s–e43s

PULMONARY EMBOLUS (PE)

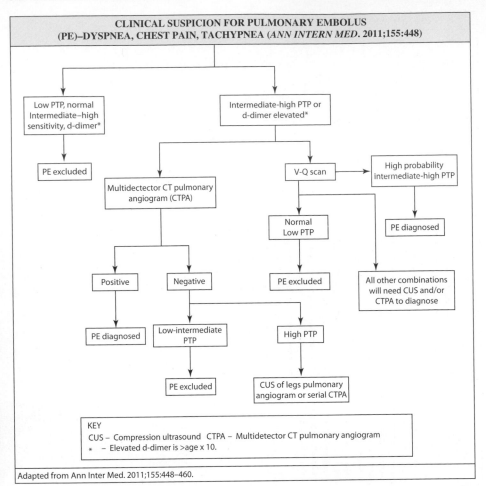

CLINICAL SUSPICION FOR PULMONARY EMBOLUS
(PE)–DYSPNEA, CHEST PAIN, TACHYPNEA (*ANN INTERN MED.* 2011;155:448)

Low PTP, normal
Intermediate–high
sensitivity, d-dimer*

PE excluded

Intermediate-high PTP or
d-dimer elevated*

Multidectector CT pulmonary
angiogram (CTPA)

V-Q scan

High probability
intermediate-high PTP

Normal
Low PTP

PE diagnosed

Positive

Negative

PE excluded

All other combinations
will need CUS and/or
CTPA to diagnose

PE diagnosed

Low-intermediate
PTP

High PTP

PE excluded

CUS of legs pulmonary
angiogram or serial CTPA

KEY
CUS – Compression ultrasound   CTPA – Multidetector CT pulmonary angiogram
*   – Elevated d-dimer is >age x 10.

Adapted from Ann Inter Med. 2011;155:448–460.

Table 1

NEW ORAL ANTICOAGULANTS[a] AND WARFARIN

Agent	Target	Dosing	Monitoring	Half-life	Time to Peak Plasma Concentration
Warfarin[b]	Vitamin K epoxide	Once daily	INR–adjusted	40 h	72–96 h
Dabigatran[a,c]	Thrombin	Fixed—once or twice daily	None	14–17 h	2 h
Rivaroxaban[c]	Factor Xa	Fixed—once or twice daily	None	5–9 h (50 y old) 9–13 h (elderly)	2.5–4 h
Apixaban[c]	Factor Xa	Fixed twice daily	None	8–15 h	3 h

[a]Do not use new oral anticoagulants in patients with mechanical valves. Warfarin is superior. Warfarin is likely superior to new oral anticoagulants in patients with anti-phospholipid antibody syndrome.
[b]If significant bleed on warfarin, give vitamin K, and four factor prothrombin complex concentrate (PCC) or recombinant FVIIa if not controlled.
[c]If significant bleed, no standard of care. Aggressively treat source of bleed; consider 4 factor PCC or recombinant FVIIa. Agents to reverse anticoagulation with new oral anticoagulants will be available soon.

	VITAMIN DEFICIENCIES				

Disease Management	Organization	Date	Population	Recommendations	Comments	Source
Vitamin Deficiencies	BCSH	2014	All patients with or suspected of having serum cobalamin and folate deficiency	1. Serum cobalamin less than 200 ng/L suggests cobalamin deficiency. 2. Patients with normal cobalamin level but high suspicion of cobalamin deficiency should undergo methylmalonic acid (MMA) testing. 3. Patients with cobalamin deficiency or unexplained anemia, neuropathy, or glossitis (regardless of cobalamin level) should have an anti-intrinsic factor antibody test to rule out pernicious anemia. 4. Initial therapy for cobalamin deficiency is vitamin B_{12} 1 mg IM TIW for 3 wk and then maintenance therapy. 5. Maintenance therapy is either 1 mg IM every 3 mo (if no neurologic symptoms) or every 2 mo (if neurologic symptoms) or vitamin B_{12} 2 mg PO daily. 6. Serum folate level <7 nmol/L (<3 μg/L) indicates folate deficiency.	Recommend against anti-parietal cell antibody to test for pernicious anemia.	http://www.guideline.gov/content.aspx?id=48197

VALVULAR ADULT HEART DISEASE
2014 ACC/AHA GUIDELINES

AORTIC STENOSIS (AS)

- Transthoracic echocardiogram (TTE) is recommended as initial evaluation with known or suspected aortic stenosis to establish the diagnosis and to determine the severity of the stenosis.
- Exercise treadmill testing is rarely indicated but helpful to evaluate patients who have discordant echo/clinical findings (ie, moderate or severe stenosis in the absence of expected symptoms). Previously undetected symptoms of chest pain, shortness of breath, exertional dizziness, or syncope may be identified to prevent sudden death.
- Hypertension should be treated in the present of significant AS.
- Statin therapy does not prevent the progression of the AS.
- No medical therapy is available to address symptoms or disease progression.
- Aortic valve replacement (AVR) is indicated in symptomatic patients with a mean gradient ≥40 mm Hg; aortic valve replacement is indicated in asymptomatic patients with decreased systolic function (EF50%) and mean gradient ≥40 mm Hg (valve gradient is underestimated with systolic dysfunction).
- Transcatheter aortic valve replacement (TAVR) should be considered in patients with a high surgical risk, marked frailty, associated comorbidities, and minimal associated coronary artery disease who have the same indication for AVR and have a 12-mo life expectancy.
- Percutaneous aortic balloon dilation procedure: should be considered a "bridging therapy" to AVR or TAVR therapy.

AORTIC INSUFFICIENCY (AI)

- Transthoracic echocardiogram is recommended as initial evaluation with known or suspected aortic insufficiency to establish the diagnosis and to determine the severity if the insufficiency.
- Cardiac magnetic resonance (CMR) is an alternative form of evaluation if the TTE is nondiagnostic or suboptimal.
- Hypertension should be treated to keep SBP <140 mm Hg with nondihydropyridine calcium channel blocker, ACE inhibitor, or ARB agent.
- Aortic valve replacement: symptomatic person with severe AI regardless of the systolic function; asymptomatic patient with severe AI and systolic dysfunction <50% or with end systolic volume (ESD) >50 mm.

MITRAL STENOSIS (MS)

- Transthoracic echocardiogram is recommended as initial evaluation with known or suspected mitral stenosis to establish the diagnosis and to determine the severity if the stenosis.
- Transesophageal echocardiogram (TEE) should be considered prior to sending the patient for percutaneous mitral balloon commissurotomy (PMBC) to exclude the presence of left atrial thrombus.
- Warfarin is indicated in patients with mitral stenosis and atrial fibrillation, prior embolic event or intracardiac thrombus.
- Heart rate control in atrial fibrillation is imperative to allow optimal diastolic filling time across the stenotic valve.
- PMBC is indicated in symptomatic patients with severe mitral stenosis (MVA ≤1.5 cm²) with no atrial thrombus and no or minimal mitral insufficiency.
- Mitral valve replacement is indicated if balloon commissurotomy is contraindicated in a patient with severe symptoms and severe mitral stenosis.

MITRAL REGURGITATION (MR)

- Transthoracic echocardiogram is recommended as initial evaluation with known or suspected mitral regurgitation to establish the diagnosis and to determine the severity if the insufficiency, left atrial and ventricular size and right ventricular function.
- Cardiac magnetic resonance (CMR) is an alternative form of evaluation if the TTE is nondiagnostic or suboptimal.
- Mitral valve replacement or repair is indicated in a symptomatic patient with severe regurgitation if the systolic function (EF) is >30%.
- Mitral valve replacement is indicated in an asymptomatic patient with severe mitral regurgitation if the systolic function (EF) is between 30% and 60% or the left ventricular end systolic dimension (LVESD) ≥40%.

Source: Nishimura RA, Otto CM, Bonow RO. 2014 AHA/ACC Guidelines for the Management of Patients With Valvular Heart Disease: A Report of the American College of Cardiology/American Heart Association Task Force on Practice Guidelines. *J Am Coll Cardiol.* June 10, 2014;63(22):e57. doi:10.1016/jack.2014.02.536.

VERTIGO, BENIGN PAROXYSMAL POSITIONAL (BPPV)

Disease Management	Organization	Date	Population	Recommendations	Comments	Source
Vertigo, Benign Paroxysmal Positional (BPPV)	AAO-HNS	2008	Adults	1. Recommends the Dix-Hallpike maneuver to diagnose posterior semicircular canal BPPV. 2. Recommends treatment of posterior semicircular canal BPPV with a particle repositioning maneuver. 3. If the Dix-Hallpike test result is negative, recommends a supine roll test to diagnose lateral semicircular canal BPPV. 4. Recommends offering vestibular rehabilitation exercises for the initial treatment of BPPV. 5. Recommends evaluating patients for an underlying peripheral vestibular or central nervous system disorder if they have an initial treatment failure of presumed BPPV. 6. Recommends against routine radiologic imaging for patients with BPPV. 7. Recommends against routine vestibular testing for patients with BPPV. 8. Recommends against routine use of antihistamines or benzodiazepines for patients with BPPV.	BPPV is the most common vestibular disorder in adults, afflicting 2.4% of adults at some point during their lives.	http://www.guideline.gov/content.aspx?id=13403

4
Appendices

SCREENING INSTRUMENTS: ALCOHOL ABUSE

SENSITIVITY AND SPECIFICITY OF SCREENING TESTS FOR PROBLEM DRINKING

Instrument Name	Screening Questions/Scoring	Threshold Score	Sensitivity/Specificity (%)	Source
CAGE[a]	See page 385	>1 >2 >3	77/58 53/81 29/92	*Am J Psychiatry.* 1974;131:1121 *J Gen Intern Med.* 1998;13:379
AUDIT	See page 385	>4 >5 >6	87/70 77/84 66/90	*BMJ.* 1997;314:420 *J Gen Intern Med.* 1998;13:379

[a]The CAGE may be less applicable to binge drinkers (e.g., college students), the elderly, and minority populations.

SCREENING INSTRUMENTS: ALCOHOL ABUSE

SCREENING PROCEDURES FOR PROBLEM DRINKING

1. CAGE screening test[a]

Have you ever felt the need to	**C**ut down on drinking?
Have you ever felt	**A**nnoyed by criticism of your drinking?
Have you ever felt	**G**uilty about your drinking?
Have you ever taken a morning	**E**ye opener?

INTERPRETATION: Two "yes" answers are considered a positive screen. One "yes" answer should arouse a suspicion of alcohol abuse.

2. The Alcohol Use Disorder Identification Test (AUDIT)[b] (Scores for response categories are given in parentheses. Scores range from 0 to 40, with a cutoff score of ≥5 indicating hazardous drinking, harmful drinking, or alcohol dependence.)

1) How often do you have a drink containing alcohol?

   (0) Never (1) Monthly or less (2) Two to four times a month (3) Two or three times a week (4) Four or more times a week

2) How many drinks containing alcohol do you have on a typical day when you are drinking?

   (0) 1 or 2 (1) 3 or 4 (2) 5 or 6 (3) 7 to 9 (4) 10 or more

3) How often do you have 6 or more drinks on 1 occasion?

   (0) Never (1) Less than monthly (2) Monthly (3) Weekly (4) Daily or almost daily

4) How often during the last year have you found that you were not able to stop drinking once you had started?

   (0) Never (1) Less than monthly (2) Monthly (3) Weekly (4) Daily or almost daily

5) How often during the last year have you failed to do what was normally expected of you because of drinking?

   (0) Never (1) Less than monthly (2) Monthly (3) Weekly (4) Daily or almost daily

6) How often during the last year have you needed a first drink in the morning to get yourself going after a heavy drinking session?

   (0) Never (1) Less than monthly (2) Monthly (3) Weekly (4) Daily or almost daily

7) How often during the last year have you had a feeling of guilt or remorse after drinking?

   (0) Never (1) Less than monthly (2) Monthly (3) Weekly (4) Daily or almost daily

8) How often during the last year have you been unable to remember what happened the night before because you had been drinking?

   (0) Never (1) Less than monthly (2) Monthly (3) Weekly (4) Daily or almost daily

9) Have you or has someone else been injured as a result of your drinking?

   (0) No (2) Yes, but not in the last year (4) Yes, during the last year

10) Has a relative or friend or a doctor or other health worker been concerned about your drinking or suggested you cut down?

   (0) No (2) Yes, but not in the last year (4) Yes, during the last year

[a]Modified from Mayfield D, McLeod G, Hall P. The CAGE questionnaire: validation of a new alcoholism screening instrument. *Am J Psychiatry.* 1974;131:1121.

[b]From Piccinelli M, Tessari E, Bortolomasi M, et al. Efficacy of the alcohol use disorders identification test as a screening tool for hazardous alcohol intake and related disorders in primary care: a validity study. *BMJ.* 1997;314:420.

SCREENING INSTRUMENTS: DEPRESSION

SCREENING TESTS FOR DEPRESSION

Instrument Name	Screening Questions/Scoring	Threshold Score	Source
Beck Depression Inventory (short form)	See page 389	0–4: None or minimal depression 5–7: Mild depression 8–15: Moderate depression >15: Severe depression	*Postgrad Med.* 1972;Dec:81
Geriatric Depression Scale	See page 390	≥15: Depression	*J Psychiatr Res.* 1983;17:37
PRIME-MD® (mood questions)	1. During the last month, have you often been bothered by feeling down, depressed, or hopeless? 2. During the last month, have you often been bothered by little interest or pleasure in doing things?	"Yes" to either question[a]	*JAMA.* 1994;272:1749 *J Gen Intern Med.* 1997;12:439
Patient Health Questionnaire (PHQ-9)®	http://www.pfizer.com/phq-9/ See pages 387–388	*Major depressive syndrome:* if answers to #1a or b and ≥5 of #1a–i are at least "More than half the days" (count #1i if present at all) *Other depressive syndrome:* if #1a or b and 2–4 of #1a–i are at least "More than half the days" (count #1i if present at all) 5–9: mild depression 10–14: moderate depression 15–19: moderately severe depression 20–27: severe depression	*JAMA.* 1999;282:1737 *J Gen Intern Med.* 2001;16:606

[a]Sensitivity 86%–96%; specificity 57%–75%.
®Pfizer Inc.

SCREENING INSTRUMENTS: DEPRESSION

PHQ-9 DEPRESSION SCREEN, ENGLISH

Over the past 2 weeks, how often have you been bothered by any of the following problems?

	Not at all	Several days	>Half the days	Nearly every day
a. Little interest or pleasure in doing things	0	1	2	3
b. Feeling down, depressed, or hopeless	0	1	2	3
c. Trouble falling or staying asleep, or sleeping too much	0	1	2	3
d. Feeling tired or having little energy	0	1	2	3
e. Poor appetite or overeating	0	1	2	3
f. Feeling bad about yourself—or that you are a failure or that you have let yourself or your family down	0	1	2	3
g. Trouble concentrating on things, such as reading the newspaper or watching television	0	1	2	3
h. Moving or speaking so slowly that other people could have noticed? Or the opposite—being so fidgety or restless that you have been moving around a lot more than usual?	0	1	2	3
i. Thoughts that you would be better off dead or of hurting yourself in some way	0	1	2	3
For office coding: Total Score	— =	— +	— +	—

Major depressive syndrome: If ≥5 items present scored ≥2 and one of the items is depressed mood (b) or anhedonia (a). If item "i" is present, then this counts, even if score = 1.
Depressive screen positive: If at least one item ≥2 (or item "i" is ≥1).

Source: From the Primary Care Evaluation of Mental Disorders Patient Health Questionnaire (PRIME-MD PHQ). The PHQ was developed by Drs. Robert L., et al. For research information, contact Dr. Spitzer at rls8@columbia.edu. PRIME-MD® is a trademark of Pfizer Inc. Copyright © 1999 Pfizer Inc. All rights reserved. Reproduced with permission. For office coding: Maj Dep Syn if answer to #2a or b and ≥5 of #2a–i are at least "More than half the days" (count #2i if present at all). Other Dep Syn if #2a or b and 2, 3, or 4 of #2a–i are at least "More than half the days" (count #2i if present at all).

SCREENING INSTRUMENTS: DEPRESSION

PHQ-9 DEPRESSION SCREEN, SPANISH

Durante las últimas 2 semanas, ¿con qué frecuencia le han molestado los siguientes problemas?

	Nunca	Varios dias	>La mitad de los dias	Casi todos los dias
a. Tener poco interés o placer en hacer las cosas	0	1	2	3
b. Sentirse desanimada, deprimida, o sin esperanza	0	1	2	3
c. Con problemas en dormirse o en mantenerse dormida, o en dormir demasiado	0	1	2	3
d. Sentirse cansada o tener poca energía	0	1	2	3
e. Tener poco apetito o comer cn exceso	0	1	2	3
f. Sentir falta de amor propio—o qe sea un fracaso o que decepcionara a sí misma o a su familia	0	1	2	3
g. Tener dificultad para concentrarse en cosas tales como leer el periódico o mirar la televisión	0	1	2	3
h. Se mueve o habla tan lentamente que otra gente se podría dar cuenta—o de lo contrario, está tan agitada o inquieta que se mueve mucho más de lo acostumbrado	0	1	2	3
i. Se le han ocurrido pensamientos de que se haría daño de alguna manera	0	1	2	3
For office coding: Total Store	—	=	—	+	—	+	—

Source: From the Primary Care Evaluation of Mental Disorders Patient Health Questionnaire (PRIME-MD PHQ). The PHQ was developed by Drs. Robert L., et al. For research information, contact Dr. Spitzer at rls8@columbia.edu. PRIME-MD® is a trademark of Pfizer Inc. Copyright © 1999 Pfizer Inc. All rights reserved. Reproduced with permission. For office coding: Maj Dep Syn if answer to #2a or b and ≥5 of #2a–i are at least "More than half the days" (count #2i if present at all). Other Dep Syn if #2a or b and 2, 3, or 4 of #2a–i are at least "More than half the days" (count #2i if present at all).

SCREENING INSTRUMENTS: DEPRESSION

BECK DEPRESSION INVENTORY, SHORT FORM

Instructions: This is a questionnaire. On the questionnaire are groups of statements. Please read the entire group of statements in each category. Then pick out the one statement in that group that best describes the way you feel today, that is, right now! Circle the number beside the statement you have chosen. If several statements in the group seem to apply equally well, circle each one. Sum all numbers to calculate a score.

Be sure to read all the statements in each group before making your choice.

A. Sadness
3 I am so sad or unhappy that I can't stand it.
2 I am blue or sad all the time and I can't snap out of it.
1 I feel sad or blue.
0 I do not feel sad.

B. Pessimism
3 I feel that the future is hopeless and that things cannot improve.
2 I feel I have nothing to look forward to.
1 I feel discouraged about the future.
0 I am not particularly pessimistic or discouraged about the future.

C. Sense of failure
3 I feel I am a complete failure as a person (parent, husband, wife).
2 As I look back on my life, all I can see is a lot of failures.
1 I feel I have failed more than the average person.
0 I do not feel like a failure.

D. Dissatisfaction
3 I am dissatisfied with everything.
2 I don't get satisfaction out of anything anymore.
1 I don't enjoy things the way I used to.
0 I am not particularly dissatisfied.

E. Guilt
3 I feel as though I am very bad or worthless.
2 I feel quite guilty.
1 I feel bad or unworthy a good part of the time.
0 I don't feel particularly guilty.

F. Self-dislike
3 I hate myself.
2 I am disgusted with myself.
1 I am disappointed in myself.
0 I don't feel disappointed in myself.

G. Self-harm
3 I would kill myself if I had the chance.
2 I have definite plans about committing suicide.
1 I feel I would be better off dead.
0 I don't have any thoughts of harming myself.

H. Social withdrawal
3 I have lost all of my interest in other people and don't care about them at all.
2 I have lost most of my interest in other people and have little feeling for them.
1 I am less interested in other people than I used to be.
0 I have not lost interest in other people.

I. Indecisiveness
3 I can't make any decisions at all anymore.
2 I have great difficulty in making decisions.
1 I try to put off making decisions.
0 I make decisions about as well as ever.

J. Self-image change
3 I feel that I am ugly or repulsive looking.
2 I feel that there are permanent changes in my appearance and they make me look unattractive.
1 I am worried that I am looking old or unattractive.
0 I don't feel that I look worse than I used to.

K. Work difficulty
3 I can't do any work at all.
2 I have to push myself very hard to do anything.
1 It takes extra effort to get started at doing something.
0 I can work about as well as before.

L. Fatigability
3 I get too tired to do anything.
2 I get tired from doing anything.
1 I get tired more easily than I used to.
0 I don't get any more tired than usual.

M. Anorexia
3 I have no appetite at all anymore.
2 My appetite is much worse now.
1 My appetite is not as good as it used to be.
0 My appetite is no worse than usual.

Source: Reproduced with permission from Beck AT, Beck RW. Screening depressed patients in family practice: a rapid technic. *Postgrad Med.* 1972;52:81.

GERIATRIC DEPRESSION SCALE

Choose the best answer for how you felt over the past week

1. Are you basically satisfied with your life?	yes / no
2. Have you dropped many of your activities and interests?	yes / no
3. Do you feel that your life is empty?	yes / no
4. Do you often get bored?	yes / no
5. Are you hopeful about the future?	yes / no
6. Are you bothered by thoughts you can't get out of your head?	yes / no
7. Are you in good spirits most of the time?	yes / no
8. Are you afraid that something bad is going to happen to you?	yes / no
9. Do you feel happy most of the time?	yes / no
10. Do you often feel helpless?	yes / no
11. Do you often get restless and fidgety?	yes / no
12. Do you prefer to stay at home, rather than going out and doing new things?	yes / no
13. Do you frequently worry about the future?	yes / no
14. Do you feel you have more problems with memory than most?	yes / no
15. Do you think it is wonderful to be alive now?	yes / no
16. Do you often feel downhearted and blue?	yes / no
17. Do you feel pretty worthless the way you are now?	yes / no
18. Do you worry a lot about the past?	yes / no
19. Do you find life very exciting?	yes / no
20. Is it hard for you to get started on new projects?	yes / no
21. Do you feel full of energy?	yes / no
22. Do you feel that your situation is hopeless?	yes / no
23. Do you think that most people are better off than you are?	yes / no
24. Do you frequently get upset over little things?	yes / no
25. Do you frequently feel like crying?	yes / no
26. Do you have trouble concentrating?	yes / no
27. Do you enjoy getting up in the morning?	yes / no
28. Do you prefer to avoid social gatherings?	yes / no
29. Is it easy for you to make decisions?	yes / no
30. Is your mind as clear as it used to be?	yes / no

One point for each response suggestive of depression. (Specifically "no" responses to questions 1, 5, 7, 9, 15, 19, 21, 27, 29, and 30, and "yes" responses to the remaining questions are suggestive of depression.)

A score of ≥15 yields a sensitivity of 80% and a specificity of 100%, as a screening test for geriatric depression. *Clin Gerontol.* 1982;1:37.

Source: Reproduced with permission from Yesavage JA, Brink TL, Rose TL, et al. Development and validation of a geriatric depression screening scale: a preliminary report. *J Psychiatr Res.* 1982–1983;17:37.

FUNCTIONAL ASSESSMENT SCREENING IN THE ELDERLY

Target Area	Assessment Procedure	Abnormal Result	Suggested Intervention
Vision	Inquire about vision changes, Snellen chart testing.	Presence of vision changes; inability to read >20/40	Refer to ophthalmologist.
Hearing	Whisper a short, easily answered question such as "What is your name?" in each ear while the examiner's face is out of direct view. Use audioscope set at 40 dB; test using 1000 and 2000 Hz. Brief hearing loss screener.	Inability to answer question Inability to hear 1000 or 2000 Hz in both ears or inability to hear frequencies in either ear Brief hearing loss screen score ≥3	Examine auditory canals for cerumen and clean if necessary. Repeat test; if still abnormal in either ear, refer for audiometry and possible prosthesis.
Balance and gait	Observe the patient after instructing as follows: "Rise from your chair, walk 10 ft, return, and sit down." Check orthostatic blood pressure and heart rate.	Inability to complete task in 15 s	Performance-Oriented Mobility Assessment (POMA). Consider referral for physical therapy.
Continence of urine	Ask, "Do you ever lose your urine and get wet?" If yes, then ask, "Have you lost urine on at least 6 separate days?"	"Yes" to both questions	Ascertain frequency and amount. Search for remediable causes, including local irritations, polyuric states, and medications. Consider urologic referral.
Nutrition	Ask, "Without trying, have you lost 10 lb or more in the last 6 months?" Weigh the patient. Measure height.	"Yes" or weight is below acceptable range for height	Do appropriate medical evaluation.
Mental status	Instruct as follows: "I am going to name three objects (pencil, truck, and book). I will ask you to repeat their names now and then again a few minutes from now."	Inability to recall all three objects after 1 minute	Administer Folstein Mini-Mental State Examination. If score is <24, search for causes of cognitive impairment. Ascertain onset, duration, and fluctuation of overt symptoms. Review medications. Assess consciousness and affect. Do appropriate laboratory tests.
Depression	Ask, "Do you often feel sad or depressed?" or "How are your spirits?"	"Yes" or "Not very good, I guess"	Administer Geriatric Depression Scale or PHQ-9. If positive, check for antihypertensive, psychotropic, or other pertinent medications. Consider appropriate pharmacologic or psychiatric treatment.
ADL-IADL[a]	Ask, "Can you get out of bed yourself?" "Can you dress yourself?" "Can you make your own meals?" "Can you do your own shopping?"	"No" to any question	Corroborate responses with patient's appearance; question family members if accuracy is uncertain. Determine reasons for the inability (motivation compared with physical limitation). Institute appropriate medical, social, or environmental interventions.
Home environment	Ask, "Do you have trouble with stairs inside or outside of your home?" Ask about potential hazards inside the home with bathtubs, rugs, or lighting.	"Yes"	Evaluate home safety and institute appropriate countermeasures.
Social support	Ask, "Who would be able to help you in case of illness or emergency?"	—	List identified persons in the medical record. Become familiar with available resources for the elderly in the community.
Pain	Inquire about pain.	Presence of pain	Pain inventory.
Dentition	Oral examination.	Poor dentition	Dentistry referral.
Falls	Inquire about falls in past year and difficulty with walking or balance.	Presence of falls or gait/balance problems	Falls evaluation (see page 12

[a]Activities of Daily Living–Instrumental Activities of Daily Living.
Source: Modified from Fleming KC, Evans JM, Weber DC, Chutka DS. Practical functional assessment of elderly persons: a primary-c approach. *Mayo Clin Proc.* 1995;70(9):890–910.

SCREENING AND PREVENTION GUIDELINES IN PERSPECTIVE: PGPC 2012

The following tables highlight areas where differences exist between various organizations' guideline recommendations and areas where a new direction appears to be developing as a result of new or updated guidelines.

1. Areas of significant difference in guideline recommendations

Guidelines	Organization	Recommendations
Adolescent Alcohol Abuse	USPSTF/AAFP	Evidence insufficient
	Bright Futures/NIAAA	Screen annually
Breast CA Screening, Women age 40–49 y	UK-NHS	Routine screening not recommended
	ACP	Mammogram and CBE yearly starting at age 40 y—high-risk patients (>20% lifetime risk of breast CA) add annual MRI
	USPSTF/AAFP	Mammography ± breast examination every 2 y beginning at age 50 y and stop at age 75. In women age 40–50 y, counsel regarding risks and benefits; it should no longer be done routinely
Breast CA Screening, Women age 50–70 y	UK-NHS	Mammography screening every 3 y
	USPSTF/AAFP	Mammography screening every 2 y
	ACS	Annual mammography screening
Cervical CA Screening, Women age <50 y	UK-NHS	Begin screening every 3 y after age 25 y
	ACS	Screen beginning at age 21 y no matter when sexual activity started; screen annually (or every 2 y if liquid-based Pap smear) until age 30, then every 3 y if consecutive negative Pap smear results. HPV testing can be added after age 30 y. If Pap smears and HPV testing are both negative, the frequency of testing can be every 5 y
Prostate CA Screening, Men age >50 y	USPSTF/AAFP	Do not use PSA-based screening for prostate cancer at any age—evidence suggests harms outweigh benefits
	UK-NHS	Informed decision making
	ACS	Discuss screening PSA and digital rectal examination. Discuss risks and benefits including treatment options and side effects of treatment. Do not do PSA screen unless patient desires
Testicular CA Screening	USPSTF/AAFP	Recommend against screening
	ACS	Perform testicular examination as part of routine CA-related checkup
Depression, Children and Adolescents	USPSTF/AAFP/CTF/NICE	Insufficient evidence to recommend for or against screening
	Bright Futures	Annual screening for behaviors/emotions that indicate depression or risk of suicide
Family Violence and Abuse, Children and Adolescents	USPSTF/AAFP	Insufficient evidence to recommend for or against screening
	Family Violence Prevention Fund	Assess caregivers/parents and adolescent patients at least annually
Hearing Loss, Newborns	USPSTF/AAFP	Insufficient evidence to recommend for or against screening during the postpartum hospitalization
	Joint Committee on Infant Hearing	All infants should be screened for neonatal or congenital hearing loss
Thyroid Screening, Adults	USPSTF/AAFP	Evidence insufficient to recommend for or against screening
	ATA	Screen all women age >35 y at 5-y intervals
Glaucoma, Adults	USPSTF/AAFP	Evidence insufficient to recommend for or against screening
	AOA	Comprehensive eye examination every 2 y ages 18–60 y, then every year age >60
Diabetes Mellitus, Gestational	USPSTF/AAFP	Evidence insufficient to recommend for or against screening asymptomatic pregnant women
	ADA	Risk assess all women at first prenatal visit

y directions resulting from new or updated guidelines

ening: Opt-out screening for practically everyone, actively recommended against written informed consent.

prophylaxis: Now targets those at increased risk of complications from endocarditis, rather than risk of endocarditis.

guidelines: New data have emerged on beta blockade that is not reflected in current guidelines. Two randomized trials of metoprolol found that perioperative metoprolol does not appear to be effective in reducing postoperative death rates cted patients.

Risk Algorithm (FRAX) developed to calculate the 1-y probability of fracture to guide treatment decisions.
mmendations for men.
to measure and supplement serum 25-OH vitamin D levels.
ention: New recommendation to consider metformin for those at very high risk of developing diabetes.

nical breast examination; HIV, human immunodeficiency syndrome; HPV, human papillomavirus; MRI, naging; PSA, prostate-specific antigen.

95TH PERCENTILE OF BLOOD PRESSURE FOR BOYS

Age (y)	Systolic Blood Pressure (mm Hg) by Percentile of Height							Diastolic Blood Pressure (mm Hg) by Percentile of Height						
	5%	10%	25%	50%	75%	90%	95%	5%	10%	25%	50%	75%	90%	95%
3	104	105	107	109	110	112	113	63	63	64	65	66	67	67
4	106	107	109	111	112	114	115	66	67	68	69	70	71	71
5	108	109	110	112	114	115	116	69	70	71	72	73	74	74
6	109	110	112	114	115	117	117	72	72	73	74	75	76	76
7	110	111	113	115	117	113	119	74	74	75	76	77	78	78
8	111	112	114	116	118	119	120	75	76	77	78	79	79	80
9	113	114	116	118	119	121	121	76	76	78	79	80	81	81
10	115	116	117	119	121	122	123	77	78	79	80	81	81	82
11	117	118	119	121	123	124	125	78	78	79	80	81	82	82
12	119	120	122	123	125	127	127	78	79	80	81	82	82	83
13	121	122	124	126	128	129	130	79	79	80	81	82	83	83
14	124	125	127	128	130	132	132	80	80	81	82	83	84	84
15	126	127	129	131	133	134	135	81	81	82	83	84	85	85
16	129	130	132	134	135	137	137	82	83	83	84	85	86	87
17	131	132	134	136	138	139	140	84	85	86	87	87	88	89

95TH PERCENTILE OF BLOOD PRESSURE FOR GIRLS

Age (y)	Systolic Blood Pressure (mm Hg) by Percentile of Height							Diastolic Blood Pressure (mm Hg) by Percentile of Height						
	5%	10%	25%	50%	75%	90%	95%	5%	10%	25%	50%	75%	90%	95%
3	104	104	105	107	108	109	110	65	66	66	67	68	68	69
4	105	106	107	108	110	111	112	68	68	69	70	71	71	72
5	107	107	108	110	111	112	113	70	71	71	72	73	73	74
6	108	109	110	111	113	114	115	72	72	73	74	74	75	76
7	110	111	112	113	115	116	116	73	74	74	75	76	76	77
8	112	112	114	115	116	118	118	75	75	75	76	77	78	78
9	114	114	115	117	118	119	120	76	76	76	77	78	79	79
10	116	116	117	119	120	121	122	77	77	77	78	79	80	80
11	118	118	119	121	122	123	124	78	78	78	79	80	81	81
12	119	120	121	123	124	125	126	79	79	79	80	81	82	82
13	121	122	123	124	126	127	128	80	80	80	81	82	83	83
14	123	123	125	126	127	129	129	81	81	81	82	83	84	84
15	124	125	126	127	129	130	131	82	82	82	83	84	85	85
16	125	126	127	128	130	131	132	82	82	83	84	85	85	86
17	125	126	127	129	130	131	132	82	83	83	84	85	85	86

Source: Blood Pressure Tables for Children and Adolescents from the *Fourth Report on the Diagnosis, Evaluation, and Treatment of High Blood Pressure in Children and Adolescents.* http://www.nhlbi.nih.gov/guidelines/hypertension/child_tbl.htm. Accessed June 3, 2008.

BODY MASS INDEX (BMI) CONVERSION TABLE

Height in inches (cm)	BMI 25 kg/m^2	BMI 27 kg/m^2	BMI 30 kg/m^2
	Body weight in pounds (kg)		
58 (147.32)	119 (53.98)	129 (58.51)	143 (64.86)
59 (149.86)	124 (56.25)	133 (60.33)	148 (67.13)
60 (152.40)	128 (58.06)	138 (62.60)	153 (69.40)
61 (154.94)	132 (59.87)	143 (64.86)	158 (71.67)
62 (157.48)	136 (61.69)	147 (66.68)	164 (74.39)
63 (160.02)	141 (63.96)	152 (68.95)	169 (76.66)
64 (162.56)	145 (65.77)	157 (71.22)	174 (78.93)
65 (165.10)	150 (68.04)	162 (73.48)	180 (81.65)
66 (167.64)	155 (70.31)	167 (75.75)	186 (84.37)
67 (170.18)	159 (72.12)	172 (78.02)	191 (86.64)
68 (172.72)	164 (74.39)	177 (80.29)	197 (89.36)
69 (175.26)	169 (76.66)	182 (82.56)	203 (92.08)
70 (177.80)	174 (78.93)	188 (85.28)	207 (93.90)
71 (180.34)	179 (81.19)	193 (87.54)	215 (97.52)
72 (182.88)	184 (83.46)	199 (90.27)	221 (100.25)
73 (185.42)	189 (85.73)	204 (92.53)	227 (102.97)
74 (187.96)	194 (88.00)	210 (95.26)	233 (105.69)
75 (190.50)	200 (90.72)	216 (97.98)	240 (108.86)
76 (193.04)	205 (92.99)	221 (100.25)	246 (111.59)

Metric conversion formula = weight (kg)/height (m^2)
Example of BMI calculation:
A person who weighs 78.93 kg and is 177 cm tall has a BMI of 25:
weight (78.93 kg)/height (1.77 m^2) = **25**

BMI categories:
Underweight = <18.5
Normal weight = 18.5–24.9
Overweight = 25–29.9
Obesity = ≥30

Nonmetric conversion formula = [weight (lb)/height (in^2)] × 704.5
Example of BMI calculation:
A person who weighs 164 lb and is 68 in (or 5′8″) tall has a BMI of 25:
[weight (164 lb)/height (68 in^2)] × 704.5 = 25

Source: Adapted from NHLBI Obesity Guidelines in Adults. http://www.nhlbi.nih.gov/guidelines/obesity/bmi_tbl.htm. Accessed October 13, 2011. BMI online calculator. http://www.nhlbisupport.com/bmi/bmicalc.htm. Accessed October 13, 2011.

ESTIMATE OF 10-y CARDIAC RISK FOR MEN[a]

Age (y)	Points
20–34	–9
35–39	–4
40–44	0
45–49	3
50–54	6
55–59	8
60–64	10
65–69	11
70–74	12
75–79	13

Total Cholesterol	Points				
	Age 20–39	Age 40–19	Age 50–59	Age 60–69	Age 70–79
<160	0	0	0	0	0
160–199	4	3	2	1	0
200–239	7	5	3	1	0
240–279	9	6	4	2	1
≥280	11	8	5	3	1

	Points				
	Age 20–39	Age 40–49	Age 50–59	Age 60–69	Age 70–79
Nonsmoker	0	0	0	0	0
Smoker	8	5	3	1	1

High-Density Lipoprotein (mg/dL)	Points
≥60	–1
50–59	0
40–49	1
<40	2

Systolic Blood Pressure (mm Hg)	If Untreated	If Treated
<120	0	0
120–129	0	1
130–139	1	2
140–159	1	2
≥160	2	3

Point Total	10-y Risk %	Point Total	10-y Risk %	
<0	<1	9	5	
0	1	10	6	
1	1	11	8	
2	1	12	10	
3	1	13	12	
4	1	14	16	
5	2	15	20	
6	2	16	25	
7	3	≥17	≥30	10-y Risk _____ %
8	4			

[a]Framingham point scores.

Source: U.S. Department of Health and Human Services, Public Health Service, National Institutes of Health, National Heart, Lung, and Blood Institute. NIH Publication No. 01-3305, May 2001.
Online risk calculator. http://hp2010.nhlbihin.net/atpiii/calculator.asp.

ESTIMATE OF 10-y CARDIAC RISK FOR WOMEN[a]

Age (y)	Points
20–34	−7
35–39	−3
40–44	0
45–49	3
50–54	6
55–59	8
60–64	10
65–69	12
70–74	14
75–79	16

Total Cholesterol	Points				
	Age 20–39	Age 40–19	Age 50–59	Age 60–69	Age 70–79
<160	0	0	0	0	0
160–199	4	3	2	1	1
200–239	8	6	4	2	1
240–279	11	8	5	3	2
≥280	13	10	7	4	2

	Points				
	Age 20–39	Age 40–49	Age 50–59	Age 60–69	Age 70–79
Nonsmoker	0	0	0	0	0
Smoker	9	7	4	2	1

High-Density Lipoprotein (mg/dL)	Points
≥60	−1
50–59	0
40–49	1
<40	2

Systolic Blood Pressure (mm Hg)	If Untreated	If Treated
<120	0	0
120–129	1	3
130–139	2	4
140–159	3	5
≥160	4	6

Point Total	10-y Risk %	Point Total	10-y Risk %
<9	<1	17	5
9	1	18	6
10	1	19	8
11	1	20	11
12	1	21	14
13	2	22	17
14	2	23	22
15	3	24	27
16	4	≥25	≥30

10-y Risk_____%

[a]Framingham point scores.

Source: U.S. Department of Health and Human Services, Public Health Service, National Institutes of Health, National Heart, Lung, and Blood Institute. NIH Publication No. 01-3305, May 2001.
Online risk calculator. http://hp2010.nhlbihin.net/atpiii/calculator.asp.

ESTIMATE OF 10-y STROKE RISK FOR MEN

Age (y)	Points	Untreated Systolic Blood Pressure (mm Hg)	Points
54–56	0	97–105	0
57–59	1	106–115	1
60–62	2	116–125	2
63–65	3	126–135	3
66–68	4	136–145	4
69–72	5	146–155	5
73–75	6	156–165	6
76–78	7	166–175	7
79–81	8	176–185	8
82–84	9	186–195	9
85	10	196–205	10

Treated Systolic Blood Pressure (mm Hg)	Points	History of Diabetes	Points
97–105	0	No	0
106–112	1	Yes	2
113–117	2		
118–123	3		
124–129	4		
130–135	5		
136–142	6		
143–150	7		
151–161	8		
162–176	9		
177–205	10		

Cigarette Smoking	Points	Cardiovascular Disease	Points
No	0	No	0
Yes	3	Yes	4

Atrial Fibrillation	Points	Left Ventricular Hypertrophy on Electrocardiogram	Points
No	0	No	0
Yes	4	Yes	5

Point Total	10-y Risk %	Point Total	10-y Risk %
1	3	16	22
2	3	17	26
3	4	18	29
4	4	19	33
5	5	20	37
6	5	21	42
7	6	22	47
8	7	23	52
9	8	24	57
10	10	25	63
11	11	26	68
12	13	27	74
13	15	28	79
14	17	29	84
15	20	30	88

10-y Risk _____%

Source: Modified Framingham Stroke Risk Profile. *Circulation.* 2006;113:e873–e923.

ESTIMATE OF 10-y STROKE RISK FOR WOMEN

Age (y)	Points	Untreated Systolic Blood Pressure (mm Hg)	Points
54–56	0	95–106	1
57–59	1	107–118	2
60–62	2	119–130	3
63–64	3	131–143	4
65–67	4	144–155	5
68–70	5	156–167	6
71–73	6	168–180	7
74–76	7	181–192	8
77–78	8	193–204	9
79–81	9	205–216	10
82–84	10		

Treated Systolic Blood Pressure (mm Hg)	Points	History of Diabetes	Points
95–106	1	No	0
107–113	2	Yes	3
114–119	3		
120–125	4		
126–131	5		
132–139	6		
140–148	7		
149–160	8		
161–204	9		
205–216	10		

Cigarette Smoking	Points	Cardiovascular Disease	Points
No	0	No	0
Yes	3	Yes	2

Atrial Fibrillation	Points	Left Ventricular Hypertrophy on Electrocardiogram	Points
No	0	No	0
Yes	6	Yes	4

Point Total	10-y Risk %	Point Total	10-y Risk %
1	1	16	19
2	1	17	23
3	2	18	27
4	2	19	32
5	2	20	37
6	3	21	43
7	4	22	50
8	4	23	57
9	5	24	64
10	6	25	71
11	8	26	78
12	9	27	84
13	11	28	
14	13	29	
15	16	30	

10-y Risk_____%

Source: Modified Framingham Stroke Risk Profile. *Circulation.* 2006;113:e873-e923.

Figure 1. Recommended immunization schedule for persons aged 0 through 18 years – United States, 2015.

(FOR THOSE WHO FALL BEHIND OR START LATE, SEE THE CATCH-UP SCHEDULE [FIGURE 2]).

These recommendations must be read with the footnotes that follow. For those who fall behind or start late, provide catch-up vaccination at the earliest opportunity as indicated by the green bars in Figure 1. To determine minimum intervals between doses, see the catch-up schedule (Figure 2). School entry and adolescent vaccine age groups are shaded.

Vaccine	Birth	1 mo	2 mos	4 mos	6 mos	9 mos	12 mos	15 mos	18 mos	19–23 mos	2-3 yrs	4-6 yrs	7-10 yrs	11-12 yrs	13-15 yrs	16–18 yrs
Hepatitis B¹ (HepB)	1st dose	←—— 2nd dose ——→			←——————————— 3rd dose ———————————→											
Rotavirus² (RV) RV1 (2-dose series); RV5 (3-dose series)			1st dose	2nd dose	See footnote 2											
Diphtheria, tetanus, & acellular pertussis³ (DTaP: <7 yrs)			1st dose	2nd dose	3rd dose		←————— 4th dose —————→					5th dose				
Tetanus, diphtheria, & acellular pertussis⁴ (Tdap: ≥7 yrs)														(Tdap)		
Haemophilus influenzae type b⁵ (Hib)			1st dose	2nd dose	See footnote 5		←— 3rd or 4th dose, See footnote 5 —→									
Pneumococcal conjugate⁶ (PCV13)			1st dose	2nd dose	3rd dose		←————— 4th dose —————→									
Pneumococcal polysaccharide⁶ (PPSV23)												4th dose				
Inactivated poliovirus⁷ (IPV: <18 yrs)			1st dose	2nd dose	←————————— 3rd dose —————————→							4th dose				
Influenza⁸ (IIV; LAIV) 2 doses for some: See footnote 8					Annual vaccination (IIV only) 1 or 2 doses						Annual vaccination (LAIV or IIV) 1 or 2 doses			Annual vaccination (LAIV or IIV) 1 dose only		
Measles, mumps, rubella⁹ (MMR)							←—— 1st dose ——→					2nd dose				
Varicella¹⁰ (VAR)							←—— 1st dose ——→					2nd dose				
Hepatitis A¹¹ (HepA)							←——— 2-dose series, See footnote 11 ———→									
Human papillomavirus¹² (HPV2: females only; HPV4: males and females)														(3-dose series)		
Meningococcal¹³ (Hib-MenCY ≥ 6 weeks; MenACWY-D ≥9 mos; MenACWY-CRM ≥ 2 mos)							See footnote 13							1st dose		Booster

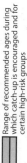

Range of recommended ages for all children

Range of recommended ages for catch-up immunization

Range of recommended ages for certain high-risk groups

Range of recommended ages during which catch-up is encouraged and for certain high-risk groups

Not routinely recommended

This schedule includes recommendations in effect as of January 1, 2015. Any dose not administered at the recommended age should be administered at a subsequent visit, when indicated and feasible. The use of a combination vaccine generally is preferred over separate injections of its equivalent component vaccines. Vaccination providers should consult the relevant Advisory Committee on Immunization Practices (ACIP) statement for detailed recommendations, available online at http://www.cdc.gov/vaccines/hcp/acip-recs/index.html. Clinically significant adverse events that follow vaccination should be reported to the Vaccine Adverse Event Reporting System (VAERS) online (http://www.vaers.hhs.gov) or by telephone (800-822-7967). Suspected cases of vaccine-preventable diseases should be reported to the state or local health department. Additional information, including precautions and contraindications for vaccination, is available from CDC online (http://www.cdc.gov/vaccines/recs/vac-admin/contraindications.htm) or by telephone (800-CDC-INFO [800-232-4636]).

This schedule is approved by the Advisory Committee on Immunization Practices (http://www.cdc.gov/vaccines/acip), the American Academy of Pediatrics (http://www.aap.org), the American Academy of Family Physicians (http://www.aafp.org), and the American College of Obstetricians and Gynecologists (http://www.acog.org).

NOTE: The above recommendations must be read along with the footnotes of this schedule.

FIGURE 2. Catch-up immunization schedule for persons aged 4 months through 18 years who start late or who are more than 1 month behind —United States, 2015.
The figure below provides catch-up schedules and minimum intervals between doses for children whose vaccinations have been delayed. A vaccine series does not need to be restarted, regardless of the time that has elapsed between doses. Use the section appropriate for the child's age. Always use this table in conjunction with Figure 1 and the footnotes that follow.

Vaccine	Minimum Age for Dose 1	Minimum Interval Between Doses			
		Children age 4 months through 6 years			
		Dose 1 to Dose 2	Dose 2 to Dose 3	Dose 3 to Dose 4	Dose 4 to Dose 5
Hepatitis B[1]	Birth	4 weeks	8 weeks *and* at least 16 weeks after first dose. Minimum age for the final dose is 24 weeks.		
Rotavirus[2]	6 weeks	4 weeks	4 weeks[2]		
Diphtheria, tetanus, and acellular pertussis[3]	6 weeks	4 weeks	4 weeks	6 months	6 months[3]
Haemophilus influenzae type b[4]	6 weeks	4 weeks if first dose was administered before the 1ˢᵗ birthday. 8 weeks (as final dose) if first dose was administered at age 12 through 14 months. No further doses needed if first dose was administered at age 15 months or older.	4 weeks[4] if current age is younger than 12 months **and** first dose was administered at younger than age 7 months, **and** at least 1 previous dose was PRP-T (ActHib, Pentacel) or unknown. 8 weeks *and age* 12 through 59 months (as final dose)[4] • if current age is younger than 12 months **and** first dose was administered at age 7 through 11 months; OR • if current age is 12 through 59 months **and** first dose was administered before the 1ˢᵗ birthday, **and** second dose administered at younger than 15 months; OR • if both doses were PRP-OMP (PedvaxHIB; Comvax) **and** were administered before the 1ˢᵗ birthday. No further doses needed if previous dose was administered at age 15 months or older.	8 weeks (as final dose) This dose only necessary for children age 12 through 59 months who received 3 doses before the 1ˢᵗ birthday.	
Pneumococcal[5]	6 weeks	4 weeks if first dose administered before the 1ˢᵗ birthday. 8 weeks (as final dose for healthy children) if first dose was administered at the 1ˢᵗ birthday or after. No further doses needed for healthy children if first dose administered at age 24 months or older.	4 weeks if current age is younger than 12 months and previous dose given at <7months old. 8 weeks (as final dose for healthy children) if previous dose given between 7-11 months (wait until at least 12 months old); OR if current age is 12 months or older and at least 1 dose was given before age 12 months. No further doses needed for healthy children if previous dose administered at age 24 months or older.	8 weeks (as final dose) This dose only necessary for children aged 12 through 59 months who received 3 doses before age 12 months or for children at high risk who received 3 doses at any age.	
Inactivated poliovirus[7]	6 weeks	4 weeks[7]	4 weeks[7]	6 months[7] (minimum age 4 years for final dose).	
Meningococcal[13]	6 weeks	8 weeks[13]	See footnote 13	See footnote 13	
Measles, mumps, rubella[9]	12 months	4 weeks			
Varicella[10]	12 months	3 months			
Hepatitis A[11]	12 months	6 months			

			Children and adolescents age 7 through 18 years	
Tetanus, diphtheria; tetanus, diphtheria, and acellular pertussis⁶	7 years⁴	4 weeks	4 weeks if first dose of DTaP/DT was administered before the 1st birthday. 6 months (as final dose) if first dose of DTaP/DT was administered at or after the 1st birthday.	6 months if first dose of DTaP/DT was administered before the 1st birthday.
Human papillomavirus¹²	9 years		Routine dosing intervals are recommended.¹²	
Hepatitis A¹¹	Not applicable (N/A)	6 months		
Hepatitis B¹	N/A	4 weeks	8 weeks **and** at least 16 weeks after first dose.	
Inactivated poliovirus⁷	N/A	4 weeks	4 weeks⁷	6 months⁷
Meningococcal¹³	N/A	8 weeks¹³		
Measles, mumps, rubella⁹	N/A	4 weeks		
Varicella¹⁰	N/A	3 months if younger than age 13 years. 4 weeks if age 13 years or older.		

NOTE: The above recommendations must be read along with the footnotes of this schedule.

Footnotes — Recommended immunization schedule for persons aged 0 through 18 years—United States, 2015

For further guidance on the use of the vaccines mentioned below, see: http://www.cdc.gov/vaccines/hcp/acip-recs/index.html.

For vaccine recommendations for persons 19 years of age and older, see the Adult Immunization Schedule.

Additional information

- For contraindications and precautions to use of a vaccine and for additional information regarding that vaccine, vaccination providers should consult the relevant ACIP statement available online at http://www.cdc.gov/vaccines/hcp/acip-recs/index.html.
- For purposes of calculating intervals between doses, 4 weeks = 28 days. Intervals of 4 months or greater are determined by calendar months.
- Vaccine doses administered 4 days or less before the minimum interval are considered valid. Doses of any vaccine administered ≥5 days earlier than the minimum interval or minimum age should not be counted as valid doses and should be repeated as age-appropriate. The repeat dose should be spaced after the invalid dose by the recommended minimum interval. For further details, see *MMWR, General Recommendations on Immunization and Reports / Vol. 60 / No. 2; Table 1. Recommended and minimum ages and intervals between vaccine doses* available online at http://www.cdc.gov/mmwr/pdf/rr/rr6002.pdf.
- Information on travel vaccine requirements and recommendations is available at http://wwwnc.cdc.gov/travel/destinations/list.
- For vaccination of persons with primary and secondary immunodeficiencies, see Table 13, *"Vaccination of persons with primary and secondary immunodeficiencies,"* in *General Recommendations on Immunization* (ACIP), available at http://www.cdc.gov/mmwr/pdf/rr/rr6002.pdf; and American Academy of Pediatrics. "Immunization in Special Clinical Circumstances," in Pickering LK, Baker CJ, Kimberlin DW, Long SS eds. *Red Book: 2012 report of the Committee on Infectious Diseases. 29th ed.* Elk Grove Village, IL: American Academy of Pediatrics.

1. Hepatitis B (HepB) vaccine. (Minimum age: birth)

Routine vaccination:

At birth:

- Administer monovalent HepB vaccine to all newborns before hospital discharge.
- For infants born to hepatitis B surface antigen (HBsAg)-positive mothers, administer HepB vaccine and 0.5 mL of hepatitis B immune globulin (HBIG) within 12 hours of birth. These infants should be tested for HBsAg and antibody to HBsAg (anti-HBs) 1 to 2 months after completion of the HepB series at age 9 through 18 months (preferably at the next well-child visit).
- If mother's HBsAg status is unknown, within 12 hours of birth administer HepB vaccine regardless of birth weight. For infants weighing less than 2,000 grams, administer HBIG in addition to HepB vaccine within 12 hours of birth. Determine mother's HBsAg status as soon as possible and, if mother is HBsAg-positive, also administer HBIG for infants weighing 2,000 grams or more as soon as possible, but no later than age 7 days.

Doses following the birth dose:

- The second dose should be administered at age 1 or 2 months. Monovalent HepB vaccine should be used for doses administered before age 6 weeks.
- Infants who did not receive a birth dose should receive 3 doses of a HepB-containing vaccine on a schedule of 0, 1 to 2 months, and 6 months starting as soon as feasible. See Figure 2.
- Administer the second dose 1 to 2 months after the first dose (minimum interval of 4 weeks); administer the third dose at least 8 weeks after the second dose AND at least 16 weeks after the **first** dose. The final (third or fourth) dose in the HepB vaccine series should be administered **no earlier than age 24 weeks.**
- Administration of a total of 4 doses of HepB vaccine is permitted when a combination vaccine containing HepB is administered after the birth dose.

Catch-up vaccination:

- Unvaccinated persons should complete a 3-dose series.
- A 2-dose series (doses separated by at least 4 months) of adult formulation Recombivax HB is licensed for use in children aged 11 through 15 years.
- For other catch-up guidance, see Figure 2.

3. Diphtheria and tetanus toxoids and acellular pertussis (DTaP) vaccine (cont'd)

Catch-up vaccination:

- The fifth dose of DTaP vaccine is not necessary if the fourth dose was administered at age 4 years or older.
- For other catch-up guidance, see Figure 2.

4. Tetanus and diphtheria toxoids and acellular pertussis (Tdap) vaccine. (Minimum age: 10 years for both Boostrix and Adacel)

Routine vaccination:

- Administer 1 dose of Tdap vaccine to all adolescents aged 11 through 12 years.
- Tdap may be administered regardless of the interval since the last tetanus and diphtheria toxoid-containing vaccine.
- Administer 1 dose of Tdap vaccine to pregnant adolescents during each pregnancy (preferred during 27 through 36 weeks gestation) regardless of time since prior Td or Tdap vaccination.

Catch-up vaccination:

- Persons aged 7 years and older who are not fully immunized with DTaP vaccine should receive Tdap vaccine as 1 dose (preferably the first) in the catch-up series; if additional doses are needed, use Td vaccine. For children 7 through 10 years who receive a dose of Tdap as part of the catch-up series, an adolescent Tdap vaccine dose at age 11 through 12 years should NOT be administered. Td should be administered instead 10 years after the Tdap dose.
- Persons aged 11 through 18 years who have not received Tdap vaccine should receive a dose followed by tetanus and diphtheria toxoid (Td) booster doses every 10 years thereafter.
- Inadvertent doses of DTaP vaccine:
  - If administered inadvertently to a child aged 7 through 10 years may count as part of the catch-up series. This dose may count as the adolescent Tdap dose, or the child can later receive a Tdap booster dose at age 11 through 12 years.
  - If administered inadvertently to an adolescent aged 11 through 18 years, the dose should be counted as the adolescent Tdap booster.
- For other catch-up guidance, see Figure 2.

2. Rotavirus (RV) vaccines. (Minimum age: 6 weeks for both RV1 [Rotarix] and RV5 [RotaTeq])

Routine vaccination:

Administer a series of RV vaccine to all infants as follows:

1. If Rotarix is used, administer a 2-dose series at 2 and 4 months of age.
2. If RotaTeq is used, administer a 3-dose series at ages 2, 4, and 6 months.
3. If any dose in the series was RotaTeq or vaccine product is unknown for any dose in the series, a total of 3 doses of RV vaccine should be administered.

Catch-up vaccination:

- The maximum age for the first dose in the series is 14 weeks, 6 days; vaccination should not be initiated for infants aged 15 weeks, 0 days or older.
- The maximum age for the final dose in the series is 8 months, 0 days.
- For other catch-up guidance, see Figure 2.

3. Diphtheria and tetanus toxoids and acellular pertussis (DTaP) vaccine. (Minimum age: 6 weeks. Exception: DTaP-IPV [Kinrix]: 4 years)

Routine vaccination:

- Administer a 5-dose series of DTaP vaccine at ages 2, 4, 6, 15 through 18 months, and 4 through 6 years. The fourth dose may be administered as early as age 12 months, provided at least 6 months have elapsed since the third dose. However, the fourth dose of DTaP need not be repeated if it was administered at least 4 months after the third dose of DTaP.

5. Haemophilus influenzae type b (Hib) conjugate vaccine (cont'd)

Catch-up vaccination:

- If dose 1 was administered at ages 12 through 14 months, administer a second (final) dose at least 8 weeks after dose 1, regardless of Hib vaccine used in the primary series.
- If both doses were PRP-OMP (PedvaxHIB or COMVAX), and were administered before the first birthday, the third (and final) dose should be administered at age 12 through 59 months and at least 8 weeks after the second dose.
- If the first dose was administered at age 7 through 11 months, administer the second dose at least 4 weeks later and a third (and final) dose at age 12 through 15 months or 8 weeks after second dose, whichever is later.
- If first dose is administered before the first birthday and second dose administered at younger than 15 months, a third (and final) dose should be given 8 weeks later.
- For unvaccinated children aged 15 months or older, administer only 1 dose.
- For other catch-up guidance, see Figure 2. For catch-up guidance related to MenHibrix, please see the meningococcal vaccine footnotes and also MMWR February 28, 2014 / 63(RR01);1-13, available at http://www.cdc.gov/mmwr/PDF/rr/rr6301.pdf.

Vaccination of persons with high-risk conditions:

- Children aged 12 through 59 months who are at increased risk for Hib disease, including chemotherapy recipients and those with anatomic or functional asplenia (including sickle cell disease), human immunodeficiency virus (HIV) infection, immunoglobulin deficiency, or early component complement deficiency, who have received either no doses or only 1 dose of Hib vaccine before 12 months of age, should receive 2 additional doses of Hib vaccine 8 weeks apart; children who received 2 or more doses of Hib vaccine before 12 months of age should receive 1 additional dose.
- For patients younger than 5 years of age undergoing chemotherapy or radiation treatment who received a Hib vaccine dose(s) within 14 days of starting therapy or during therapy, repeat the dose(s) at least 3 months following therapy completion.
- Recipients of hematopoietic stem cell transplant (HSCT) should be revaccinated with a 3-dose regimen

5. Haemophilus influenzae type b (Hib) conjugate vaccine. (Minimum age: 6 weeks for PRP-T [ACTHIB, DTaP-IPV/Hib (Pentacel) and Hib-MenCY (MenHibrix)], PRP-OMP [PedvaxHIB or COMVAX], 12 months for PRP-T [Hiberix])

Routine vaccination:

- Administer a 2- or 3-dose Hib vaccine primary series and a booster dose (dose 3 or 4 depending on vaccine used in primary series) at age 12 through 15 months to complete a full Hib vaccine series.
- The primary series with ActHIB, MenHibrix, or Pentacel consists of 3 doses and should be administered at 2, 4, and 6 months of age. The primary series with PedvaxHib or COMVAX consists of 2 doses and should be administered at 2 and 4 months of age; a dose at age 6 months is not indicated.
- One booster dose (dose 3 or 4 depending on vaccine used in primary series) of any Hib vaccine should be administered at age 12 through 15 months. An exception is Hiberix vaccine. Hiberix should only be used for the booster (final) dose in children aged 12 months through 4 years who have received at least 1 prior dose of Hib-containing vaccine.
- For recommendations on the use of MenHibrix in patients at increased risk for meningococcal disease, please refer to the meningococcal vaccine footnotes and also to MMWR February 28, 2014 / 63(RR01);1-13, available at http://www.cdc.gov/mmwr/PDF/rr/rr6301.pdf.

For further guidance on the use of the vaccines mentioned below, see: http://www.cdc.gov/vaccines/hcp/acip-recs/index.html.

6. Pneumococcal vaccines (cont'd)

- For children aged 6 through 18 years who have cerebrospinal fluid leak; cochlear implant; sickle cell disease and other hemoglobinopathies; anatomic or functional asplenia; congenital or acquired immunodeficiencies; HIV infection; chronic renal failure; nephrotic syndrome; diseases associated with treatment with immunosuppressive drugs or radiation therapy, including malignant neoplasms, leukemias, lymphomas, and Hodgkin's disease; generalized malignancy; solid organ transplantation; or multiple myeloma:

  1. If neither PCV13 nor PPSV23 has been received previously, administer 1 dose of PCV13 now and 1 dose of PPSV23 at least 8 weeks later.
  2. If PCV13 has been received previously but PPSV23 has not, administer 1 dose of PPSV23 at least 8 weeks after the most recent dose of PCV13.
  3. If PPSV23 has been received but PCV13 has not, administer 1 dose of PCV13 at least 8 weeks after the most recent dose of PPSV23.

- For children aged 6 through 18 years with chronic heart disease (particularly cyanotic congenital heart disease and cardiac failure), chronic lung disease (including asthma if treated with high-dose oral corticosteroid therapy), diabetes mellitus, alcoholism, or chronic liver disease, who have not received PPSV23, administer 1 dose of PPSV23. If PCV13 has been received previously, then PPSV23 should be administered at least 8 weeks after any prior PCV13 dose.
- A single revaccination with PPSV23 should be administered 5 years after the first dose to children with sickle cell disease or other hemoglobinopathies; anatomic or functional asplenia; congenital or acquired immunodeficiencies; HIV infection; chronic renal failure; nephrotic syndrome; diseases associated with treatment with immunosuppressive drugs or radiation therapy, including malignant neoplasms, leukemias, lymphomas, and Hodgkin's disease; generalized malignancy; solid organ transplantation; or multiple myeloma.

7. Inactivated poliovirus vaccine (IPV). (Minimum age: 6 weeks)

Routine vaccination:

- Administer a 4-dose series of IPV at ages 2, 4, 6 through 18 months, and 4 through 6 years. The final dose in the of Hib vaccine starting 6 to 12 months after successful transplant, regardless of vaccination history; doses should be administered at least 4 weeks apart.

- A single dose of any Hib-containing vaccine should be administered to unimmunized* children and adolescents 15 months of age and older undergoing an elective splenectomy; if possible, vaccine should be administered at least 14 days before procedure.
- Hib vaccine is not routinely recommended for patients 5 years or older. However, 1 dose of Hib vaccine should be administered to unimmunized* persons aged 5 years or older who have anatomic or functional asplenia (including sickle cell disease) and unvaccinated persons 5 through 18 years of age with human immunodeficiency virus (HIV) infection.

Patients who have not received a primary series and booster dose or at least 1 dose of Hib vaccine after 14 months of age are considered unimmunized.

6. **Pneumococcal vaccines. (Minimum age: 6 weeks for PCV13, 2 years for PPSV23)**
Routine vaccination with PCV13:
- Administer a 4-dose series of PCV13 vaccine at ages 2, 4, and 6 months and at age 12 through 15 months.
- For children aged 14 through 59 months who have received an age-appropriate series of 7-valent PCV (PCV7), administer a single supplemental dose of 13-valent PCV (PCV13).

Catch-up vaccination with PCV13:
- Administer 1 dose of PCV13 to all healthy children aged 24 through 59 months who are not completely vaccinated for their age.
- For other catch-up guidance, see Figure 2.

Vaccination of persons with high-risk conditions with PCV13 and PPSV23:
- All recommended PCV13 doses should be administered prior to PPSV23 vaccination if possible.
- For children 2 through 5 years of age with any of the following conditions: chronic heart disease (particularly cyanotic congenital heart disease and cardiac failure); chronic lung disease (including asthma if treated with high-dose oral corticosteroid therapy); diabetes mellitus; cerebrospinal fluid leak; cochlear implant; sickle cell disease and other hemoglobinopathies; anatomic or functional asplenia; HIV infection; chronic renal failure; nephrotic syndrome; diseases associated with treatment with immunosuppressive drugs or radiation therapy, including malignant neoplasms, leukemias, lymphomas, and Hodgkin's disease; solid organ transplantation; or congenital immunodeficiency:
  1. Administer 1 dose of PCV13 if any incomplete schedule of 3 doses of PCV (PCV7 and/or PCV13) were received previously.
  2. Administer 2 doses of PCV13 at least 8 weeks apart if unvaccinated or any incomplete schedule of fewer than 3 doses of PCV (PCV7 and/or PCV13) were received previously.
  3. Administer 1 supplemental dose of PCV13 if 4 doses of PCV7 or other age-appropriate complete PCV7 series was received previously.
  4. The minimum interval between doses of PCV (PCV7 or PCV13) is 8 weeks.
  5. For children with no history of PPSV23 vaccination, administer PPSV23 at least 8 weeks after the most recent dose of PCV13.

series should be administered on or after the fourth birthday and at least 6 months after the previous dose.

Catch-up vaccination:
- In the first 6 months of life, minimum age and minimum intervals are only recommended if the person is at risk of imminent exposure to circulating poliovirus (i.e., travel to a polio-endemic region or during an outbreak).
- If 4 or more doses are administered before age 4 years, an additional dose should be administered at age 4 through 6 years and at least 6 months after the previous dose.
- A fourth dose is not necessary if the third dose was administered at age 4 years or older and at least 6 months after the previous dose.
- If both OPV and IPV were administered as part of a series, a total of 4 doses should be administered, regardless of the child's current age. IPV is not routinely recommended for U.S. residents aged 18 years or older.
- For other catch-up guidance, see Figure 2.

8. **Influenza vaccines. (Minimum age: 6 months for inactivated influenza vaccine [IIV], 2 years for live, attenuated influenza vaccine [LAIV])**
Routine vaccination:
- Administer influenza vaccine annually to all children beginning at age 6 months. For most healthy, nonpregnant persons aged 2 through 49 years, either LAIV or IIV may be used. However, LAIV should NOT be administered to some persons, including 1) persons who have experienced severe allergic reactions to LAIV, any of its components, or to a previous dose of any other influenza vaccine; 2) children 2 through 17 years receiving aspirin or aspirin-containing products; 3) persons who are allergic to eggs; 4) pregnant women; 5) immunosuppressed persons; 6) children 2 through 4 years of age with asthma or who had wheezing in the past 12 months; or 7) persons who have taken influenza antiviral medications in the previous 48 hours. For all other contraindications and precautions to use of LAIV, see *MMWR* August 15, 2014 / 63(32);691–697 [40 pages] available at http://www.cdc.gov/mmwr/pdf/wk/mm6332.pdf.

For children aged 6 months through 8 years:
- For the 2014-15 season, administer 2 doses (separated by at least 4 weeks) to children who are receiving influenza vaccine for the first time. Some children in this age group who have been vaccinated previously will also need 2 doses. For additional guidance, follow dosing guidelines in the 2014-15 ACIP influenza vaccine recommendations, *MMWR* August 15, 2014 / 63(32);691–697 [40 pages] available at http://www.cdc.gov/mmwr/pdf/wk/mm6332.pdf.
- For the 2015–16 season, follow dosing guidelines in the 2015 ACIP influenza vaccine recommendations.

For persons aged 9 years and older:
- Administer 1 dose.

For further guidance on the use of the vaccines mentioned below, see: http://www.cdc.gov/vaccines/hcp/acip-recs/index.html.

13. **Meningococcal conjugate vaccines. (Minimum age: 6 weeks for Hib-MenCY [MenHibrix], 9 months for MenACWY-D [Menactra], 2 months for MenACWY-CRM [Menveo])**
Routine vaccination:
- Administer a single dose of Menactra or Menveo vaccine at age 11 through 12 years, with a booster dose at age 16 years.
- Adolescents aged 11 through 18 years with human immunodeficiency virus (HIV) infection should receive a 2-dose primary series of Menactra or Menveo with at least 8 weeks between doses.
- For children aged 2 months through 18 years with high-risk conditions, see below.

9. **Measles, mumps, and rubella (MMR) vaccine. (Minimum age: 12 months for routine vaccination)**
Routine vaccination:
- Administer a 2-dose series of MMR vaccine at ages 12 months and 4 through 6 years. The second dose may be administered before age 4 years, provided at least 4 weeks have elapsed since the first dose.
- Administer 1 dose of MMR vaccine to infants aged 6 through 11 months before departure from the United States for international travel. These children should be revaccinated with 2 doses of MMR vaccine, the first at age 12 through 15 months (12 months if the child remains in an area where disease risk is high), and the

second dose at least 4 weeks later.

- Administer 2 doses of MMR vaccine to children aged 12 months and older before departure from the United States for international travel. The first dose should be administered on or after age 12 months and the second dose at least 4 weeks later.

Catch-up vaccination:

- Ensure that all school-aged children and adolescents have had 2 doses of MMR vaccine, the minimum interval between the 2 doses is 4 weeks.

10. Varicella (VAR) vaccine. (Minimum age: 12 months)

Routine vaccination:

- Administer a 2-dose series of VAR vaccine at ages 12 through 15 months and 4 through 5 years. The second dose may be administered before age 4 years, provided at least 3 months have elapsed since the first dose. If the second dose was administered at least 4 weeks after the first dose, it can be accepted as valid.

Catch-up vaccination:

- Ensure that all persons aged 7 through 18 years without evidence of immunity (see *MMWR* 2007 / 56 [No. RR-4], available at http://www.cdc.gov/mmwr/pdf/rr/rr5604.pdf) have 2 doses of varicella vaccine. For children aged 7 through 12 years, the recommended minimum interval between doses is 3 months (if the second dose was administered at least 4 weeks after the first dose, it can be accepted as valid); for persons aged 13 years and older, the minimum interval between doses is 4 weeks.

11. Hepatitis A (HepA) vaccine. (Minimum age: 12 months)

Routine vaccination:

- Initiate the 2-dose HepA vaccine series at 12 through 23 months; separate the 2 doses by 6 to 18 months.
- Children who have received 1 dose of HepA vaccine before age 24 months should receive a second dose 6 to 18 months after the first dose.
- For any person aged 2 years and older who has not already received the HepA vaccine series, 2 doses of HepA vaccine separated by 6 to 18 months may be administered if immunity against hepatitis A virus infection is desired.

Catch-up vaccination:

- The minimum interval between the two doses is 6 months.

Special populations:

- Administer 2 doses of HepA vaccine at least 6 months apart to previously unvaccinated persons who live in areas where vaccination programs target older children, or who are at increased risk for infection. This includes persons travelling to or working in countries that have high or intermediate endemicity of infection; men having sex with men; users of injection and non-injection illicit drugs; persons who work with HAV-infected primates or with HAV in a research laboratory; persons with clotting-factor disorders; persons with chronic liver disease; and persons who anticipate close personal contact (e.g. household or regular babysitting) with an international adoptee during the first 60 days after arrival in the United States from a country with high or intermediate endemicity. The first dose should be administered as soon as the adoption is planned, ideally 2 or more weeks before the arrival of the adoptee.

12. Human papillomavirus (HPV) vaccines. (Minimum age: 9 years for HPV2 [Cervarix] and HPV4 [Gardasil])

Routine vaccination:

- Administer a 3-dose series of HPV vaccine on a schedule of 0, 1-2, and 6 months to all adolescents aged 11 through 12 years. Either HPV4 or HPV2 may be used for females, and only HPV4 may be used for males.
- The vaccine series may be started at age 9 years.
- Administer the second dose 1 to 2 months after the first dose (minimum interval of 4 weeks); administer the third dose 24 weeks after the first dose and 16 weeks after the second dose (minimum interval of 12 weeks).

Catch-up vaccination:

- Administer the vaccine series to females (either HPV2 or HPV4) and males (HPV4) at age 13 through 18 years if not previously vaccinated.
- Use recommended routine dosing intervals (see Routine vaccination above) for vaccine series catch-up.

Catch-up vaccination:

- Administer Menactra or Menveo vaccine at age 13 through 18 years if not previously vaccinated.
- If the first dose is administered at age 13 through 15 years, a booster dose should be administered at age 16 through 18 years with a minimum interval of at least 8 weeks between doses.
- If the first dose is administered at age 16 years or older, a booster dose is not needed.
- For other catch-up guidance, see Figure 2.

Vaccination of persons with high-risk conditions and other persons at increased risk of disease:

- Children with anatomic or functional asplenia (including sickle cell disease):
  1. Menveo
     o *Children who initiate vaccination at 8 weeks through 6 months:* Administer doses at 2, 4, 6, and 12 months of age.
     o *Unvaccinated children 7 through 23 months:* Administer 2 doses, with the second dose administered at least 12 weeks after the first dose AND after the first birthday.
     o *Children 24 months and older who have not received a complete series:* Administer 2 primary doses at least 8 weeks apart.
  2. MenHibrix
     o *Children 6 weeks through 18 months:* Administer doses at 2, 4, 6, and 12 through 15 months of age.
     o If the first dose of MenHibrix is given at or after 12 months of age, a total of 2 doses should be given at least 8 weeks apart to ensure protection against serogroups C and Y meningococcal disease.
  3. Menactra
     o *Children 24 months and older who have not received a complete series:* Administer 2 primary doses at least 8 weeks apart. If Menactra is administered to a child with asplenia (including sickle cell disease), do not administer Menactra until 2 years of age and at least 4 weeks after the completion of all PCV13 doses.
- Children with persistent complement component deficiency:
  1. Menveo
     o *Children who initiate vaccination at 8 weeks through 6 months:* Administer doses at 2, 4, 6, and 12 months of age.
     o *Unvaccinated children 7 through 23 months:* Administer 2 doses, with the second dose administered at least 12 weeks after the first dose AND after the first birthday.
     o *Children 24 months and older who have not received a complete series:* Administer 2 primary doses at least 8 weeks apart.
  2. MenHibrix
     o *Children 6 weeks through 18 months:* Administer doses at 2, 4, 6, and 12 through 15 months of age.
     o If the first dose of MenHibrix is given at or after 12 months of age, a total of 2 doses should be given at least 8 weeks apart to ensure protection against serogroups C and Y meningococcal disease.
  3. Menactra
     o *Children 9 through 23 months:* Administer 2 primary doses at least 12 weeks apart.
     o *Children 24 months and older who have not received a complete series:* Administer 2 primary doses at least 8 weeks apart.
- For children who travel to or reside in countries in which meningococcal disease is hyperendemic or epidemic, including countries in the African meningitis belt or the Hajj, administer an age-appropriate formulation and series of Menactra or Menveo for protection against serogroups A and W meningococcal disease. Prior receipt of MenHibrix is not sufficient for children traveling to the meningitis belt or the Hajj because it does not contain serogroups A or W.
- For children at risk during a community outbreak attributable to a vaccine serogroup, administer or complete an age- and formulation-appropriate series of MenHibrix, Menactra, or Menveo.
- For booster doses among persons with high-risk conditions, refer to *MMWR* 2013 / 62(RR02):1-22, available at http://www.cdc.gov/mmwr/preview/mmwrhtml/rr6202a1.htm.

For other catch-up recommendations for these persons, and complete information on use of meningococcal vaccines, including guidance related to vaccination of persons at increased risk of infection, see *MMWR* March 22, 2013 ; 62(RR02);1-22, available at http://www.cdc.gov/mmwr/pdf/rr/rr6202.pdf.

Recommended Adult Immunization Schedule—United States - 2015

Note: These recommendations must be read with the footnotes that follow containing number of doses, intervals between doses, and other important information.

Figure 1. Recommended adult immunization schedule, by vaccine and age group[1]

VACCINE ▼ / AGE GROUP ▶	19-21 years	22-26 years	27-49 years	50-59 years	60-64 years	≥65 years
Influenza[*,2]	1 dose annually					
Tetanus, diphtheria, pertussis (Td/Tdap)[*,3]	Substitute 1-time dose of Tdap for Td booster; then boost with Td every 10 yrs					
Varicella[*,4]	2 doses					
Human papillomavirus (HPV) Female[*,5]	3 doses	3 doses				
Human papillomavirus (HPV) Male[*,5]	3 doses	3 doses				
Zoster[6]					1 dose	1 dose
Measles, mumps, rubella (MMR)[*,7]	1 or 2 doses					
Pneumococcal 13-valent conjugate (PCV13)[*,8]						1-time dose
Pneumococcal polysaccharide (PPSV23)[8]			1 or 2 doses			1 dose
Meningococcal[*,9]	1 or more doses					
Hepatitis A[*,10]	2 doses					
Hepatitis B[*,11]	3 doses					
Haemophilus influenzae type b (Hib)[*,12]	1 or 3 doses					

Legend:
- For all persons in this category who meet the age requirements and who lack documentation of vaccination or have no evidence of previous infection; zoster vaccine recommended regardless of prior episode of zoster
- Recommended if some other risk factor is present (e.g., on the basis of medical, occupational, lifestyle, or other indication)
- No recommendation

*Covered by the Vaccine Injury Compensation Program

Report all clinically significant postvaccination reactions to the Vaccine Adverse Event Reporting System (VAERS). Reporting forms and instructions on filing a VAERS report are available at www.vaers.hhs.gov or by telephone, 800-822-7967.

Information on how to file a Vaccine Injury Compensation Program claim is available at www.hrsa.gov/vaccinecompensation or by telephone, 800-338-2382. To file a claim for vaccine injury, contact the U.S. Court of Federal Claims, 717 Madison Place, N.W., Washington, D.C. 20005; telephone, 202-357-6400.

Additional information about the vaccines in this schedule, extent of available data, and contraindications for vaccination is also available at www.cdc.gov/vaccines or from the CDC-INFO Contact Center at 800-CDC-INFO (800-232-4636) in English and Spanish, 8:00 a.m. - 8:00 p.m. Eastern Time, Monday - Friday, excluding holidays.

Use of trade names and commercial sources is for identification only and does not imply endorsement by the U.S. Department of Health and Human Services.

The recommendations in this schedule were approved by the Centers for Disease Control and Prevention's (CDC) Advisory Committee on Immunization Practices (ACIP), the American Academy of Family Physicians (AAFP), the American College of Physicians (ACP), American College of Obstetricians and Gynecologists (ACOG) and American College of Nurse-Midwives (ACNM).

Figure 2. Vaccines that might be indicated for adults based on medical and other indications[1]

VACCINE ▼ / INDICATION ▶	Pregnancy	Immuno-compromising conditions (excluding human immunodeficiency virus [HIV]) [4,6,7,8,13]	HIV infection CD4+ T lymphocyte count [4,6,7,8,13] < 200 cells/µL	HIV infection CD4+ T lymphocyte count ≥ 200 cells/µL	Men who have sex with men (MSM)	Kidney failure, end-stage renal disease, receipt of hemodialysis	Heart disease, chronic lung disease, chronic alcoholism	Asplenia (including elective splenectomy and persistent complement component deficiencies) [8,12]	Chronic liver disease	Diabetes	Healthcare personnel
Influenza[*,2]	1 dose IIV annually				1 dose IIV or LAIV annually						1 dose IIV or LAIV annually
Tetanus, diphtheria, pertussis (Td/Tdap)[*,3]	1 dose Tdap each pregnancy	Substitute 1-time dose of Tdap for Td booster; then boost with Td every 10 yrs									
Varicella[*,4]	Contraindicated	Contraindicated		2 doses							
Human papillomavirus (HPV) Female[*,5]	3 doses through age 26 yrs	3 doses through age 26 yrs						3 doses through age 26 yrs			
Human papillomavirus (HPV) Male[*,5]	3 doses through age 26 yrs	3 doses through age 26 yrs						3 doses through age 21 yrs			
Zoster[6]	Contraindicated	Contraindicated						1 dose			
Measles, mumps, rubella (MMR)[*,7]	Contraindicated	Contraindicated						1 or 2 doses			
Pneumococcal 13-valent conjugate (PCV13)[8]						1 dose					
Pneumococcal polysaccharide (PPSV23)[8]						1 or 2 doses					
Meningococcal[*,9]						1 or more doses					
Hepatitis A[*,10]						2 doses					
Hepatitis B[*,11]						3 doses					
Haemophilus influenzae type b (Hib)[12]	post-HSCT recipients only					1 or 3 doses					

[*] Covered by the Vaccine Injury Compensation Program

For all persons in this category who meet the age requirements and who lack documentation of vaccination or have no evidence of previous infection; zoster vaccine recommended regardless of prior episode of zoster

Recommended if some other risk factor is present (e.g., on the basis of medical, occupational, lifestyle, or other indications)

No recommendation

U.S. Department of Health and Human Services
Centers for Disease Control and Prevention

These schedules indicate the recommended age groups and medical indications for which administration of currently licensed vaccines is commonly recommended for adults ages 19 years and older, as of February 1, 2015. For all vaccines being recommended on the Adult Immunization Schedule: a vaccine series does not need to be restarted, regardless of the time that has elapsed between doses. Licensed combination vaccines may be used whenever any components of the combination are indicated and when the vaccine's other components are not contraindicated. For detailed recommendations on all vaccines, including those used primarily for travelers or that are issued during the year, consult the manufacturers' package inserts and the complete statements from the Advisory Committee on Immunization Practices (www.cdc.gov/vaccines/hcp/acip-recs/index.html). Use of trade names and commercial sources is for identification only and does not imply endorsement by the U.S. Department of Health and Human Services.

Footnotes—Recommended Immunization Schedule for Adults Aged 19 Years or Older: United States, 2015

1. Additional information

- Additional guidance for the use of the vaccines described in this supplement is available at www.cdc.gov/vaccines/hcp/acip-recs/index.html.
- Information on vaccination recommendations when vaccination status is unknown and other general immunization information can be found in the General Recommendations on Immunization at www.cdc.gov/mmwr/preview/mmwrhtml/rr6002a1.htm.
- Information on travel vaccine requirements and recommendations (e.g., for hepatitis A and B, meningococcal, and other vaccines) is available at wwwnc.cdc.gov/travel/destinations/list.
- Additional information and resources regarding vaccination of pregnant women can be found at www.cdc.gov/vaccines/adults/rec-vac/pregnant.html.

2. Influenza vaccination

- Annual vaccination against influenza is recommended for all persons aged 6 months or older.
- Persons aged 6 months or older, including pregnant women and persons with hives-only allergy to eggs can receive the inactivated influenza vaccine (IIV). An age-appropriate IIV formulation should be used.
- Adults aged 18 years or older can receive the recombinant influenza vaccine (RIV) (FluBlok). RIV does not contain any egg protein and can be given to age-appropriate persons with egg allergy of any severity.
- Healthy, nonpregnant persons aged 2 to 49 years without high-risk medical conditions can receive either intranasally administered live, attenuated influenza vaccine (LAIV) (FluMist) or IIV.
- Health care personnel who care for severely immunocompromised persons who require care in a protected environment should receive IIV or RIV; health care personnel who receive LAIV should avoid providing care for severely immunosuppressed persons for 7 days after vaccination.
- The intramuscularly or intradermally administered IIV are options for adults aged 18 through 64 years.
- Adults aged 65 years or older can receive the standard-dose IIV or the high-dose IIV (Fluzone High-Dose).
- A list of currently available influenza vaccines can be found at www.cdc.gov/flu/protect/vaccine/vaccines.htm.

- For males, HPV4 is recommended in a 3-dose series for routine vaccination at age 11 or 12 years and for those aged 13 through 21 years, if not previously vaccinated. Males aged 22 through 26 years may be vaccinated.
- HPV4 is recommended for men who have sex with men through age 26 years for those who did not get any or all doses when they were younger.
- Vaccination is recommended for immunocompromised persons (including those with HIV infection) through age 26 years for those who did not get any or all doses when they were younger.
- A complete series for either HPV4 or HPV2 consists of 3 doses. The second dose should be administered 4 to 8 weeks (minimum interval of 4 weeks) after the first dose; the third dose should be administered 24 weeks after the first dose and 16 weeks after the second dose (minimum interval of at least 12 weeks).
- HPV vaccines are not recommended for use in pregnant women. However, pregnancy testing is not needed before vaccination. If a woman is found to be pregnant after initiating the vaccination series, no intervention is needed; the remainder of the 3-dose series should be delayed until completion or termination of pregnancy.

6. Zoster vaccination

- A single dose of zoster vaccine is recommended for adults aged 60 years or older regardless of whether they report a prior episode of herpes zoster. Although the vaccine is licensed by the U.S. Food and Drug Administration for use among and can be administered to persons aged 50 years or older, ACIP recommends that vaccination begin at age 60 years.
- Persons aged 60 years or older with chronic medical conditions may be vaccinated unless their condition constitutes a contraindication, such as pregnancy or severe immunodeficiency.

7. Measles, mumps, rubella (MMR) vaccination

- Adults born before 1957 are generally considered immune to measles and mumps. All adults born in 1957 or later should have documentation of 1 or more doses of MMR vaccine unless they have a medical contraindication to the vaccine or laboratory evidence of immunity to each of the three diseases. Documentation of provider-diagnosed disease is not considered acceptable evidence of immunity for measles, mumps, or rubella.

3. Tetanus, diphtheria, and acellular pertussis (Td/Tdap) vaccination

- Administer 1 dose of Tdap vaccine to pregnant women during each pregnancy (preferably during 27 to 36 weeks' gestation) regardless of interval since prior Td or Tdap vaccination.
- Persons aged 11 years or older who have not received Tdap vaccine or for whom vaccine status is unknown should receive a dose of Tdap followed by tetanus and diphtheria toxoids (Td) booster doses every 10 years thereafter. Tdap can be administered regardless of interval since the most recent tetanus or diphtheria-toxoid containing vaccine.
- Adults with an unknown or incomplete history of completing a 3-dose primary vaccination series with Td-containing vaccines should begin or complete a primary vaccination series including a Tdap dose.
- For unvaccinated adults, administer the first 2 doses at least 4 weeks apart and the third dose 6 to 12 months after the second.
- For incompletely vaccinated (i.e., less than 3 doses) adults, administer remaining doses.
- Refer to the ACIP statement for recommendations for administering Td/Tdap as prophylaxis in wound management (see footnote 1).

4. Varicella vaccination

- All adults without evidence of immunity to varicella (as defined below) should receive 2 doses of single-antigen varicella vaccine or a second dose if they have received only 1 dose.
- Vaccination should be emphasized for those who have close contact with persons at high risk for severe disease (e.g., health care personnel and family contacts of persons with immunocompromising conditions) or are at high risk for exposure or transmission (e.g., teachers; child care employees; residents and staff members of institutional settings, including correctional institutions; college students; military personnel; adolescents and adults living in households with children; nonpregnant women of childbearing age; and international travelers).
- Pregnant women should be assessed for evidence of varicella immunity. Women who do not have evidence of immunity should receive the first dose of varicella vaccine upon completion or termination of pregnancy and before discharge from the health care facility. The second dose should be administered 4 to 8 weeks after the first dose.
- Evidence of immunity to varicella in adults includes any of the following:
  — documentation of 2 doses of varicella vaccine at least 4 weeks apart;
  — U.S.-born before 1980, except health care personnel and pregnant women;
  — history of varicella based on diagnosis or verification of varicella disease by a health care provider;

Measles component:

- A routine second dose of MMR vaccine, administered a minimum of 28 days after the first dose, is recommended for adults who:
  — are students in postsecondary educational institutions,
  — work in a health care facility, or
  — plan to travel internationally.
- Persons who received inactivated (killed) measles vaccine or measles vaccine of unknown type during 1963–1967 should be revaccinated with 2 doses of MMR vaccine.

Mumps component:

- A routine second dose of MMR vaccine, administered a minimum of 28 days after the first dose, is recommended for adults who:
  — are students in a postsecondary educational institution,
  — work in a health care facility, or
  — plan to travel internationally.
- Persons vaccinated before 1979 with either killed mumps vaccine or mumps vaccine of unknown type who are at high risk for mumps infection (e.g., persons who are working in a health care facility) should be considered for revaccination with 2 doses of MMR vaccine.

Rubella component:

- For women of childbearing age, regardless of birth year, rubella immunity should be determined. If there is no evidence of immunity, women who are not pregnant should be vaccinated. Pregnant women who do not have evidence of immunity should receive MMR vaccine upon completion or termination of pregnancy and before discharge from the health care facility.

Health care personnel born before 1957:

- For unvaccinated health care personnel born before 1957 who lack laboratory evidence of measles, mumps, and/or rubella immunity or laboratory confirmation of disease, health care facilities should consider vaccinating personnel with 2 doses of MMR vaccine at the appropriate interval for measles and mumps or 1 dose of MMR vaccine for rubella.

8. Pneumococcal (13-valent pneumococcal conjugate vaccine [PCV13] and 23-valent pneumococcal polysaccharide vaccine [PPSV23]) vaccination

- General information
  — When indicated, only a single dose of PCV13 is recommended for adults.
  — No additional dose of PPSV23 is indicated for adults vaccinated with PPSV23 at or after age 65 years.
  — When both PCV13 and PPSV23 are indicated, PCV13 should be administered first; PCV13 and PPSV23 should not be administered during

— history of herpes zoster based on diagnosis or verification of herpes zoster disease by a health care provider; or

— laboratory evidence of immunity or laboratory confirmation of disease.

5. Human papillomavirus (HPV) vaccination

• Two vaccines are licensed for use in females, bivalent HPV vaccine (HPV2) and quadrivalent HPV vaccine (HPV4), and one HPV vaccine for use in males (HPV4).

• For females, either HPV4 or HPV2 is recommended in a 3-dose series for routine vaccination at age 11 or 12 years and for those aged 13 through 26 years, if not previously vaccinated.

Footnotes—Recommended Immunization Schedule for Adults Aged 19 Years or Older: United States, 2015

8. Pneumococcal vaccination (continued)

— Have not received PCV13 but have received 1 or more doses of PPSV23 before age 65: Administer PCV13 at least 1 year after the most recent dose of PPSV23; administer a dose of PPSV23 6 to 12 months after PCV13, or as soon as possible if this time window has passed, and at least 5 years after the most recent dose of PPSV23.

— Have received PCV13 but not PPSV23 before age 65: Administer PPSV23 6 to 12 months after PCV13 or as soon as possible if this time window has passed.

— Have received PCV13 and 1 or more doses of PPSV23 before age 65 years: Administer PPSV23 6 to 12 months after PCV13, or as soon as possible if this time window has passed, and at least 5 years after the most recent dose of PPSV23.

• Adults aged 19 through 64 years with immunocompromising conditions or anatomical or functional asplenia (defined below) who

— Have not received PCV13 or PPSV23: Administer PCV13 followed by PPSV23 at least 8 weeks after PCV13; administer a second dose of PPSV23 at least 5 years after the first dose of PPSV23.

— Have not received PCV13 but have received 1 dose of PPSV23: Administer PCV13 at least 1 year after the PPSV23; administer a second dose of PPSV23 at least 8 weeks after PCV13 and at least 5 years after the first dose of PPSV23.

— Have not received PCV13 but have received 2 doses of PPSV23: Administer PCV13 at least 1 year after the most recent dose of PPSV23.

— Have received PCV13 but not PPSV23: Administer PPSV23 at least 8 weeks after PCV13; administer a second dose of PPSV23 at least 5 years after the first dose of PPSV23.

the same visit.

— When indicated, PCV13 and PPSV23 should be administered to adults whose pneumococcal vaccination history is incomplete or unknown.

• Adults aged 65 years or older who

— Have not received PCV13 or PPSV23: Administer PCV13 followed by PPSV23 in 6 to 12 months.

— Have not received PCV13 but have received a dose of PPSV23 at age 65 years or older: Administer PCV13 at least 1 year after the dose of PPSV23 received at age 65 years or older.

10. Hepatitis A vaccination

• Vaccinate any person seeking protection from hepatitis A virus (HAV) infection and persons with any of the following indications:

— men who have sex with men and persons who use injection or noninjection illicit drugs;

— persons working with HAV-infected primates or with HAV in a research laboratory setting;

— persons with chronic liver disease and persons who receive clotting factor concentrates;

— persons traveling to or working in countries that have high or intermediate endemicity of hepatitis A; and

— unvaccinated persons who anticipate close personal contact (e.g., household or regular babysitting) with an international adoptee during the first 60 days after arrival in the United States from a country with high or intermediate endemicity. (See footnote 1 for more information on travel recommendations.) The first dose of the 2-dose hepatitis A vaccine series should be administered as soon as adoption is planned, ideally 2 or more weeks before the arrival of the adoptee.

• Single-antigen vaccine formulations should be administered in a 2-dose schedule at either 0 and 6 to 12 months (Havrix), or 0 and 6 to 18 months (Vaqta). If the combined hepatitis A and hepatitis B vaccine (Twinrix) is used, administer 3 doses at 0, 1, and 6 months; alternatively, a 4-dose schedule may be used, administered on days 0, 7, and 21 to 30 followed by a booster dose at month 12.

11. Hepatitis B vaccination

• Vaccinate persons with any of the following indications and any person seeking protection from hepatitis B virus (HBV) infection:

— sexually active persons who are not in a long-term, mutually monogamous relationship (e.g., persons with more than 1 sex partner during the previous 6 months); persons seeking evaluation or treatment for a sexually transmitted disease (STD); current or recent injection drug users; and men who have sex with men;

— health care personnel and public safety workers who are potentially exposed to blood or other infectious body fluids;

— persons with diabetes who are younger than age 60 years as soon as feasible after diagnosis; persons with diabetes who are age 60 years or older at the discretion of the treating clinician based on the likelihood of acquiring HBV infection, including the risk posed by an increased need for assisted blood glucose monitoring in long-term care facilities, the likelihood of experiencing chronic sequelae if infected with HBV, and the likelihood of immune response to vaccination;

— persons with end-stage renal disease, including patients receiving hemodialysis, persons with HIV infection, and persons with chronic liver disease;

— household contacts and sex partners of hepatitis B surface antigen–positive persons, clients and staff members of institutions for persons with developmental disabilities, and international travelers to countries with high or intermediate prevalence of chronic HBV infection; and

— all adults in the following settings: STD treatment facilities, HIV testing and treatment facilities, facilities providing drug abuse treatment and prevention services, health care settings targeting services to injection drug users or men who have sex with men, correctional facilities, end-stage renal disease programs and facilities for chronic hemodialysis patients, and institutions and nonresidential day care facilities for persons with developmental disabilities.

• Administer missing doses to complete a 3-dose series of hepatitis B vaccine to those persons not vaccinated or not completely vaccinated. The second dose should be administered 1 month after the first dose; the third dose should be given at least 2 months after the second dose (and at least 4 months after the first dose). If the combined hepatitis A and hepatitis B vaccine (Twinrix) is used, give 3 doses at 0, 1, and 6 months; alternatively, a 4-dose Twinrix schedule, administered on days 0, 7, and 21 to 30 followed by a booster dose at month 12 may be used.

• Adult patients receiving hemodialysis or with other immunocompromising conditions should receive 1 dose of 40 mcg/mL (Recombivax HB) administered on a 3-dose schedule at 0, 1, and 6 months or 2 doses of 20 mcg/mL (Engerix-B) administered simultaneously on a 4-dose schedule at 0, 1, 2, and 6 months.

— Have received PCV13 and 1 dose of PPSV23: Administer a second dose of PPSV23 at least 5 years after the first dose of PPSV23.

• Adults aged 19 through 64 years with cerebrospinal fluid leaks or cochlear implants: Administer PCV13 followed by PPSV23 at least 8 weeks after PCV13.

• Adults aged 19 through 64 years with chronic heart disease (including congestive heart failure and cardiomyopathies, excluding hypertension), chronic lung disease (including chronic obstructive lung disease, emphysema, and asthma), chronic liver disease (including cirrhosis), alcoholism, or diabetes mellitus: Administer PPSV23.

• Adults aged 19 through 64 years who smoke cigarettes or reside in nursing home or long-term care facilities: Administer PPSV23.

• Routine pneumococcal vaccination is not recommended for American Indian/Alaska Native or other adults unless they have the indications as above; however, public health authorities may consider recommending the use of pneumococcal vaccines for American Indians/Alaska Natives or other adults who live in areas with increased risk for invasive pneumococcal disease.

• Immunocompromising conditions that are indications for pneumococcal vaccination are: Congenital or acquired immunodeficiency (including B- or T-lymphocyte deficiency, complement deficiencies, and phagocytic disorders excluding chronic granulomatous disease), HIV infection, chronic renal failure, nephrotic syndrome, leukemia, lymphoma, Hodgkin disease, generalized malignancy, multiple myeloma, solid organ transplant, and iatrogenic immunosuppression (including long-term systemic corticosteroids and radiation therapy).

• Anatomical or functional asplenia that are indications for pneumococcal vaccination are: Sickle cell disease and other hemoglobinopathies, congenital or acquired asplenia, splenic dysfunction, and splenectomy. Administer pneumococcal vaccines at least 2 weeks before immunosuppressive therapy or an elective splenectomy, and as soon as possible to adults who are newly diagnosed with asymptomatic or symptomatic HIV infection.

9. Meningococcal vaccination

• Administer 2 doses of quadrivalent meningococcal conjugate vaccine (MenACWY [Menactra, Menveo]) at least 2 months apart to adults of all ages with anatomical or functional asplenia or persistent complement component deficiencies. HIV infection is not an indication for routine vaccination with MenACWY. If an HIV-infected person of any age is vaccinated, 2 doses of MenACWY should be administered at least 2 months apart.

• Administer a single dose of meningococcal vaccine to microbiologists routinely exposed to isolates of *Neisseria meningitidis*, military recruits, persons at risk during an outbreak attributable to a vaccine serogroup, and persons who travel to or live in countries in which meningococcal disease is hyperendemic or epidemic.

- First-year college students up through age 21 years who are living in residence halls should be vaccinated if they have not received a dose on or after their 16th birthday.
- MenACWY is preferred for adults with any of the preceding indications who are aged 55 years or younger as well as for adults aged 56 years or older who a) were vaccinated previously with MenACWY and are recommended for revaccination, or b) for whom multiple doses are anticipated. Meningococcal polysaccharide vaccine (MPSV4 [Menomune]) is preferred for adults aged 56 years or older who have not received MenACWY previously and who require a single dose only (e.g., travelers).
- Revaccination with MenACWY every 5 years is recommended for adults previously vaccinated with MenACWY or MPSV4 who remain at increased risk for infection (e.g., adults with anatomical or functional asplenia, persistent complement component deficiencies, or microbiologists).

12. *Haemophilus influenzae* type b (Hib) vaccination

- One dose of Hib vaccine should be administered to persons who have anatomical or functional asplenia or sickle cell disease or are undergoing elective splenectomy if they have not previously received Hib vaccine. Hib vaccination 14 or more days before splenectomy is suggested.
- Recipients of a hematopoietic stem cell transplant (HSCT) should be vaccinated with a 3-dose regimen 6 to 12 months after a successful transplant, regardless of vaccination history; at least 4 weeks should separate doses.
- Hib vaccine is not recommended for adults with HIV infection since their risk for Hib infection is low.

13. Immunocompromising conditions

- Inactivated vaccines generally are acceptable (e.g., pneumococcal, meningococcal, and inactivated influenza vaccine) and live vaccines generally are avoided in persons with immune deficiencies or immunocompromising conditions. Information on specific conditions is available at www.cdc.gov/vaccines/hcp/acip-recs/index.html.

PROFESSIONAL SOCIETIES AND GOVERNMENTAL AGENCIES

Abbreviation	Full Name	Internet Address
AACE	American Association of Clinical Endocrinologists	http://www.aace.com
AAD	American Academy of Dermatology	http://www.aad.org
AAFP	American Academy of Family Physicians	http://www.aafp.org
AAHPM	American Academy of Hospice and Palliative Medicine	http://www.aahpm.org
AAN	American Academy of Neurology	http://www.aan.com
AAO	American Academy of Ophthalmology	http://www.aao.org
AAO-HNS	American Academy of Otolaryngology—Head and Neck Surgery	http://www.entnet.org
AAOS	American Academy of Orthopaedic Surgeons and American Association of Orthopaedic Surgeons	http://www.aaos.org
AAP	American Academy of Pediatrics	http://www.aap.org
ACC	American College of Cardiology	http://www.acc.org
ACCP	American College of Chest Physicians	http://www.chestnet.org
ACIP	Advisory Committee on Immunization Practices	http://www.cdc.gov/vaccines/acip/index.html
ACOG	American Congress of Obstetricians and Gynecologists	http://www.acog.com
ACP	American College of Physicians	http://www.acponline.org
ACR	American College of Radiology	http://www.acr.org
ACR	American College of Rheumatology	http://www.rheumatology.org
ACS	American Cancer Society	http://www.cancer.org
ACSM	American College of Sports Medicine	http://www.acsm.org
ADA	American Diabetes Association	http://www.diabetes.org
AGA	American Gastroenterological Association	http://www.gastro.org
AGS	The American Geriatrics Society	http://www. americangeriatrics.org
AHA	American Heart Association	http://www.americanheart.org
ANA	American Nurses Association	http://www.nursingworld.org
AOA	American Optometric Association	http://www.aoa.org
ASA	American Stroke Association	http://www.strokeassociation.org
ASAM	American Society of Addiction Medicine	http://www.asam.org
ASCCP	American Society for Colposcopy and Cervical Pathology	http://www.asccp.org
ASCO	American Society of Clinical Oncology	http://www.asco.org
ASCRS	American Society of Colon and Rectal Surgeons	http://www.fascrs.org
ASGE	American Society for Gastrointestinal Endoscopy	http://asge.org
ASHA	American Speech-Language-Hearing Association	http://www.asha.org
ASN	American Society of Neuroimaging	http://www.asnweb.org
ATA	American Thyroid Association	http://www.thyroid.org
ATS	American Thoracic Society	http://www.thoracic.org
AUA	American Urological Association	http://auanet.org
BASHH	British Association for Sexual Health and HIV	http://www.bashh.org
	Bright Futures	http://brightfutures.org
BGS	British Geriatrics Society	http://www.bgs.org.uk/
BSAC	British Society for Antimicrobial Chemotherapy	http://www.bsac.org.uk
CDC	Centers for Disease Control and Prevention	http://www.cdc.gov
COG	Children's Oncology Group	http://www.childrensoncologygroup.org
CSVS	Canadian Society for Vascular Surgery	http://canadianvascular.ca
CTF	Canadian Task Force on Preventive Health Care	http://canadiantaskforce.ca
EASD	European Association for the Study of Diabetes	http://www.easd.org
EAU	European Association of Urology	http://www.uroweb.org
ERS	European Respiratory Society	http://ersnet.org
ESC	European Society of Cardiology	http://www.escardio.org
ESH	European Society of Hypertension	http://www.eshonline.org

PROFESSIONAL SOCIETIES AND GOVERNMENTAL AGENCIES (CONTINUED)

Abbreviation	Full Name	Internet Address
IARC	International Agency for Research on Cancer	http://screening.iarc.fr
ICSI	Institute for Clinical Systems Improvement	http://www.icsi.org
IDF	International Diabetes Federation	http://www.idf.org
NAPNAP	National Association of Pediatric Nurse Practitioners	http://www.napnap.org
NCCN	National Comprehensive Cancer Network	http://www.nccn.org/cancer-guidelines.html
NCI	National Cancer Institute	http://www.cancer.gov/cancerinformation
NEI	National Eye Institute	http://www.nei.nih.gov
NGC	National Guideline Clearinghouse	http://www.guidelines.gov
NHLBI	National Heart, Lung, and Blood Institute	http://www.nhlbi.nih.gov
NIAAA	National Institute on Alcohol Abuse and Alcoholism	http://www.niaaa.nih.gov
NICE	National Institute for Health and Clinical Excellence	http://www.nice.org.uk
NIDCR	National Institute of Dental and Craniofacial Research	http://www.nidr.nih.gov
NIHCDC	National Institutes of Health Consensus Development Program	http://www.consensus.nih.gov
NIP	National Immunization Program	http://www.cdc.gov/vaccines
NKF	National Kidney Foundation	http://www.kidney.org
NOF	National Osteoporosis Foundation	http://www.nof.org
NTSB	National Transportation Safety Board	http://www.ntsb.gov
SCF	Skin Cancer Foundation	http://www.skincancer.org
SGIM	Society of General Internal Medicine	http://www.sgim.org
SKI	Sloan-Kettering Institute	http://www.mskcc.org/mskcc/html/5804.cfm
SVU	Society for Vascular Ultrasound	http://www.svunet.org
UK-NHS	United Kingdom National Health Service	http://www.nhs.uk
USPSTF	United States Preventive Services Task Force	http://www.ahrq.gov/clinic/uspstfix.htm
WHO	World Health Organization	http://www.who.int/en

Index